". . . here's inspiration to turn off the television and head for the hills."
—*Napa Valley Register*

"If you like to hike, make the most of your outdoor adventures by toting this handy reference guide in your backpack. With author Matt Heid's insights, you're sure to wander through some of this scenic region's most stunning backcountry."
—Southwest Airlines *Spirit* magazine

"A wonderful selection of trails, good writing, and helpful graphics make this a choice guidebook for ambles in the special places of Northern California."
—Honorable Mention, 2001 National Outdoor Book Awards

"Before heading into the backcountry, a generation or two of hikers have packed an essential piece of equipment: a trusty Wilderness Press hiking guide . . ."
—*Sacramento Bee*

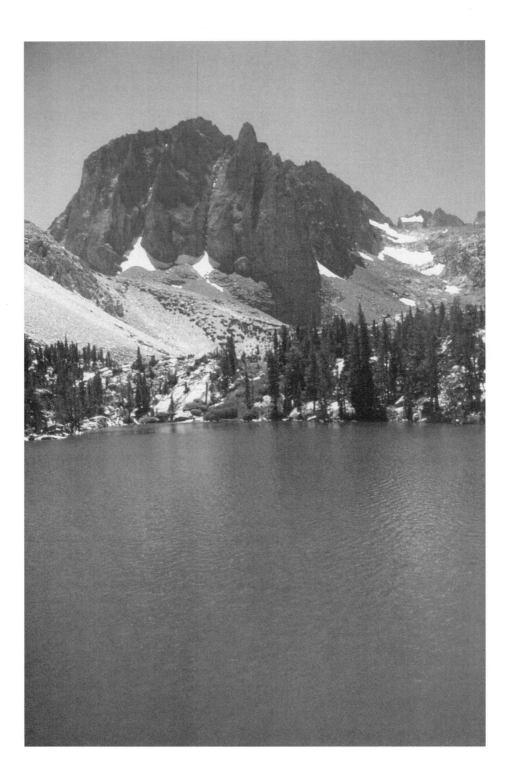

101 HIKES

in Northern California

Exploring Mountains, Valleys, and Seashore

Matt Heid

 WILDERNESS PRESS ... *on the trail since 1967*

Dedicated to the great state
of Northern California

101 Hikes in Northern California: Exploring Mountains, Valleys, and Seashore

1st EDITION December 2000
2nd EDITION October 2008
   2nd printing 2010

Copyright © 2000, 2008 by Matt Heid

Front cover photos copyright © 2008 by Matt Heid
Maps and interior photos: Matt Heid, except for the following:
   Analise Elliot Heid, pp. 19, 22, and 40; Laura Shauger, p. 121
All topographic maps © 2008 National Geographic Maps with trails added by the author
Locator map (p. viii) by Jaan Hitt and Larry B. Van Dyke
Cover, book design, and layout: Larry B. Van Dyke
Book editor: Laura Shauger

ISBN 978-0-89997-474-3

Manufactured in the United States of America

Published by: **Wilderness Press**
   c/o Keen Communications
   PO Box 43673
   Birmingham, AL 35243
   (800) 443-7227; FAX (205) 326-1012
   www.wildernesspress.com
Visit our website for a complete listing of our books and for ordering information.

Distributed by Publishers Group West

Cover photos: Table Rock in Robert Louis Stevenson State Park, Trip 38 *(background);*
   Wildcat Beach, Trip 34 *(top inset);* and Palisade Crest above Big Pine Creek,
   Trip 95 *(bottom inset)*
Frontispiece: Temple Crag rises above First Lake (Hike 95)

SAFETY NOTICE: Although Wilderness Press and the author have made every attempt to ensure that the information in this book is accurate at press time, they are not responsible for any loss, damage, injury, or inconvenience that may occur to anyone while using this book. You are responsible for your own safety and health. The fact that a trail is described in this book does not mean that it will be safe for you. Be aware that trail conditions can change from day to day. Always check local conditions and know your own limitations.

Acknowledgments

Thanks go first to the countless rangers, public land managers, and stewards of Northern California's natural treasures. They patiently answered my long lists of questions and were an invaluable resource in ensuring the accuracy of this updated guide.

Many wonderful people have joined me on these 101 hikes over the years: my wife Gretchen, brother John, father Bill, mother Jan, Joann Volinski, Sid Bean, Marsha Lewis, Lindsey Lewis, Big Tom Hruschka, Chuck Kapelke, Cindy Miner, Ben Hart, Erich von Ibsch, Leslie Rubin, Julio Gutierrez, Dan Hruschka, Sean Fitzpatrick, U. G. Stone, Mike Jones, Kara Forman (and Sonoma), Genevieve Juliard, David Doostan, Kevin Daly, Ethan Phillips, and, of course, Pogen MacNeilage, poster boy for the entire endeavor. May there be many more hikes together.

I would like to especially acknowledge Analise Elliot Heid for her support and never-ending enthusiasm. As the hiking expert on Big Sur, Analise contributed material for Hikes 1, 2, 6, and 7; she is the author of *Hiking & Backpacking Big Sur* (also published by Wilderness Press).

Thank you to Laura Shauger, who expertly shepherded this through the editing and production process; and to Roslyn Bullas, who keeps things on the right track. Thank you also to Larry Van Dyke, the soul of Wilderness Press, for his outstanding design work. Thanks to all the folks at REI. Thank you to everybody who continues to support my passions. And thanks most especially to Gretchen, my loved adventurer in life.

Matt Heid
Anchorage, Alaska
July 2008

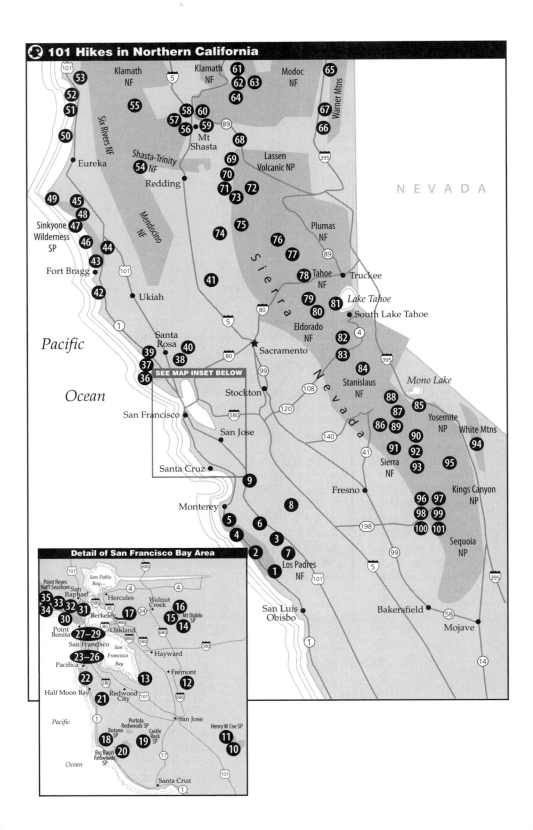

Contents

THE NORTH COAST AND KLAMATH MOUNTAINS

SHASTA AND THE MODOC PLATEAU

THE SIERRA NEVADA

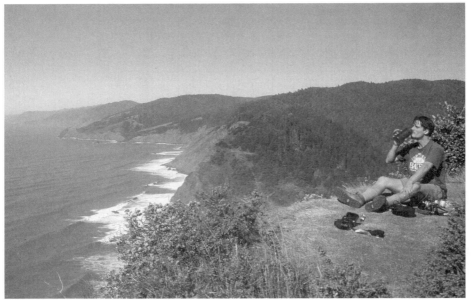

Above the Lost Coast (Hike 46)

Preface

Welcome to the total Northern California outdoor experience. Every aspect of the region's incredible natural diversity is found within these 101 hikes—the jagged granite of the High Sierra, the crashing surf of the Pacific Coast, the volcanic landscape of the Modoc Plateau, the rich diversity of the Klamath Mountains, the magnificent redwoods of the North Coast, the spectacular views of the Bay Area. Lakes, peaks, rivers, creeks, waterfalls, valleys, beaches, forests, meadows, wildlife, wildflowers, lighthouses, volcanoes . . . they can all be found within these pages.

This book describes a greater area than most Northern California guidebooks. Stretching north from Sequoia National Park through the Modoc Plateau of northeast California, it includes virtually all of the Sierra Nevada. Sweeping north along the coast from Big Sur to the Oregon border, it contains the Coast Ranges, the San Francisco Bay Area, and the Klamath Mountains. In total, this book covers the entire northern two-thirds of the state. And now this second edition opens up several new realms, with 15 entirely new trips and expanded coverage of Big Sur, the San Francisco Bay Area, and the Lost Coast.

The hikes were selected using three basic criteria, and each adventure includes some combination of:

- **Isolation:** Wilderness is freedom, an escape from the trappings of society. The fewer the people you encounter, the deeper your experience.
- **Scenic Beauty:** Sweeping 360-degree vistas, exquisite works of nature, and the splendor of Northern California
- **Unique Destinations:** Redwood forests, giant sequoias, granite domes, marble mountains, thundering waterfalls—places unlike anywhere else on Earth

While all of the hikes can be completed in a single day, more than half can also be done as overnight backpacking trips. Each hike includes summary information outlining the basics of the trip, detailed driving directions, an in-depth trail description, and the location of the nearest visitors center and campground. Backpacking information is provided for appropriate hikes. The hikes are broadly distributed across Northern California; no matter where you are, an adventure awaits nearby. Enjoy!

Hikes by Theme

Using This Book

To prepare for the total Northern California outdoors experience, first carefully read Safety, Gear, and the Wilderness Ethic (starting on p. 4). Selecting a hike can be an absorbing process. Those unfamiliar with the state or unsure about where to visit should consult Where Should I Go Hiking? (starting on p. 11). For those looking for a specific feature, the hikes are grouped by theme in the front of the book. Otherwise, just flip through the pages to your desired area and evaluate each hike based on the standard information provided.

Beginning along the Pacific shore with the Big Sur region, the hikes are organized clockwise around the state: north through the Bay Area, Coast Ranges, and Pacific Coast to the Klamath Mountains, then inland east across the Modoc Plateau, and finally south through the Sierra Nevada to end in southern Sequoia National Park.

Each hike is organized into a standard, easily understood template. Each hike includes at-a-glance summary information, detailed driving directions, a detailed hike description, and some additional information about nearby facilities:

Summary Information

Tagline. All hikes have a fun tagline for intrigue and inspiration.

Highlights. The most exciting features of a particular hike.

Distance. The total mileage of the hike as described. For point-to-point hikes, the one-way distance is listed.

Total Elevation Gain/Loss. The total amount of climbing and descending on the hike. It can be significantly greater than the difference between the hike's lowest and highest points.

Hiking Time. The total amount of time required for the hike, including time for brief rest stops and a meal break on longer trips. As this varies markedly depending on physical fitness and pace, a range of times is usually given. The lower number indicates the amount of time a fit hiker can complete the hike, pausing only briefly for short breaks. The higher number is for hikers moving at a more leisurely pace and for anybody who likes to take extended breaks over the course of a journey. Remember that these times are only rough estimates and hikes can potentially take longer for slower hikers and those with heavy backpacks.

It is important to be aware of your physical capabilities and limitations when selecting a hike. As a general rule of thumb, a reasonably fit hiker can expect to cover 2–3 miles per hour over level ground and on gradual descents, 1–2 miles per hour on gradual climbs, and only about 1 mile—or 750–1000 feet of elevation—per hour on the steepest ascents.

Optional Maps. Usually the appropriate U.S. Geological Survey 7.5-minute topographic maps but occasionally a Forest Service Wilderness map or other recommended source. Many of the hikes can be completed using only the maps in the book or those available near the trailhead, but more detailed and comprehensive maps generally provide an extra measure of safety and comfort, especially on the more difficult and remote hikes.

Most Forest Service maps are available for purchase online at www.fs.fed.us/r5. All USGS maps can be ordered online at www.usgs.gov or printed out at home using software such as National Geographic's TOPO! series.

Best Times. The best times of year to do the hike. Note that many of the hikes can be done outside of the times listed, but weather or crowds will probably make them much less appealing.

Agency. This line identifies the governing agency. Contact information is listed in the nearby facility information at the end of each description.

Difficulty. This book uses a difficulty rating system of one to five stars. While all factors contributing to the overall challenge of the hike are taken into account, some general criteria for each level are as follows:

★ *Easy.* Typically short and level, these hikes can be done by anybody and have less than 500 feet of total elevation gain.

★★ *Moderate.* Moderate. Hikes on good trails with roughly 500–1000 feet of total elevation gain. Suitable for any reasonably fit hiker.

★★★ *Strenuous.* Longer hikes with approximately 1000–2000 feet of elevation gain on trails that are often rocky and steep. Good fitness required.

★★★★ *Challenging.* A very strenuous hike with roughly 2000–3000 feet of elevation gain in often remote regions on challenging trails. Experienced wilderness users only. Many are good overnight trips.

★★★★★ *Epic.* An adventure with an elevation gain in excess of 3000 feet on rough and difficult trails. Cross-country navigation skills are often required. Only the fittest individuals can complete these hikes in a single day. Excellent for overnight trips.

Trip Type Symbols

An **out-and-back** hike that returns to the starting trailhead by retracing its route.

A **loop** or **semiloop** hike that retraces little or none of its route to return to the starting trailhead.

A **point-to-point** hike that ends at a different trailhead. A second car or a shuttle is required to return to the starting trailhead.

Other Symbols

All hikes that can be done as **overnight backpacking trips** include this symbol. Specific backpacking information is listed at the end of each hike.

A hike that requires some **travel through thick or overhanging brush**. Long pants and a long-sleeve shirt are recommended to guard against ticks and scratches.

A location that **allows dogs** in the backcountry.

A hike **well-suited for young children**. A hike bearing this symbol is short and easy and often has educational interpretive signs.

Hike Description

The body of the hike is broken down into three main sections:

The Hike. Following introductory material and background information is a brief overview of the hike discussing seasonal differences, crowds, recommended equipment, special regulations, fishing possibilities, and the availability of water both at the trailhead and along the hike.

To Reach the Trailhead. Concise driving directions to the start of the hike. This book assumes that you have a basic highway map of California. Mention is made if access requires a four-wheel-drive or high-clearance vehicle. Entrance fees are also included in this section.

Every vehicle's odometer is slightly different, especially the 1980s-era Toyota pickup trucks used to research most of these hikes. Please note your mileages may vary from those listed here; any discrepancy should be consistent throughout the book.

Description. The hike itself. Parenthetical notations such as (10,320´) indicate elevation in feet. Parenthetical notations such as (2.7/8750´) are included at important junctions or landmarks. The first number represents the total distance from the trailhead in miles. The second identifies the elevation of the location in feet.

Nearby Facilities

Information about nearby facilities is displayed in a shaded box at the end of each hike:

Nearest Visitors Center. The closest source of information to the trailhead and the best place to call for general information. Opening hours are included, but be aware that schedules are subject to regular change; these times should only be considered approximate. Unless otherwise mentioned, assume the hours are year-round.

Backpacking Information. If the hike can be done as an overnight backpacking trip, this section discusses required permits, fees, quotas, and crowds. Campsite locations may be briefly mentioned but they are not described in detail or discussed in the main body of text.

Nearest Campground. The closest organized campground to the trailhead. "Organized" means that there are at least

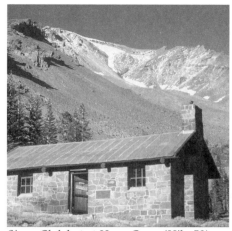

Sierra Club hut at Horse Camp (Hike 59)

picnic tables, fire rings, and toilets. Water is available at the campgrounds unless specifically mentioned otherwise. The total number of sites and camping fees are included as well. Be aware that prices always increase and that those listed should be considered approximate. All state park campgrounds operate on the same reservation system—call 1-800-444-7275 or visit www.reserveamerica.com to reserve a site.

Additional Information. Any recommended Web sites.

Maps

The maps in this book were created using TOPO! software from National Geographic Maps. Note that they are reproduced at different sizes, and scale varies from map to map. Because they are only intended to convey very basic route information, most hikers will want to purchase the optional map(s) listed in the trip summary information.

Safety, Gear, and the Wilderness Ethic

Safety

Always tell somebody where you are hiking and when you expect to return. Friends, family, rangers, and visitors centers are all valuable resources that can save you from a backcountry disaster when you fail to reappear on time.

Know your limits. Don't undertake a hike that exceeds your physical fitness or wilderness abilities.

Try not to hike alone. A hiking partner can provide the margin between life and death in the event of a serious backcountry mishap.

Be prepared. Plan appropriately for the expected terrain and weather and always carry essential survival gear.

Drink lots of water. Prevent dehydration and its accompanying dangers by consuming as much water as possible. Always purify water taken from rivers, lakes, and streams in the backcountry.

The Animal Hazards

Bears

The grizzly bear is extinct in California and only its smaller cousin the black bear still roams the mountains. Seldom dangerous, black bears will usually run away as soon as they spot you. In popular areas—Yosemite being the prime example—resident bears have learned that people mean food and exhibit no fear of humans. If a bear approaches, be loud and obnoxious, bang pots, throw small rocks, and try to frighten the animal away. Always avoid females with cubs as the maternal instinct can make her attack if she feels her young are threatened.

When you are camping in bear country, it is imperative that you safely secure food and any scented items (toothpaste, deodorant, etc.) away from the campsite. Plastic bear canisters are the most effective method and can be purchased or rented at many outdoor equipment shops; they are mandatory in some locations. Hanging your food from a nearby tree is a good option in less-traveled areas. To hang your food, divide it evenly between two stuff sacks and find a tree with a long thin branch extending at least 10 feet from the trunk and at least 20 feet from the ground. Throw a rope over the branch using a weighted object of some kind, tie one of the stuff sacks to the end, hoist it to the branch, attach the second stuff sack as far above the ground as possible on the other end of the rope, and use a stick to push the second sack upward until it is level with the first.

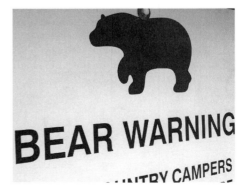

4

Rattlesnakes

Common throughout Northern California below approximately 6000 feet, these venomous snakes like to bask on hot rocks in the sun. They usually flee at the first sight of people and will only attack if threatened. Be wary when cruising off-trail and don't put your hands where you can't see them when scrambling on rocky slopes. If you are bitten, the goal is to reduce the rate at which the poison circulates through your body—try and remain calm, keep the bite site below the level of your heart, remove any constricting items (rings, watches, etc.) from the soon-to-be-swollen extremity, and do not apply ice or chemical cold to the bite as this can cause further damage to the surrounding tissue. Seek medical attention as quickly as possible.

Ticks

These parasites love brushy areas at low elevations and are common throughout the state, especially during the rainy season. Always perform regular body checks when hiking through tick country. If you find a tick attached to you, do not try to pull it out with your fingers or pinch the body; they are difficult to remove this way and it can increase the risk of infection. Using an appropriate tool instead, gently pull the tick out by lifting upward from the base of the body where it is attached to the skin. Pull straight out until the tick releases and do not twist or jerk as this may break the mouth parts off under your skin. Tweezers or a small V cut in the side of a credit card works well for this operation.

Lyme Disease

While this disease is present in Northern California, only one of the 48 tick species found in the state is capable of transmitting it—the diminutive western black-legged tick. Chances for exposure are, therefore, low. Caused by a spirochete, this potentially life-threatening disease can be hard to diagnose in its early phases. Common early symptoms include fatigue, chills and fever, headache, muscle and joint pain, swollen lymph nodes, and a blotchy skin rash that clears centrally to produce a characteristic ring shape 3–30 days after exposure. If you fear that you have been exposed to Lyme disease, consult a doctor immediately. Note that the majority of infected people never see the tick that bit them.

Giardia

Giardia lamblia is a microscopic organism occasionally found in backcountry water sources. Existing in a dormant cyst form while in the water, the critter develops in the gastrointestinal tract upon being consumed and can cause diarrhea, excessive flatulence, foul-smelling excrement, nausea, fatigue, and abdominal cramps. While the risk of contraction is very slight, the potential consequences are worth preventing. All water taken from the backcountry should be purified by boiling, chemical treatment, or the use of a filter.

Deer Mice

There is no known cure for hantavirus, a rare but usually fatal pulmonary syndrome acquired by ingesting urine, droppings, or saliva from infected rodents; or by touching your nose, mouth, or eyes after handling infected rodents, their nests, or droppings. Deer mice are 4–7 inches long, gray to brown in color with white fur on the belly, and have large ears. They are common around the state. Never handle rodent nests, avoid buildings they inhabit, and never leave food sitting out.

Mountain Lions

Common throughout the state, mountain lions are rarely seen. If you do encounter a mountain lion acting in an aggressive manner, make yourself look as large as possible and do not run away.

Plants to Avoid

Poison Oak

If you learn to identify only one plant in California, it had better be this one. Poison oak grows throughout California below approximately 4000 feet. A low-lying shrub or bush, its glossy oaklike leaves always grow in clusters of three and turn bright red in the fall before dropping off in the winter. Both the leaves and stems contain an oil that causes a strong allergic reaction in most people, creating a maddening and long-lived itchy rash that can spread across the body. Wash thoroughly after any exposure. It is mentioned in the hike description if it occurs along a given trail.

Stinging Nettle

Common along the coast, this spiny plant causes an unpleasant stinging sensation when any part of it comes in contact with your skin. It is mentioned in the hike description when it appears along a given trail.

Physical Dangers

Lightning

Thunderstorms are common during the summer months and often bring lightning, especially at higher elevations. If you see a thunderstorm approaching, avoid exposed ridges and peaks, take shelter in low places, and sit on some sort of insulating material if you feel in real danger: your backpack, sleeping pad, or anything else you might have handy.

Hypothermia

This life-threatening condition occurs when the body is unable to stay adequately warm and its core temperature begins to drop. Initial symptoms include weakness, mental confusion, and uncontrollable shivering. Cold, wet weather poses the greatest hazard as wet clothes conduct heat away from the body roughly 20 times faster than dry layers. Fatigue reduces your body's ability to produce its own heat; wind poses an increased risk as it can quickly strip away warmth. Immediate treatment is critical and entails raising the body's core temperature. Get out of the wind, take off wet clothes, drink warm beverages, eat simple energy foods, and take shelter in a warm tent or sleeping bag. Do not drink alcohol as this dilates the blood vessels and causes increased heat loss.

Heat Stroke

The opposite of hypothermia, this condition occurs when the body is unable to control its internal temperature and overheats. Usually brought on by excessive exposure to the sun and accompanying dehydration, symptoms include cramping, headache, and mental confusion. Treatment entails rapid, aggressive cooling of the body through whatever means are available—cooling the head and torso is most important—and drinking lots of fluids. Stay hydrated and be sure to carry some type of sun protection for your head if you expect to travel a hot, exposed section of trail.

Sunburn

The Northern California sun can fry you quickly—especially at higher elevations where the air filters less of the damaging rays. Always wear sunscreen of sufficiently high SPF. Wear pants and long sleeves when appropriate and a hat with a brim to protect your skin.

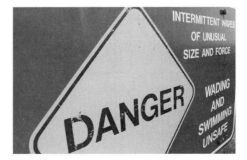

The Pacific Ocean

The dangerous waters of the Pacific are frigid, swirling with strong currents and undertows that can instantly suck the unwary out to sea. Rogue waves can always occur, sweeping the unsuspecting from seemingly safe rocks and beaches—especially during times of large swell. Unless you are confident in your abilities and knowledge of the ocean, don't tempt fate by going into the water.

Gear

Survival Essentials

You should always have:

Water. Carry at least one liter of water (preferably two), drink frequently, and have some means of purifying backcountry sources (chemical treatment or filter).

Fire. Waterproof matches to help build an emergency fire and some easy-to-light kindling to get it going; vaseline-coated cotton balls work well for this.

First-Aid Kit. A basic kit should include at least the following: some type of painkiller/swelling reducer (ibuprofen is always good), an ACE bandage, a topical antibiotic (like Neosporin), and sterile wound dressings. Prepackaged kits are readily available at any outdoor-equipment store.

Warmth. Extra clothing can be critical in the event of an unexpected night out. Always carry an additional insulating layer.

Light. A headlamp or flashlight will help you find the trail home on a hike that extends later than expected.

Knife. A good knife can be invaluable in the event of a disaster. Pocket knives and all-in-one tools have many other useful features as well.

Extra Food. An extra snack or two can be invaluable if you end up being out longer than expected.

Map and Compass. To find your way home.

For Your Feet

Your feet are the single, most important component of your total hike experience. If they are unhappy, you will be even more so. Appreciate them. Care for them.

Footwear. The appropriate hiking footwear provides stability and support for your feet and ankles while protecting them from the abuses of the environment. For most hikes in this book, a solid pair of midweight hiking boots is recommended. When selecting footwear, keep in mind that the most important feature is a good fit—your toes should not hit the front while going downhill, your heel should be locked in place inside the boot to prevent friction and blisters, and there should be minimal extra space around your foot. Stability over uneven ground is enhanced by a stiffer sole and higher ankle collar. All-leather boots last longer, have a good deal of natural water resistance, and will mold to your feet over time. Many boots have Gore-Tex, making them totally waterproof. Be sure to break in new boots before taking them on an extended hike—simply wear them around as much as possible beforehand. While many of these hikes could be completed in sandals or tennis shoes, their use increases the risk of twisting an ankle, offers minimal protection from rocks, and is generally not recommended.

Socks. After armpits, feet are the sweatiest part of the human body. Unfortunately, wet feet are much more prone to blisters. Good hiking socks will manage foot moisture, keep a dry layer next to your skin, and provide padding for your feet. Avoid cotton socks at all cost as these quickly become saturated, stay wet inside your shoes, and take forever to dry. Many socks are a confusing mix of natural and synthetic fibers. Wool provides warmth and padding and, while it does absorb roughly 30 percent of its weight in water, it is effective at keeping your feet dry. If regular wool makes your feet itch, try softer merino wool. Nylon, polyester, acrylic, and polypropylene (also called olefin) are all synthetic fibers that absorb

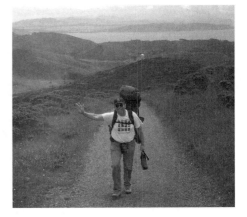

very little water, dry quickly, and add durability. Liner socks are a thin pair of socks worn underneath the principal sock designed to more effectively wick moisture away—good for really sweaty feet.

Blister Kit. As everybody knows, blisters suck. They are usually caused by friction caused by foot movement inside your shoes and are best prevented by buying properly fitting footwear, wearing appropriate socks, breaking your shoes in ahead of time, and using some simple preventive items. Always carry moleskin or the equivalent, and apply it as soon as you notice a hot spot developing.

Clothing

Although it seems like it should be easy enough to just get dressed and go, the more appropriately you dress, the more comfortable you will likely be. The following information is helpful for staying warm and dry on the trail.

The Fabrics. Cotton is generally a lousy outdoors fabric. It absorbs water quickly and takes a long time to dry, leaving a cold wet layer next to your skin when you stop hiking. In hot, dry environments, however, cotton is useful as the water it retains helps keep you cool for longer periods of time. Wool is a good natural fiber for hiking. Despite the fact that it retains up to 30 percent of its weight in water, it still insulates when wet. Polyester and nylon are two commonly used synthetic fibers

in outdoor clothing. They dry almost instantly, wick moisture effectively, and are generally much lighter weight than natural fibers. They will melt quickly, however, if placed in contact with a heat source (camp stove, fire, sparks, etc.) and tend to retain funky odors with extended use.

Raingear and Windgear. There are three types available: waterproof/breathable, waterproof/nonbreathable, and water-resistant. Waterproof/breathable shells contain Gore-Tex or the equivalent and effectively keep liquid water out while still allowing water vapor (i.e. your sweat) to pass through. They keep you somewhat more comfortable during heavy exertions in the rain, but are still unable to effectively transfer the amount of moisture you produce at a full sweat. Waterproof/nonbreathable shells are typically rubber or coated nylon and keep water out but hold all your sweat in. Seams must be taped for them to be completely waterproof. Although wearing these while hiking strenuously is a hot and sticky experience, they are inexpensive and often very lightweight. Water-resistant shells are typically lightweight nylon windbreakers coated with a water repellent that wears away with use. They will keep you dry for a short period of time but will quickly soak through in a heavy rain. Soft shells also fall into this category. Highly breathable and water-resistant, they will keep you dry in all but the wettest conditions. Unless you are planning some rainy winter hikes, a simple coated waterproof/nonbreathable nylon shell should be more than adequate and can remain hidden in your pack until the day you need it.

Keeping Your Head and Neck Warm. The three most important parts of the body to keep warm are the torso, neck, and head. Your body will strive to keep these a constant temperature at all times. Without any insulation, the heat coursing through your neck to your brain radiates out into space and is lost. Warmth that might have been directed to your extremities is instead spent replacing the heat lost from your head. A warm hat and neck gaiter are small items, weigh almost nothing, and are more effective at keeping you warm than an extra sweater.

Keeping Your Hands Warm. Hiking in cold and damp conditions will often chill your hands unpleasantly. A lightweight pair of polypropylene liner gloves will do wonders.

Important Hiking Equipment

Backpack. The ideal daypack is big enough to easily carry everything you need and should have between roughly 1000 and 2000 cubic inches of volume. For shorter dayhikes a large fanny pack is often adequate. For overnight trips, a pack with at least 3000 cubic inches is required. The pack should ride principally on your hips, not on your shoulders—look for a comfortable hip belt that effectively transfers loads to the lower body. Outside water-bottle pockets and an abundance of compartments are nice.

Flashlight. Hiking after dark is no fun without a flashlight. Even if you plan to return well before sundown, unexpected delays and extended periods of enjoyment can result in you hiking past dusk. Headlamps keep your hands free and are recommended.

Trekking Poles. Spare your knees. Trekking poles are highly recommended for steep descents, river crossings, and rough off-trail adventures. They provide stability, transfer some shock absorption to the upper body, and protect your knees.

Essential Overnight Equipment

Sleeping Bag. Nights are surprisingly cold in Northern California, especially at high elevations. Down sleeping bags offer the highest warmth-to-weight ratio and are incredibly compressible. However, down loses all its insulating ability when wet and takes forever to dry. Synthetic-fill sleeping bags retain their insulating ability even when wet but the increased bulk and weight are drawbacks. A temperature rating of 20°F or lower is recommended

for most hikes—keep in mind that the bag will lose some of its loft and insulating ability over time.

Sleeping Pad. Inflatable pads are the most compact and comfortable to sleep on, but a minor pain to inflate and deflate. Foam pads are lightweight, cheap, instantly available, and virtually indestructible, but are bulky.

Tent or Tarp? During the Northern California summer, a tent offers little more than privacy. Rains are very infrequent—especially in the Sierra Nevada and Modoc Plateau—and there is little to prevent you from sleeping under the stars. Thunderstorms do occur but are usually short-lived. A large tarp is always useful: emergency tent, sunshade, groundcover, rain shelter . . . but don't forget the rope! Due to fog and wind, a tent is always advisable along the coast. In winter and spring, a tent is essential across the state.

The Kitchen Sink. All your cooking and eating supplies: stove, fuel, cooking gear, silverware, dish (a Frisbee or gold pan is good), mug, pots (at least one big one), pans, lighter or matches, spices, oil, and plenty of food!

Campwear. Time to kick it. A nice pair of thick fleece pants, sandals/camp shoes, warm long underwear, and collapsible furniture are all highly recommended.

Other Good Stuff. A collapsible water bag (5 liters or more), sun hat, sunglasses, sunscreen, waterproof backpack cover, towel, toiletries, Ziplock bags, garbage bags, scissors, duct tape (you can store it taped around your water bottle), and trowel.

Fun Equipment

Still have room in your pack?

Camera. Make sure it is ready for outdoor abuse. Protective camera bags cost much less than new cameras. A polarizing filter is good for taking outdoor pictures with lots of sky and water. Shady forests are challenging to photograph when the sun is out—wait for foggy and overcast days.

Fishing Equipment. Fly-fish or use very lightweight spinning tackle in the mountain lakes and streams. A valid fishing license is required for all anglers 16 or older and can be purchased at just about any store that sells outdoor equipment.

Altimeter. A useful gadget for tracking your progress and identifying your location. While they are generally accurate to within 100 feet, greater precision requires constant recalibration. Elevation is measured by change in barometric pressure, and regular fluctuations in air pressure make it necessary to input a known elevation at least once a day to maintain accuracy.

Other Fun Stuff. You can see more with binoculars and play more with a Hacky Sack, Frisbee, or cards.

The Wilderness Ethic

In order to preserve the wilderness for future generations, follow some simple guidelines to leave no trace of your passage:

Do Not Scar the Land. Do not cut switchbacks. Stay on the trail as much as possible.

Camping. Camp at established sites. Select a location that has adequate water runoff, and do not dig ditches around your tent. Keep your camp clean and never leave food out.

Fires. Campfires should always be made in a fire ring. Use preexisting rings if available; otherwise, scatter the stones and ashes before you leave. Keep fires small and use only material that is already dead and down. Avoid making campfires in heavy use areas and at high elevations where firewood is scarce. Make sure the fire is completely out before leaving.

Sanitation. Choose a spot at least 200 feet away from trails, water sources, and campsites. Dig a cat hole six inches deep, make your deposit, and cover it with the soil you removed. Do not bury toilet paper.

Garbage. Carry out all garbage and burn only paper.

Group Size. Keep groups small to minimize impact. Maximum group size allowed varies by location but is usually 10 or less.

Animals. Do not feed wild animals.

Noise. Be respectful of other wilderness users. Listen to the sounds of nature.

Meeting Stock on the Trail. Move off the trail on the downhill side and stand still until the animals pass by.

Where Should I Go Hiking?

Because these hikes range from supremely easy to incredibly difficult, you should be able to find a hike that fulfills your personal sense of adventure in the region you wish to visit. For an overview of the difficulty rating system, please see How to Use This Book on p. 1. For those looking for a specific trail feature, the hikes are organized by theme beginning on p. xiv. Those unfamiliar with Northern California's geography and weather patterns should read on.

California Dreaming

For the purposes of this book, Northern California can be divided into four regions that share similar characteristics. Each is described briefly below.

The Central Coast, Bay Area, and Coast Ranges (Hikes 1–44)

Stretching from Silver Peak Wilderness on the southern end of Big Sur to the northern end of Highway 1 in Mendocino County, this region encompasses the

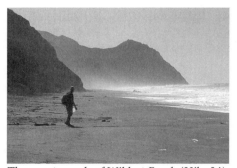

The remote sands of Wildcat Beach (Hike 34)

stretch of coastline accessible from Highway 1, all of the Bay Area, and the interior Coast Ranges. The overall topography is one of low mountain ranges divided by broad valleys—interrupted by the unique world of the San Francisco Bay Area. While the coastline is generally rocky and characterized by steep bluffs and headlands, beaches are also common.

Annual precipitation is high on the coast but diminishes rapidly as you go inland, creating habitat for lush redwood and mixed-evergreen forests near the Pacific, and extensive oak woodlands farther east. Going from south to north, precipitation generally increases while average temperatures decrease, leaving the southern regions hotter and drier for most of the year. Dense fog is common along the coast during the summer months, snow seldom falls anywhere in the region, and most of these hikes can be done year-round. Highlights of the region include rolling oak woodlands flushed green in spring, foaming surf on the dramatic Pacific Coast, lush redwood forests, and the endless variety of hikes and views available in the Bay Area.

The North Coast and Klamath Mountains (Hikes 45–58)

Stretching from the Lost Coast north to the Oregon border and east to Mt. Shasta, this region includes the hard-to-access strip of coastline north of Highway 1, the magnificent old-growth redwood forests along Highway 101, and the convoluted ranges of the Klamath Mountains. The coastal topography is usually rocky and often dominated by sheer cliffs. Inland, the Klamath Mountains compose a variety of

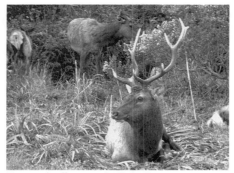

Roosevelt elk roam the Lost Coast.

smaller ranges incised by deep river canyons. Elevations rarely exceed 8000 feet. The Trinity Alps and Marble Mountains are two of the more notable subranges.

Annual precipitation is high throughout the entire region and creates thick forests that blanket all but the tallest ridges and peaks. Snow occurs down to 3000 feet in the winter and dense fog envelops the coast during the summer. Highlights include remote locations, luxuriant forests, and some of California's choicest wilderness.

Shasta and the Modoc Plateau (Hikes 59–74)

Including all of northeast California from Mt. Shasta east to Nevada and Lassen Peak north to Oregon, this region is a starkly different place. The landscape is entirely volcanic, an extensive plateau averaging around 4000 feet in elevation dominated by two active volcanoes—Mt.

Shasta and Lassen Peak. Cinder cones, defunct volcanoes, lava flows, and the notable Warner Mountains add a distinctive topography to the land.

Annual precipitation is low and summer temperatures are high, creating deserts and dry forests. Snow falls across the plateau in the winter. Highlights include the volcanic wonderlands of Mt. Shasta and Lassen Peak, the Warner Mountains, and some of the emptiest corners in the state.

The Sierra Nevada (Hikes 75–101)

For the purposes of this book, the Sierra Nevada stretches north from southern Sequoia National Park to the edge of the Modoc Plateau near Lake Almanor, and includes a few locations east of the range. Ranging in height from over 14,000 feet at its southern end to barely 7000 feet at its northern terminus, the range is characterized by jagged peaks, major rivers, and countless alpine lakes. While naked granite composes much of the range, a more complicated geologic mix is prevalent in the northern regions.

Annual precipitation is high and arrives in the form of heavy winter snows that melt throughout the summer, creating a broad forest belt that extends upward to about 10,000 feet. The highest elevations support only bare expanses of rock, snow, and hardy low-lying plants. Highlights include spectacular alpine scenery, unique landforms, deep river canyons, and the magnificent giant sequoia.

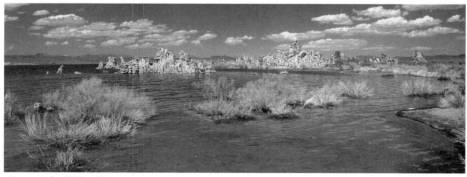

Mono Lake (Hike 85)

Northern California Weather

The overall weather in California is closely linked to the sun's relative position with the Earth. As the sun's rays strike more directly north of the equator in spring, the air it warms in the tropics rises into the upper atmosphere and moves north over the Pacific Ocean. Cooled as it travels, the air sinks back down to the surface to form an area of high pressure over the north Pacific known as the Pacific High. As the summer progresses, the high becomes increasingly stable and prevents low-pressure storm fronts in the Gulf of Alaska from reaching Northern California. As a consequence, summers are almost entirely devoid of rain. Localized thunderstorms do occur—especially in the high mountains—but generally the entire state basks in never-ending blue skies and sunshine. Summers on the coast are remarkably different, however. The same Pacific High that keeps storms away also creates northwest winds that almost continually buffet the shoreline. Warm moisture-laden summer air condenses into fog over the cold Pacific waters, which is then pushed onshore by wind and the land/sea temperature differential. Summer on the coast can seem a lot like winter.

As the sun begins to strike north of the equator more obliquely in October, the entrenched Pacific High keeps storms away for most of the month while the decreasing temperatures greatly reduce the incidence of fog. It is California's choicest month of weather. Storms return by November, striking the North Coast first and then gradually reaching farther south as the Pacific High deteriorates. By January, storm after storm is hitting the state, inundating it with heavy rainfall and deep snow. Sunny breaks do occur between storms, but they are generally short-lived. February is the wettest month and storms can continue well into April, although sunny spring days usually begin to occur in March. As a more direct angle of sunlight hits the north once again, the cycle repeats itself.

A Month-by-Month Playbook

The following is a brief description of the hiking opportunities available each month. Bear in mind that many hikes can be done year-round or at times not explicitly mentioned below.

January

Winter storms begin drenching the cold state and only low-elevation regions near the coast are free from snow. Last year's brown slopes begin to explode with green grass and powerful winter waves often break, making a coastal trip very worthwhile during sunny spells. The storms also cleanse the pollution from the air, making this the start of prime hiking season for views in the Bay Area—try Morgan Territory (Hike 14), Mt. Diablo (Hike 15), San Bruno Mountain (Hike 26), or Mt. Tamalpais (Hike 32). Redwood forests are always open for hiking on rainy days. Crowds are all but nonexistent.

February

The wettest month of the year hammers at the state and hiking is challenging. Stay coastal and in the Bay Area if the weather breaks. Pinnacles National Monument (Hike 8) is a great place to visit on sunny days. The adventurous can go looking for bald eagles around Cache Creek (Hike 40), at Gray Lodge Wildlife Area in the Great Central Valley (Hike 41), or at Tule Lake (Hike 61). Crowds remain absent.

March

A highly variable month, March can continue to bring wintry storms or break into long stretches of warm sunshine. Regardless of how frequently they come, the first spring days arrive this month and herald the start of wildflower season. Open slopes along the coast burst with color, views remain generally clear throughout the Bay Area, and oak woodlands flourish green. Big Sur (Hikes 1–7) can be downright hot during sunny spells.

April

Though much like March, April has increasing sunshine and warm weather. Fog can already begin to reappear on the coast, making this the last good month for fog-free coastal adventuring. Oak woodlands explode with wildflowers and Henry W. Coe State Park (Hikes 10–11) is a choice destination. Bidwell Park and Ishi Wilderness (Hikes 73–74) make a great combination trip. This is also a great time to tackle the North Coast (Hikes 45–53). Pummeled by rain and/or fog much of the year, the region experiences some of its nicest weather this month, when tourist crowds are absent.

May

The winter snowpack begins to melt at higher elevations and hikes below 5000 feet open for the season. Mountain rivers rage with snowmelt, the waterfalls of Yosemite Valley are spectacular (Hike 86), and deep river canyons offer summer heat and wildflowers. Warm sunny days on the coast are intermittent as the fog begins to increase, hills in the Coast Ranges begin to brown, and summer haze begins to collect, ending the prime Bay Area hiking season.

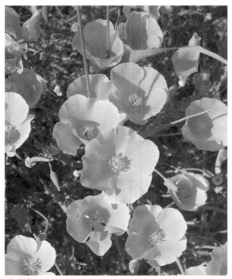

California poppies

Crowds remain surprisingly light until Memorial Day, when the summer hordes instantaneously appear.

June

The winter snowpack continues to melt, but hikes above 8000 feet usually remain snow-covered and inaccessible all month. The cable route on Half Dome (Hike 87) is usually put up early in the month, and Sequoia and Kings Canyon national parks (Hikes 95–101) offer great early summer adventures. Coastal fog continues to increase, and heat in the Coast Ranges and Sierra foothills starts to become oppressive. The summer crowds are out in force at popular destinations.

July

Unless it has been an unusually heavy winter, virtually all hikes are open by July and the three-month high-elevation season has begun. While the Sierra Nevada is the destination of choice with its wide variety of alpine hikes, also consider a trip north to Mt. Shasta and the Klamath Mountains (Hikes 54–60). Wildflower season begins to taper off as the month progresses. Fog and crowds are heavy along the coast. Avoid the Fourth of July weekend if at all possible.

August

Though much like July, the very highest elevation hikes to Palisade Glacier (Hike 95) and Sawtooth Peak (Hike 101) sometimes don't become snow-free until this time. Coastal fog is as thick as it gets, statewide temperatures max out, and crowds remain heavy all month long.

September

This is a great month to be anywhere in the mountains. Summer vacation ends for a lot of people on Labor Day and crowds suddenly vanish, yet the weather remains absolutely ideal across the state. It's a good time to visit Lake Tahoe (Hikes 80–81) or the Trinity Alps (Hike 54). Coastal fog begins to diminish, and high elevations become increasingly cold at night.

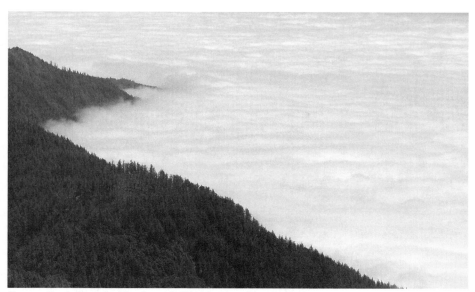

Fog routinely laps the Northern California coast in summer.

October

This is a great month to be anywhere in California. It is the month of Indian summer when the sun shines day in and day out, coastal fog finally disappears for the season, and fall colors fluoresce in the mountains. Hot summer weather lingers on a tour of the Modoc Plateau (Hikes 61–65) and the aspens of empty South Warner Wilderness (Hikes 66–67) rustle gold in the breeze. Higher elevation hikes usually remain open but nighttime temperatures often drop below freezing. Be aware that hunting season opens early in the month on National Forest lands; wearing bright colors is a good idea. Near the end of the month, temperatures begin to swing markedly and the first rogue winter storm often strikes the state.

November

Much of California closes to hiking as snow begins falling in the mountains and a chill sets in at higher elevations. Intermittent winter storms occur and air quality and visibility start to improve in the Bay Area. Fall lingers in the low-elevation foothills of the Sierra Nevada for the first half of the month—Rubicon River (Hike 79) is a pleasant destination. Stay coastal or in the Bay Area otherwise.

December

Daylight dwindles to a minimum as California slips into the depths of winter and hiking days are short. Weather is variable; long stretches of rain, cold snaps, and sunshine can all occur. Remain strictly coastal or enjoy views in the Bay Area.

The Different Governing Agencies

This book visits a wide variety of parks and forests managed by several different governing agencies. Rules and regulations often vary by location, but generally are the same within each group. The four most commonly visited areas in this book are national parks, state parks, national forests, and wilderness areas managed by national forests. A miscellany of other governing agencies occurs as well, including the Bureau of Land Management and various city and county parks.

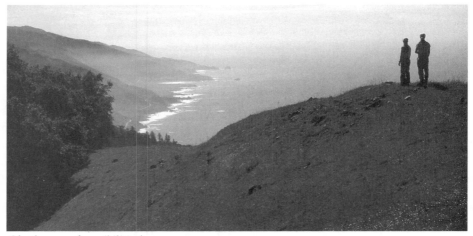

Oh, the seas of possibilities!

National Parks

Run by the federal government (Department of the Interior), national parks are designated to preserve and protect unique natural features and wilderness. Generally very user-friendly, they tend to draw the largest crowds and often have amenities like small stores, hot showers, and well-maintained campgrounds. Free park maps are handed out and driving is easy. Regulations are generally strict—car camping is permitted only in designated sites, wilderness permits are always required for overnight trips into the backcountry, trail quotas are common, and dogs are never permitted on the trail. Entrance fees are charged for all national parks.

State Parks

Run by the state of California, state parks are generally small and protect a wide variety of natural features. They are common along the coast and tend to be the most costly places to visit—day-use fees are always charged, campgrounds are expensive, and even park maps (when available) cost a few dollars. Regulations are generally strict—car camping is permitted only in designated campgrounds, backcountry camping (when possible) is usually allowed only at designated trail camps, and dogs are never allowed

in the backcountry. All state park campgrounds operate on the same reservation system; call 1-800-444-7275 or visit www.reserveamerica.com to reserve a site.

In 2009, a significant state budget shortfall prompted the state park system to increase its fees dramatically. Expect state park campgrounds and entrance fees to be more expensive than those listed in the trip descriptions. In addition, several state parks have reduced the open seasons for their campgrounds and backcountry trail camps. In some cases, entire parks have closed during the off-season (typically November–April). The situation is fluid and will likely change in the months and years ahead. Call ahead to check current park status, especially if you're planning a visit during the off-season.

National Forests

As "the land of many uses," national forests are America's playgrounds. Run by the federal government (Department of Agriculture), the U.S. Forest Service manages the land for a wide variety of purposes—logging, ranching, hunting, and hiking are all permitted—and regulations are generally few. Dogs are allowed, camping is permitted virtually anywhere, wilderness permits are not required for backcountry camping, and there are no use fees. A campfire permit is required for the use of stoves and campfires, obtainable free from any Forest Service ranger station and valid across the state for the entire year. Roads are generally poor, commonly unpaved, and often challenging and confusing to navigate. National forest maps are usually remarkably accurate, indicate areas of private property, and are all but essential for road navigation. Organized national forest campgrounds are plentiful across the state and tend to be inexpensive or even free, but generally lack amenities (pit toilets are common).

Wilderness Areas

Managed to protect the land's wilderness aspects, designated wilderness areas are much like national forests but with a few more restrictions. No roads exist, all motorized vehicles are prohibited, and logging is not permitted. Wilderness permits are required in all but the most remote areas and can be obtained free at any nearby ranger station. Due to heavy use, the wilderness areas in the Sierra Nevada are more heavily managed, and trail quotas are often in effect for backpackers. Dogs are usually allowed and backcountry camping is permitted almost anywhere. Facilities and amenities are nonexistent—come prepared.

Other Agencies

City and county parks are common in the Bay Area and are almost all day-use only. Entrance fees are usually charged. Dogs are generally not permitted, but there are some exceptions, most notably

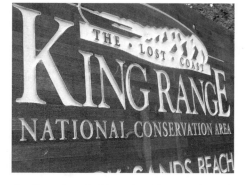

the Bay Area's East Bay Regional Park District. The Bureau of Land Management manages a few regions covered by the book. Much like national forests, they have few regulations and almost no amenities or facilities. Dogs are permitted.

Other Factors

Children

While this book is not designed for families with young children, several short hikes are perfectly suitable for the youngest hikers; look for the symbol in the trip header or the complete list in Hikes by Theme on p. xiv.

Campgrounds

Campgrounds vary markedly depending on location. State and national park campgrounds are generally the most luxurious, but are often expensive and crowded. Forest Service campgrounds are usually much more basic, smaller, cheaper, and good if you can cope with pit toilets.

101 Hikes...

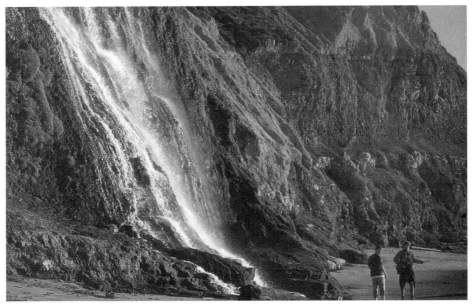

Alamere Falls, Point Reyes National Seashore (Hike 34)

HIKE 1

Upper Salmon Creek Falls

Hi Ho Silver

Highlights	Waterfalls, woodlands, and wildflowers
Distance	5.2 miles round-trip
Total Elevation Gain/Loss	1000'/1000'
Hiking Time	3–5 hours
Optional Maps	*Big Sur and Ventana Wilderness* by Wilderness Press, USGS 7.5-min. *Villa Creek* and *Burro Mountain*
Best Times	Year-round
Agency	Silver Peak Wilderness
Difficulty	★★★

On the southern edge of the Big Sur region, a little-traveled pocket of coastal mountain grandeur awaits within Silver Peak Wilderness. Far-reaching vistas look out across the ocean, perennial streams swirl beneath lush forest, and several quiet backcountry campsites entice you to spend the night.

The Hike first ascends to nearby Salmon Creek Falls, a dramatic cascade within eyeshot of Hwy. 1, and then travels along the mossy corridor of Salmon Creek to reach Upper Salmon Creek Falls. An iridescent pool shimmers at the base of this misty gem, a refreshing swimming spot on hot summer days. Fog can be thick in the summer months and poison oak is ubiquitous year-round. No water is available at the trailhead, though Salmon Creek is regularly accessible.

To Reach the Trailhead: Follow Hwy. 1 to the signed Salmon Creek Trailhead, located at a tight bend in the highway 8 miles south of Gorda, 7 miles north of Ragged Point, and 1.5 miles north of the posted San Luis Obispo County line. Park in the wide turnouts on either side of the highway.

Description: From the trailhead, follow Salmon Creek Trail as it climbs a moderate grade along the south bank of

Salmon Creek. The falls are clearly audible and you quickly reach an unmarked junction leading downward to the base of the cascade (0.1/230'). A side trip not to be missed, the 200-foot spur drops past fragrant bays and mossy boulders to reach the mist-cloaked cascade.

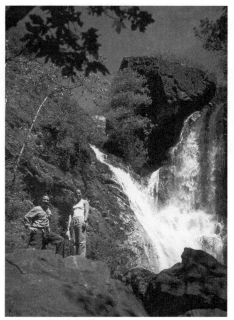

Salmon Creek Falls

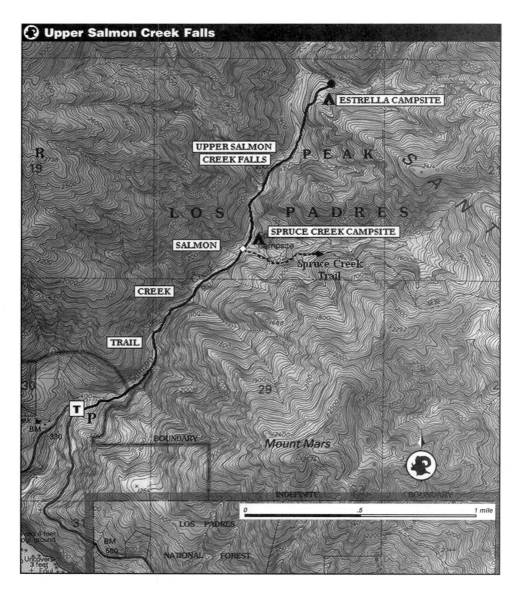

After exploring the falls, don't be taken in by the heavily used, steep spur that continues up Salmon Creek to rocky promontories above the falls. Many hikers mistake this spur for the Salmon Creek Trail, following it until it disappears into oblivion a mile upstream. Instead, carefully retrace your steps to the earlier junction, bear left, and continue climbing a moderate grade up the south canyon wall. The trail soon switchbacks past a seasonal creek and reaches a rocky viewpoint (0.3/760′) overlooking the lower Salmon Creek drainage.

Notice the diverse plant life and dramatic shift in vegetation in the surrounding canyon. A lush riparian forest of alders, maples, and bays lines the ravine's floor but quickly transitions to a drier coastal scrub zone of sagebrush, sticky monkey-flower, and coffeeberry bushes. Higher up, a rocky arid zone is populated by hardy succulents such as Our Lord's candle, a yucca that dies soon after sprouting its large stalk of cream-colored blossoms.

Onward, the trail switchbacks past a conspicuous mound of light green, slippery serpentine (0.5/760´), California's state rock. Formed atop ancient seafloors that tectonic activity later smashed into Big Sur, serpentine produces nutrient-poor soils that are inhospitable to most plant life. A few "serpentine endemics" have adapted, however, including California poppies, yucca, and other tenacious succulents.

The trail passes several unobstructed ocean views as it climbs the north-facing slopes, winding through dense coastal shrub and beneath shady live oaks and bays. Fragrant black sage and sagebrush thickets line the trail, as do mats of hedge nettles boasting deep lavender blossoms in spring. Just past a dry creekbed, you reach a crest (1.5/1050´) then gradually descend past groves of Douglas fir, tanoak, and bay amid dense huckleberry bushes. The trail contours along the south canyon wall, hopping across two seasonal creeks. Fifty feet past the last creek, you reach the signed junction for Spruce Creek Trail (1.8/1010´).

Bear left to continue on Salmon Creek Trail as it heads steadily downslope past large old-growth Douglas firs and vine-like poison oak. You soon reach Spruce Creek Camp (2.0/750´), where three idyllic campsites line the confluence of Salmon and Spruce creeks. Do not use the abandoned pit toilet 100 feet downstream along Salmon Creek; the steep topography and winter runoff are not very environmentally friendly.

Past the camp, the hike begins a moderate climb of the north-facing slopes in the shade of young Douglas firs, bays, oaks, and ceanothus, which fills the spring air with a lilac aroma from profuse blue flowers. The trail skirts high above the creek past small rapids and swirling emerald pools; a few small washouts require careful footing.

To reach Upper Salmon Creek Falls, watch for a steep spur on your left, located just before a bend in the trail (2.6/1140´). More reminiscent of a deer trail, the steep and precarious path drops 150 feet over loose rock and past poison oak to reach the base of the falls, a refreshing grotto of mist and spray that is well worth the effort. After a refreshing dip, retrace your steps to the trailhead. Alternatively, you can continue another 0.6 mile along Salmon Creek Trail and ascend 300 feet to Estrella Camp, where two pleasant campsites perch along the banks of Estrella Creek.

Nearest Visitors Center: Big Sur Station, (831) 667-2315, located just south of Pfeiffer Big Sur State Park on Hwy. 1, is open daily 8 AM–6 PM Memorial Day through Labor Day; the rest of the year it's open daily 8 AM–4:30 PM. Also try King City Ranger Station, (831) 385-5434, located at 406 S. Mildred Ave. in King City; take the Canal off-ramp from Hwy. 101, go east on Canal, right on Division, and left on Mildred. It's open 8 AM–4:30 PM Monday through Friday.

Backpacking Information: Spruce Creek and Estrella Camp are both ideally situated for an overnight trip. Several sites feature picnic tables and fire rings. A valid campfire permit is required.

Nearest Campground: Plaskett Creek Campground (43 sites, $22) is located 4 miles north of Gorda along Hwy. 1. Half the sites are reservable year-round; call (800) 444-7275 or visit www.reserveamerica.com.

Additional Information: www.fs.fed.us/r5/lospadres

HIKE 2

Vicente Flat

Flat Out

Highlights	Golden coastal bluffs and ancient redwoods
Distance	10.4 miles round-trip
Total Elevation Gain/Loss	2000´/2000´
Hiking Time	6–10 hours
Optional Maps	*Big Sur and Ventana Wilderness* by Wilderness Press, USGS 7.5-min. *Cone Peak* and *Lopez Point*
Best Times	Year-round
Agency	Ventana Wilderness
Difficulty	★★★

Extreme topography defines the coastal flanks of Cone Peak, where soaring ridges and chasmic valleys crease the mountainside. The area is also known for its exceptional biodiversity, from wildflower-painted grasslands to yucca-studded chaparral, fluttering oak woodland to towering old-growth redwood forest. And don't forget the sweeping ocean views, which look out for miles across a glittering aquamarine sea.

The Hike ascends nearly 2000 feet above the wave-swept coast and then traverses inland to reach Vicente Flat along redwood-lined Hare Creek. Open terrain allows dramatic coastal and canyon vistas as the trail initially climbs the grassy slopes, then heads inland through an increasingly lush forest to reach Vicente Flat, which offers campsites in a sun-drenched meadow or beneath old-growth trees. Spring welcomes a profusion of wildflowers to the otherwise golden slopes. Summer brings view-shrouding fog and the majority of visiting hikers. At other times of the year, you may have the trail entirely to yourself. Water is available near the trailhead in adjacent Kirk Creek Campground.

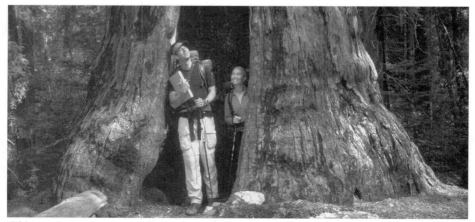

Old growth dreams—an ancient redwood tree at Vicente Flat

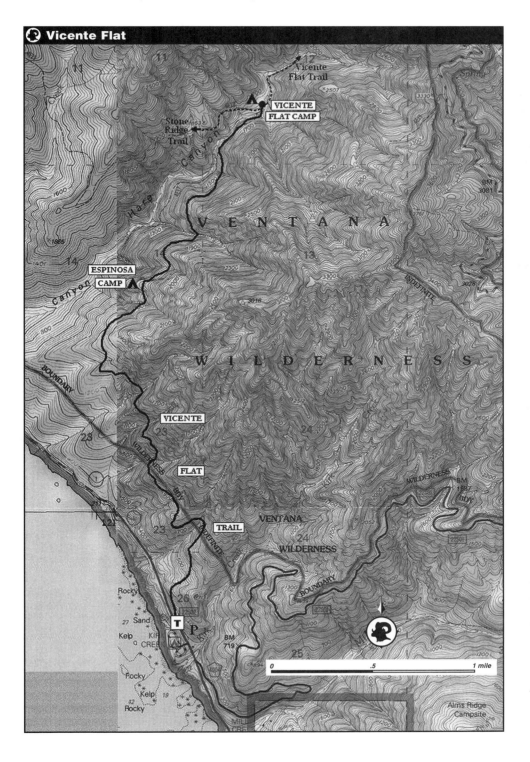

To Reach the Trailhead: Take Hwy. 1 to Kirk Creek Campground, located 38 miles south of Pfeiffer Big Sur State Park and 36 miles north of Hearst Castle. The trailhead is on the east side of Hwy. 1, across the road from the campground.

Description: From Hwy. 1 (0.0/190′), Vicente Flat Trail quickly climbs a series of switchbacks past coastal scrub. Flowering lupines, poppies, sticky monkeyflowers, and sagebrush highlight the hillside in spring. In 0.3 mile you cross a minor gully, head toward a minor saddle, then turn north across rolling grasslands and coastal chaparral. After crossing a gully choked with invasive blackberry and broom species, listen for water trickling from a nearby spring (0.9/700′).

The grade steepens as the trail passes scattered yuccas, spiny testaments to the aridity of these exposed slopes. You next reach a ridge (1.4/1000′) offering spectacular views of the convergence of land and sea. Continuing, the trail quickly enters the Ventana Wilderness and reaches shade beneath a canopy of oaks, madrones, and bays. You follow the ridgeline through four gullies and past a dense band of redwoods, then climb steeply to a prominent ridge (2.9/1610′), where exceptional views entice you to linger. To the east, 5155-foot Cone Peak (Hike 3) and its neighbor, double-notched Twin Peak, loom over Hare and Limekiln creeks. Hare Canyon is one of the state's deepest gorges; Limekiln Canyon boasts the steepest coastal slope in the Lower 48.

The trail now descends off the ridge, veering northeast through varied microclimates that support a range of drought-tolerant and moisture-loving plants. The contrast is stark—yuccas dot the arid slopes, while moisture-reliant redwoods cluster nearby in damp gullies. You next reach a short spur to Espinosa Camp (3.4/1660′), marked by a large fallen redwood 100 yards past a major gully.

The spur leads 100 feet to several small campsites atop a minor ridge in the shade of live oaks, bays, redwoods, and rare, endemic Santa Lucia firs. Rock outcrops offer unobstructed views toward the coast. This is an excellent picnic or overnight spot, though the nearby gully is usually dry. The continuing hike contours inland along the slopes, rounds a prominent ridge, and reaches the first reliable water source, a creeklet cascading past redwoods and ferns. Open grassy slopes return as the trail tops out at 1860 feet and begins a gentle descent to Vicente Flat.

You cross three rubble-strewn gullies (4.1/1800′), their adjacent marble faces misted in winter by a seasonal flow. After the next dry redwood gully, the trail contours north and enters dense woods a quarter mile before reaching Hare Creek and several large redwoods. A few feet farther, a spur cuts upstream to a pair of sites in the open meadow of Vicente Flat itself. The main trail continues a short distance to the Stone Ridge Trail junction (5.2/1620′); beyond lay many beautiful campsites in the redwoods.

Nearest Visitors Center: Big Sur Station, (831) 667-2315, located just south of Pfeiffer Big Sur State Park on Hwy. 1, is open daily 8 AM–6 PM Memorial Day through Labor Day; the rest of the year it's open daily 8 AM–4:30 PM.

Backpacking Information: No wilderness permit is needed but a valid campfire permit is required. The established tent sites of Espinosa and Vicente Flat camps are exceptional places to spend the night.

Nearest Campground: Kirk Creek Campground (33 sites, $16) is located at the junction of Hwy. 1 and Nacimiento Rd. Half the sites are reservable year-round; call (800) 444-7275 or visit www.reserveamerica.com.

Additional Information: www.fs.fed.us/r5/lospadres

HIKE 3

Cone Peak

Burnt

Highlights	Unobstructed views atop the highest coastal summit in California
Distance	4.0 miles round-trip
Total Elevation Gain/Loss	1400′/1400′
Hiking Time	2–3 hours
Optional Maps	*Ventana Wilderness* by the U.S. Forest Service, *Big Sur and Ventana Wilderness* by Wilderness Press, USGS 7.5-min. *Chews Ridge*
Best Times	April through November
Agency	Ventana Wilderness
Difficulty	★★★

Three miles from the ocean, Cone Peak rises a mile to the sky. In summer 1999, most of Ventana Wilderness burned. Cone Peak, the dominant mountain of the southern wilderness, burned with it. Life has since rebounded on these sheer slopes, yet does little to hide the seamless joining of ocean and sky, the towering coastal vistas, or the sweeping panorama of the Santa Lucia Mountains.

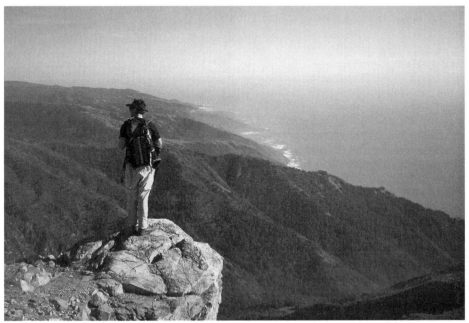

Looking south from mile-high Cone Peak

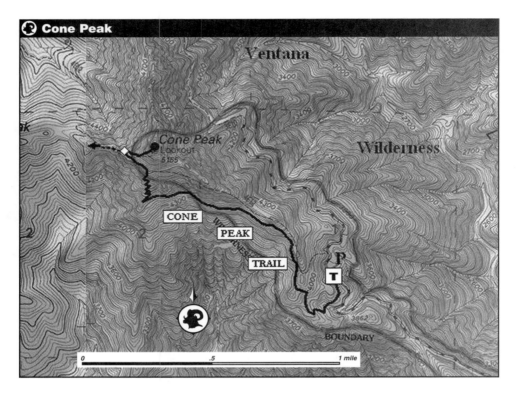

The Hike climbs to the fire lookout atop Cone Peak (5155´) on steep but short Cone Peak Trail. It's important to time your visit correctly. The 5-mile dirt access road closes after the first heavy winter rains (typically in December) and usually reopens in March, though this varies from year-to-year; call ahead to check if you're planning a trip in early spring or late fall. Crowds and coastal fog are heaviest in the summer. No water is available at the trailhead.

To Reach the Trailhead: Take Nacimiento Rd. east from Hwy. 1—the turnoff is by Kirk Creek Campground 4 miles south of Lucia. Be aware that Hwy. 1 is subject to washouts and closures, especially in the winter. Follow sinuous Nacimiento Rd. as it climbs 2800 feet in 8 miles to the divide, and turn north on rough and unpaved Cone Peak Rd. Low-clearance vehicles should have no problem making it to the trailhead, located 5.2 miles down this road by a small turnout with space for up to four cars.

Approaching from the east, take Hwy. 101 to the Hwy. G14/Fort Hunter Liggett exit just north of King City. Follow G14 south for 19 miles and turn right (west) on Mission Rd., passing immediately through an always-open fort entrance gate. Bear left on Nacimiento Rd. 3.0 miles past the gate and left again 0.9 mile farther—be watchful as the intersection signs are not obvious. From here, it is 18 increasingly narrow miles to Cone Peak Rd., where you proceed as described above.

Description: From the trailhead, the trail initially strikes west to quickly attain a nearby saddle. The cliffs of Cone Peak and the fire lookout are clearly visible to the northwest, and Hare Canyon can be seen slicing southwest down to the ocean. Far down the canyon is a dense patch of green, a stand of coastal redwoods very near the extreme southern limit of their range. Beneath them hides Vicente Flat (Hike 2). Briefly remaining on the ridge, the trail then drops inland and passes thickets of manzanita, wartleaf, and other regenerating shrubs before switchbacking up to a second saddle (0.5/4030′).

As the trail begins its long coastside traverse to approach the peak from the west, the devastation of recent fires is evident in the bare hillsides. Fires sweep through the dry chaparral about once every 20 years as part of a natural process of plant regeneration. Known as the Kirk Creek Fires, the 1999 blaze began during a dry lightning storm in September and eventually consumed 90,000 acres—more than half the area of Ventana Wilderness.

Only a few scraggly oaks survived the blaze and Coulter pine snags still protrude from the slopes like old burnt matchsticks. The exposed trail traverses below the sum-mit cliffs before beginning a tightly switch-backing ascent along a steep and rocky spur ridgeline. A small patch of unburned forest grows below the trail as it climbs to a junction with the Gamboa Trail immedi-ately below the summit (1.8/4830′).

The walkway surrounding the lookout is usually open to the public, though the views are equally tremendous on the sum-mit itself. Looking southwest, the scale of land and sea is distorted by your eleva-tion—notice the tiny bridge of Hwy. 1 at Limekiln State Park far below. Turning northeast, the tall rise of 5862-foot Juni-pero Serra Peak (Hike 7) is one of the few distinguishing peaks in this land of sheer, naked topography. Southeast, the broad valley of Fort Hunter Liggett can be dis-tinguished beyond the low nearby ridges. Heading downhill, you return the way you came.

Nearest Visitors Center: Big Sur Station, (831) 667-2315, 10 miles north of the entrance for Julia Pfeiffer Burns State Park and just south of Pfeiffer Big Sur State Park on Hwy. 1, is open daily 8 AM–6 PM Memorial Day through Labor Day; the rest of the year it's open daily 8 AM–4:30 PM.

Also try King City Ranger Station, (831) 385-5434, located at 406 S. Mildred Ave. in King City; take the Canal off-ramp from Hwy. 101, go east on Canal, right on Division, and left on Mildred. It's open 8 AM–4:30 PM Monday through Friday.

Backpacking Information: Backpacking is permitted along this hike, though not recommended due to the lack of campsites and water. No wilderness permit is needed but a valid campfire permit and Adventure Pass are required.

Nearest Campground: Kirk Creek Campground (33 sites, $22) is located at the junction of Hwy. 1 and Nacimiento Rd. Half of the sites are reservable year-round; call (800) 444-7275 or visit www.reserveamerica.com. Inland try Nacimiento Campground (7 sites, $12, no water), located on Nacimiento Rd. 3.5 miles east of Cone Peak Rd.

Additional Information: www.fs.fed.us/r5/lospadres

HIKE 4

Ewoldsen Trail

El Sur Grande

Highlights	Quiet redwood forest and aerial ocean views
Distance	4.5 miles
Total Elevation Gain/Loss	1500´/1500´
Hiking Time	3–4 hours
Optional Map	USGS 7.5-min. *Partington Ridge*
Best Times	September through May
Agency	Julia Pfeiffer Burns State Park
Difficulty	★★★

Big Sur is exceptional country. Open redwood forest lines creeks gurgling clear as glass, mountains rise thousands of feet above the foaming surf, and bare golden hilltops offer sweeping vistas of it all.

The Hike, a steady ascent along Ewoldsen Trail, takes you through a creekside redwood forest on your way to a view-point atop an open bluff more than 1600 feet above the sea. Crowds are constant on the Big Sur coast and—due to the limited amount of public land directly along the coast—all hiking trails receive heavy use. This is not a hike for solitude, and summer months are the worst for crowds. Water is available at the trailhead.

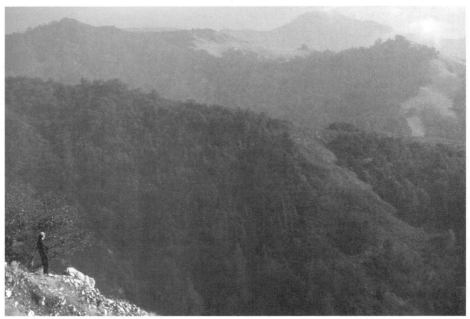

Big Sur bonanza from Ewoldsen Trail

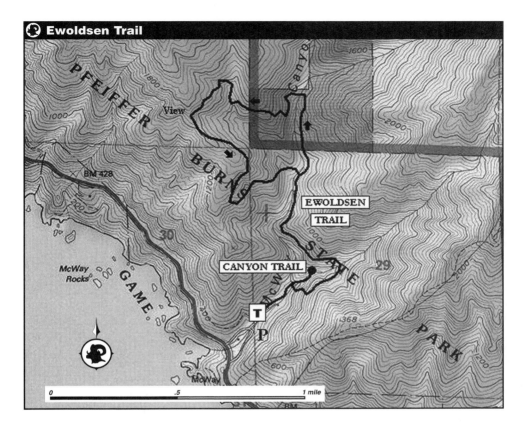

Ewoldsen Trail

To Reach the Trailhead: Take Hwy. 1 to the Julia Pfeiffer Burns State Park entrance, located 11 miles south of Pfeiffer Big Sur State Park on the central Big Sur coast. There is an $8 day-use fee, valid for all Big Sur area state parks.

Description: From the trailhead in the upper parking lot (0.0/280'), the path immediately enters the redwood forest and passes along a wooden fence before dropping down to a picnic area by McWay Creek. The open forest here is much different than the temperate rain forest more commonly associated with redwoods farther north. Here, at the southern limit of their range, the trees are only able to find adequate moisture for growth along the small creeks and rivers that slice the Big Sur coast. The drier conditions prevent the redwoods from obtaining the colossal size of their northern counterparts and

also eliminate the dense understory and thick moss normally present. A few small patches of redwood sorrel, ferns, and seasonal wildflowers can be found among the litter of the forest floor, but generally the forest is remarkably open.

Crossing the clear creek by a run-down barn, the trail begins climbing through an area good for bird-watching. American dippers can often be observed ducking in and out of the water as they look for aquatic insects and other snacks on the creek bottom. Small brown creepers are easily identified overhead by their ability to ascend trees vertically, spiraling around the trunk as they go. The junction for Canyon Trail is soon encountered (0.2/400'); it's a quick and worthwhile 0.1-mile side trip leading to a delightful bench by a cascading ribbon of water.

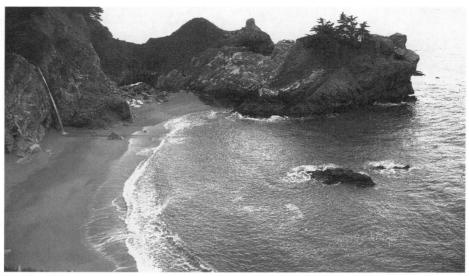

McWay Falls

Back on the main trail, you climb steeply above the canyon on a few switchbacks as tanoak begins to appear trailside. After crossing the south fork of the creek, the trail traverses the slopes and passes through a dramatic vegetation change, where redwoods suddenly disappear into thick chaparral. Large redwoods reappear as you rejoin the creek and reach a junction by a small bridge (1.6/880′). This is the start of the loop. Go right, passing several substantial trees as the trail winds along the creek. You next turn west and ascend through coast live oak and California bay to the high point of the hike where spectacular views await (2.7/1700′).

Hwy. 1 winds along the edge of the continent below and the aquamarine clarity of the ocean often allows you to distinguish a sandy bottom. Looking south, several drainages are identifiable beyond that of McWay Creek, overshadowed by peaks of the high ridge rising abruptly and paralleling the coast a short distance inland. From this viewpoint, the ridgetop is still more than 2000 feet above you, and the tallest summit visible south is nearly 4000 feet high and less than 3 miles from the ocean—imposing topography indeed. This is also

a good spot to look for red-tailed hawks and other raptors scanning the bare hillsides for lunch. From here, the trail drops behind the ridge, losing views as it makes a half-mile traverse before cutting back to quickly descend to McKay Creek and the junction at your loop's end. Head right to retrace your path to the trailhead.

Nearest Visitors Center: Big Sur Station, (831) 667-2315, located 10 miles north of this park's entrance on Hwy. 1 and just south of Pfeiffer Big Sur State Park, is open daily 8 AM–6 PM Memorial Day through Labor Day; the rest of the year it's open daily 8 AM–4:30 PM.

Nearest Campground: Pfeiffer Big Sur State Park has 218 sites ($20–$35, depending on site and time of year). Reservations are essential in the summer; visit www.reserveamerica.com or call (800) 444-7275.

Additional Information: www.parks.ca.gov

HIKE 5

Molera Beach

The Sandy Escape

Highlights	Peace and quiet on the beach
Distance	5.0 miles
Total Elevation Gain/Loss	200′/200′
Hiking Time	3–4 hours
Optional Map	USGS 7.5-min. *Big Sur*
Best Times	September through May
Agency	Andrew Molera State Park
Difficulty	★

For constantly being by the ocean, there is remarkably little coastal access from Hwy. 1 on the Big Sur coast. The jagged rocks and sheer cliffs that make the region so spectacular also make finding a beach, much less a secluded beach, a difficult proposition. Luckily there is Andrew Molera State Park and its 2-mile-long stretch of sand, whose farther end offers an opportunity to escape the crowds and commune peacefully with the sea.

The Hike explores the length of Molera Beach, traveling to its end before returning along the low bluffs. This is a tide-dependent hike and the beach is treacherous and impassable in places during high tides, making it necessary to walk along the bluffs during these times.

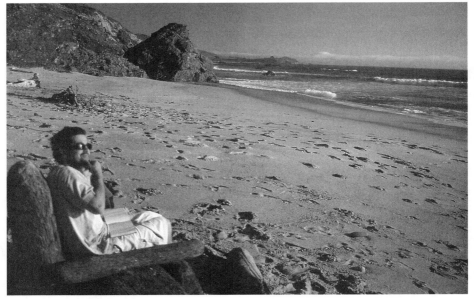

Relaxing on Molera Beach

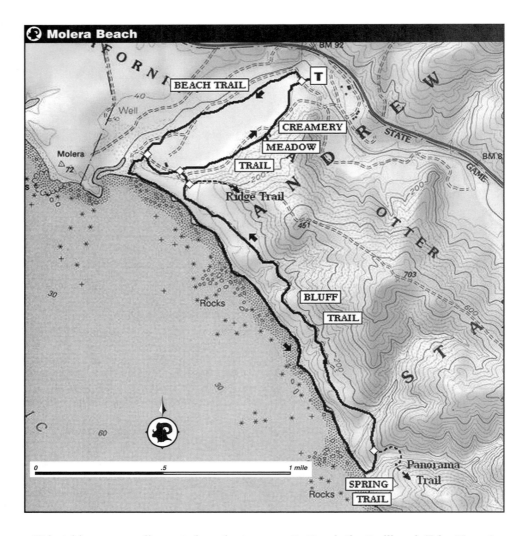

Tide tables are usually posted on the information sign in the parking lot, or you can check at Big Sur Station before heading out. Those arriving around high tide should hike first along the bluffs and return along the beach closer to low tide. Due to the treacherous nature of ocean currents here, swimming is deemed unsafe. Be aware that the seasonal, starting footbridge across Big Sur River is removed after the first heavy winter rains, making it necessary to ford the swollen river during the winter months. Water is available at the trailhead. Dogs are prohibited.

To Reach the Trailhead: Take Hwy. 1 south of Carmel for 22 miles to the park entrance and substantial parking lot. Approaching from the south, the turnoff is 4.2 miles north of the park entrance for Pfeiffer Big Sur State Park and is a hard, dog-leg left turn. There is a day-use fee of $8, valid for all Big Sur area state parks. It is possible to reach the trailhead by public transportation on Monterey-Salinas Transit Bus 22, which runs twice daily from downtown Monterey to Pfeiffer Big Sur State Park from Memorial Day to Labor Day; weekends only during the rest of the year. Call 888-678-2871 for current schedule and fare information, or visit www. mst.org.

Description: From the trailhead, cross Big Sur River on the narrow footbridge and bear right on Beach Trail. Paralleling but beyond sight of the river, you pass the Creamery, a former pasture slowly being replanted with native vegetation. Twisted sycamores, arroyo willows, black cottonwood, red alders, and a few redwoods line the river, and chest-high bush lupines dot the open meadow. Looking behind you to the east, a prominent ridge of the Santa Lucia Range is visible. Composed primarily of granite transported from the south along the San Andreas Fault, the mountain range owes much of its sheer topography to the erosion-resistant nature of its granitic rock. The Creamery is also an excellent area for birdlife—killdeer, black phoebes, and Cooper's hawks can often be spotted.

Continuing toward the beach, notice the incredibly grizzled redwood tree across the meadow on your left before you turn back toward the river. Then pass thick patches of poison oak and coffeeberry, which is easily identified by the dark black berries that ripen in the fall. Driftwood shelters and other interesting constructs fill this first sandy area where you turn south and begin the beach walk.

The low bluffs along the beach expose the variegated hues of intensely deformed rocks. While part of the Franciscan Complex, they have been more heavily metamorphosed than similar exposures found farther north in California, as a result of the numerous northwest-trending faults associated with the San Andreas Fault, which slice apart the Big Sur region and intensely shear the adjacent rock. The rare mineral almondite is exposed in places, coloring the white sand purple where it has eroded onto the beach. Rounded granite stones are also present, washed down from the Santa Lucia Mountains.

Sea lions, seals, and even sea otters can sometimes be spotted offshore as you go (barefoot) up the beach. Crowds diminish and rocky points hem in secluded stretches of sand as you continue, eventually reaching the junction for Spring Trail, your access to the return route on the bluffs above.

Eighty feet of climbing up a narrow gully brings you to Bluffs Trail—go left back the direction you came. Coyote brush, poison hemlock, California poppies, and more lupine cover the open blufftops along the trail back toward the Creamery. At the bluffs' end, the trail intersects Ridge Trail—go left again, immediately dropping down to a wide dirt road. Bearing left here returns you to the Beach Trail. Turning right down the road takes you winding along the opposite side of the Creamery close to several large coast live oaks, before the road rejoins the Beach Trail at the footbridge over Big Sur River.

Nearest Visitors Center: Big Sur Station, (831) 667-2315, located 10 miles north of the entrance of Julia Pfeiffer Burns State Park and just south of Pfeiffer Big Sur State Park on Hwy. 1, is open daily 8 AM–6 PM Memorial Day through Labor Day; the rest of the year it's open daily 8 AM–4:30 PM.

Nearest Campground: Andrew Molera State Park has 24 walk-in campsites available in a large meadow near the Big Sur River on a first-come, first-served basis ($10 per site, register at the entrance kiosk, with a maximum of four people per site and no dogs allowed). The closest developed campground is Pfeiffer Big Sur State Park (218 sites, $20–$35, depending on site and time of year). Reservations are essential in the summer; visit www.reserveamerica. com or call (800) 444-7275.

Additional Information: www. parks.ca.gov

HIKE 6

Pine Valley

Pine Away

Highlights	Sandstone cliffs, ponderosa pines, and an emerald swimming hole
Distance	12.0 miles round-trip
Total Elevation Gain/Loss	3500′/3500′
Hiking Time	6–8 hours
Optional Maps	*Ventana Wilderness* by the U.S. Forest Service, *Big Sur and Ventana Wilderness* by Wilderness Press, USGS 7.5-min. *Chews Ridge*
Best Times	September through May
Agency	Ventana Wilderness
Difficulty	★★★★

Ponderosa pines stand sentinel above wildflower-strewn meadows in the heart of Ventana Wilderness. Cliffs and stones surround this broad valley, echoing stories of the Esselen people who once called this region home. A waterfall rushes out-of-sight nearby, pouring into a glittering pool. And on the way into peaceful Pine Valley, you'll enjoy far-reaching views of the ridge-rippled landscape that defines the Santa Lucia Mountains.

As this book was going to press, the massive 2008 Basin Complex wildfire scorched virtually the entire northern half of Ventana Wilderness, including the majority of this hike. Much of central and lower Pine Valley was spared, however, including the area around Pine Falls—now more of an oasis than ever. Check with the Forest Service for the latest trail conditions before you head out.

The Hike approaches the Ventana Wilderness from the east via rough and unpaved Tassajara Road. The route first follows Pine Ridge Trail from China Camp, rising and falling along an overgrown ridgeline punctuated by several excellent views. It then turns northwest at Church Creek Divide and slowly descends

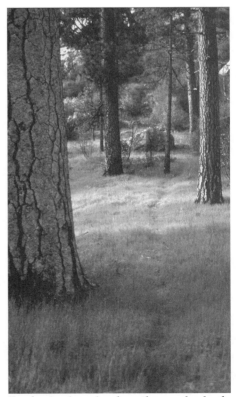

Ponderosa pines rise above the grasslands of Pine Valley.

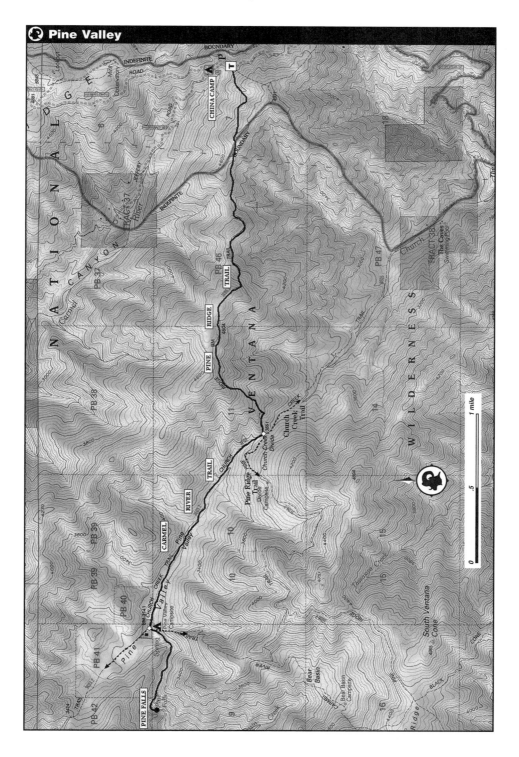

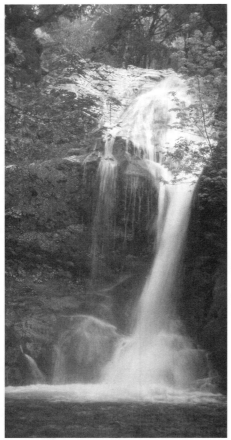

Hidden Pine Falls

China Camp entrance; the pavement ends 1.8 miles past the fork. Park at the large turnout across from the camp entrance. The trailhead is 100 feet farther south on the camp side of the road.

From points south, take Hwy. 101 to Greenfield and exit on Rte. 101 Business, the town's southernmost exit. Turn left on Elm Ave. (County Rd. G16) a half mile later and proceed 5.8 miles to Arroyo Seco Rd. (County Rd. G17). The two roads merge for 6.5 miles and then fork. Bear right and continue 17 miles on Carmel Valley Rd. to Tassajara Rd. Turn left and proceed as above.

Description: From the marked trailhead (0.0/4350′), Pine Ridge Trail gradually climbs 400 feet and then descends the same elevation through brush dominated by ceanothus and tanoak. After this scratchy welcome to the wilderness, you traverse steadily upward to emerge from the worst of the overgrown sections at the route's high point (0.6/4750′). Views look south over the Church Creek and Tassajara Creek drainages, west toward the Coast Ridge, and southeast toward 5862-foot Junipero Serra (Hike 7), which rises above the unseen Salinas Valley. Cone Peak (Hike 3) perches atop the farthest visible ridge to the south, 17 miles away.

The route cruises near the ridgeline through golden grasslands, charred forest, and thick new growth. Oak woodlands and stalks of Our Lord's candle, a large and easily distinguished yucca, punctuate the scenery as you next ascend and top a minor saddle before continuing upward to another, more prominent saddle. Views vanish briefly as the trail switchbacks southwest and then climbs north to the second highest point along the route (2.1/4740′). From this point onward, it's all downhill to Pine Valley.

The trail turns southwest on a steep grade, dropping 850 feet through open oak woodlands carpeted with spring wildflowers. A final series of switchbacks deposits you at Church Creek Divide and a four-way trail junction (3.6/3650′).

Carmel River Trail into the open terrain of Pine Valley. The route is ideal in spring and fall, when temperatures are moderate and storms infrequent. The winter months can be quite pleasant as well, though freezing temperatures and strong storms occur at times. The heat, flies, and mosquitoes of summer are best avoided. No water is available at the trailhead. Poison oak is plentiful—be watchful.

To Reach the Trailhead: From points north, follow Hwy. 1 to Carmel and take Carmel Valley Rd. (County Rd. G16) east for 23 miles to Tassajara Rd. Turn right on Tassajara Rd., bear left in 1.3 miles at the fork with Cachagua Rd., and continue on Tassajara Rd. for another 10.7 miles to the

The divide forms a deep saddle between two west-trending ridges and sits atop the 29-mile-long Church Creek Fault, a splinter fault of the greater San Andreas Fault system. The grinding faults of the area pulverize adjacent rock, which then erodes away to form distinctively straight valleys. Here the Church Creek Fault has created linear Church Creek canyon southeast of the divide, and the upper Carmel River valley (including Pine Valley) to the northwest. The divide also separates the watersheds of the Carmel River, which has its headwaters in Pine Valley, and the Salinas River, which initially flows southwest before turning north, eventually entering the sea some 80 miles north of the Carmel River mouth.

From the divide, turn north and follow Carmel River Trail toward Pine Valley. The trail slowly descends, crossing over the usually dry headwaters of the Carmel River, and then eventually levels off. As the gradient eases, sandstone cliffs appear to your right, water trickles audible off to your left, and ponderosa pines begin to rise from open meadows.

For thousands of years, Pine Valley was home to the Esselen people and provided them with fertile hunting, gathering, and living grounds. The Esselen may have used fire to clear underbrush and maintain the pine stands and broad meadow, where deer, rabbits, antelopes, and even bears once commonly grazed. In the adjacent forest, doves, quails, and other game birds flocked beneath the abundant canopy of oaks, bays, pines, and madrones. Wild roses grow in dense thickets on the east edge of the valley, perhaps cultivated by the Esselen for straight, strong arrow shafts. Beneath the sandstone cliffs, women took harvested acorns from the surrounding oak woodlands and ground the nutritious meat into flour. Their mortar holes still pepper sandstone outcrops just downstream from the Pine Valley–Pine Ridge Trail junction.

A large gate marks the official Pine Valley entrance (5.3/3140′) at a junction with the Pine Valley–Pine Ridge Trail and the route to Pine Falls. To make the trip to this waterfall oasis, be prepared for some hiking excitement—the 0.7-mile one-way journey follows a path that is narrow, overgrown, and washed out in a few precarious places. From the junction, turn left and cross the river. Head downstream a few yards and then recross the river past the first of three small unofficial campsites. The route now closely follows the river, crisscrossing it multiple times as its winds downstream through a lush riparian environment.

You eventually emerge at an overlook directly above 50-foot Pine Falls (6.0/2700′). The descent to its base can be hazardous, as you must clamber across slick boulders. Use the conveniently placed rope to negotiate the final 20 feet to the crystal clear pool. Enjoy a brisk plunge and then return the way you came.

Nearest Visitors Center: King City Ranger Station, (831) 385-5434, is located at 406 S. Mildred Ave. in King City. Take the Canal off-ramp from Hwy. 101, go east on Canal, right on Division, and left on Mildred. It's open 8 AM–4:30 PM Monday through Friday.

Backpacking Information: Campsites and water are abundant in Pine Valley. A valid campfire permit is required.

Nearest Campground: China Camp (6 sites, $5) is located adjacent to the trailhead.

Additional Information: www.fs.fed.us/r5/lospadres

HIKE 7

Junipero Serra Peak

Nemesis

Highlights	Epic panoramas from the highest peak in the Santa Lucia Range
Distance	12.4 miles round-trip
Total Elevation Gain/Loss	3900′/3900′
Hiking Time	8–12 hours
Optional Maps	*Ventana Wilderness* by the U.S. Forest Service, *Big Sur and Ventana Wilderness* by Wilderness Press, USGS 7.5-min. *Junipero Serra Peak*
Best Times	November through April
Agency	Ventana Wilderness
Difficulty	★★★★★

This monolithic mountain is draped in thick vegetation and wild coast range adventure. With a remote location, difficult trail conditions, and sustained elevation gain on the trail to its summit, 5862-foot Junipero Serra Peak rewards only the hardiest hikers. The payoff is a head-spinning vista from the highest summit in the Santa Lucia Mountains.

The Hike is a strenuous ascent of the mountain across boulder-strewn hillsides, pine groves, and blue and valley oak woodlands to the summit. Good route-finding skills are essential for this hike—the tread is faint at times and head-high brush aggressively encroaches on the trail in places. The best time to summit is during the wet season (November through April), when air quality is best and temperatures are moderate along this exposed route. Be aware, however, that snow can blanket the mountain at higher elevations after winter storms. Summer brings an onslaught of flies, scalding temperatures, and blankets of fog that obscure coastal views.

To Reach the Trailhead: Take Hwy. 101 to the Jolon Road exit, located 10 miles south of Greenfield and a mile north of the Salinas River crossing. Follow Jolon

Rd. (County Rd. G14) south for 17.8 miles, turn right onto Mission Rd., and drive 0.2 mile to the Hunter Liggett Military Reservation gate (expect to show your driver's license and vehicle registration to enter). In 4.9 miles, turn left onto Del Ventura Rd. at a four-way intersection and then bear right along the paved road 0.8 mile farther. Twelve miles past the intersection, you cross Rattlesnake Creek and enter U.S. Forest Service land. (Del Ventura Rd. becomes Milpitas Rd. somewhere along the way.) Five miles farther you reach a spur road on your right, which leads 250 feet to the gated trailhead and a large turnout for parking.

Description: From the trailhead (0.0/2090′), the broad Santa Lucia Trail heads to the east end of Santa Lucia Memorial Park through open grasslands adjacent to steep sandstone cliffs. The path ascends a minor ridge, climbs briefly northeast to arrive at a minor gap, and then continues northeast past live oaks and open terrain. Along the way you may notice the anomalous prickly pear cacti. Though Junipero Serra Peak does boast unusual and rare plant species, this cactus is not endemic to the Santa Lucia

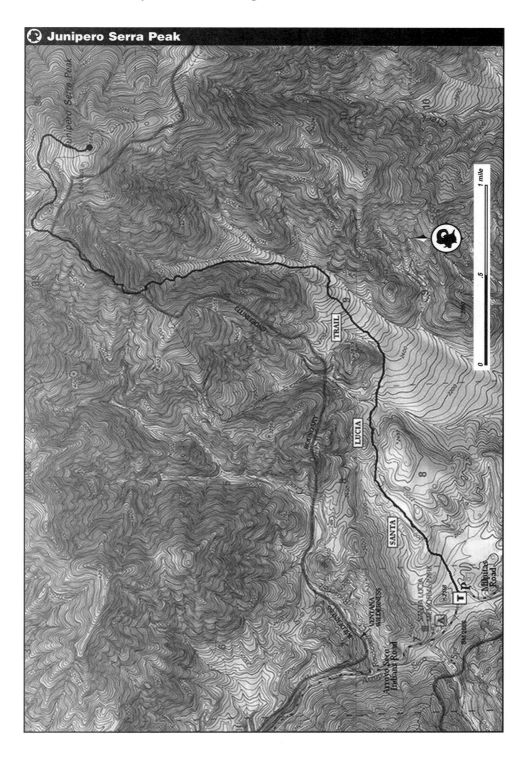

Range. Spanish missionaries brought the drought-tolerant species from Mexico as early as 1769, and modern-day specimens probably derive from stock planted by early settlers.

After attaining a scenic ridge with exceptional views, the trail turns east and climbs to a saddle (1.0/2350′). From here the route follows an abandoned road to a dry creekbed lined with willows and sycamores. In a few minutes you pass a rusty abandoned tractor (1.4/2320′). The continuing trail narrows and climbs gradually to a junction with a southbound trail (1.6/2430′). Beyond this point, the gradient markedly steepens.

Dense brush encroaches on the trail as it enters a steep-walled arroyo canyon lined with an ephemeral stream. Large granite boulders hulk in the surrounding wash,

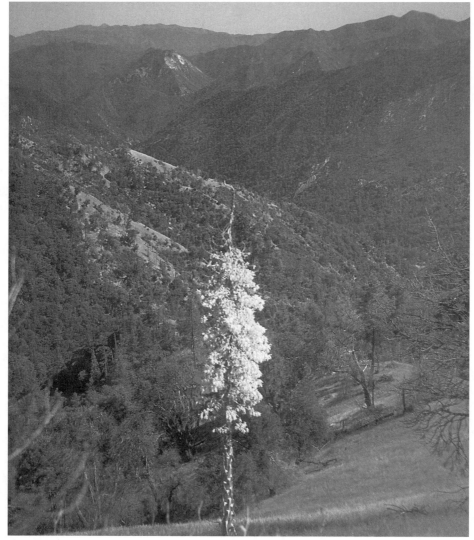

Our Lord's Candle, a yucca, commands an inspiring viewpoint.

transported here by the heavy floods that reshape this landscape about once every century. The route next follows a faint trail between two parallel washes before crossing the west wash (2.6/3170′).

The path climbs through a small meadow, past heavy chaparral thickets, and reaches a second sloping meadow. From here you switchback through head-high brush to a prominent saddle and a junction with the north-trending abandoned section of the Santa Lucia Trail (3.7/4170′), marked by a dilapidated sign that claims you're 2 miles from the summit. Forged by the U.S. Forest Service in the early 1900s, the original Santa Lucia Trail served as the only access through the eastern section of the Ventana Wilderness until Arroyo Seco Road was completed in 1939. At this point, you're more than halfway to the summit.

A faint trail leads east up the ridge from here, but your continuing route switchbacks toward the ridge along a more moderate grade. Over the next 0.8 mile, the trail tops a ridge, veers left past oak-clad slopes, and crosses through dense manzanita thickets to a notable saddle. The hike next turns east, skirting the north slopes and passing a junction for the abandoned Junipero Serra Camp Trail, located 0.4 mile and 600 feet below. Beyond the junction, enormous Coulter and sugar pines tower overhead as you climb toward a saddle between a ridge and the summit. The trail curves below the saddle and leads a quarter mile to a minor ridge, where it turns south and climbs to more open terrain. The trail makes one final push to the rounded mountaintop, where it turns south to reach an abandoned 40-foot lookout tower at the summit (6.2/5862′).

From this vantage point, you can take in a huge chunk of the Santa Lucia Mountains, including the Ventana and Silver Peak wildernesses, Hunter Liggett Military Reservation, and the Big Sur coast. To the northwest, conspicuously flat-topped Uncle Sam Mountain (4766′) and notched, barren Ventana Double Cone (4853′) rise behind Tassajara Creek and Church Creek canyons. Sixty miles of coastline spread out beyond the Coast Ridge. Looking east, Piñon Peak (5264′) caps a prominent ridge that extends east, hiding most of the Salinas Valley. To the south, 5155-foot Cone Peak (Hike 3) rises less than 3 miles from the glittering Pacific. On extremely clear days, you may even spot the high crests of the Sierra Nevada more than 150 miles east. When you're ready, return the way you came.

Nearest Visitors Center: King City Ranger Station, (831) 385-5434, located at 406 S. Mildred St. in King City. Take the Canal off-ramp from Hwy. 101, go east on Canal, right on Division, and left on Mildred. It's open 8 AM–4:30 PM Monday through Friday.

Backpacking Information: Backpacking is permitted, though the lack of water sources and quality campsites make this an unappealing option. A valid campfire permit is required.

Nearest Campground: Santa Lucia Memorial Park Campground (8 sites, free), located immediately north of the trailhead, is open year-round and doesn't have water.

Additional Information: www.fs.fed.us/r5/lospadres

HIKE 8

High Peaks Trail

The Pinnacles

Highlights	Naked monoliths of towering volcanic rock, prairie falcons, and California condors
Distance	5.3 miles
Total Elevation Gain/Loss	1650´/1650´
Hiking Time	3–4 hours
Optional Map	USGS 7.5-min. *North Chalone Peak*
Best Times	October through May
Agency	Pinnacles National Monument
Difficulty	★★★

The story of the Pinnacles began some 28 million years ago when the Pacific Tectonic Plate first made contact with North America near present-day Los Angeles, and pushed an active underwater volcanic ridge beneath the continent. Widespread geologic havoc followed, and the first strands of the San Andreas Fault began forming. Shortly after this collision, 23.5 million years ago, rising magma escaped onto the surface through one of the many newly formed fractures and created a large, short-lived stratovolcano 24 miles long and roughly 8000 feet high. Straddling the young San Andreas Fault, the volcano was quickly ripped in two as lands west of the fault were pushed northwest. The western half of the volcano was then tilted by associated splinter faults, protecting it from erosion until it was once again exposed at the surface. It slowly weathered to form the spectacularly unique peaks of the Pinnacles, 195 miles away from its eroded rock counterpart in Southern California.

While numerous volcanic rocks compose the Pinnacles, the two most common (and easily identifiable) are volcanic breccia, a mess of angular fragments welded together into the reddish rocks of the High Peaks, and flow-banded rhyolite, a fine-grained lava that preserves its original flow patterns. Several excellent sources of information on the local geology are available at the visitors center, including a guide to the Pinnacles Geological Trail, the first half of which is along this hike.

The Hike climbs from Bear Gulch Nature Center along the Condor Gulch and High Peaks trails, winding through wild volcanic formations before dropping steeply back down to Bear Gulch Picnic Area. The best time to come is February. You have to time your visit to avoid winter storms, but the reward is early wildflowers, crystalline air, flowing streams, green hillsides and, most of all, solitude. The air, the water, and the green all remain from March through May—supplemented by a greater explosion of wildflowers—but the solitude vanishes, especially on weekends. An average of 200,000 people a year visit this small monument, and most of them come during this time. In the summer months temperatures are sizzling and average almost 100°F during the day—don't bother. The fall is mild but brown and dry. Water is available at the trailhead.

To Reach the Trailhead: Take Hwy. 25 south from Hollister for 35 miles to the posted turnoff for the Pinnacles on Hwy. 146. Approaching from the south, Hwy. 25 can be accessed from Hwy. 101 via Hwy.

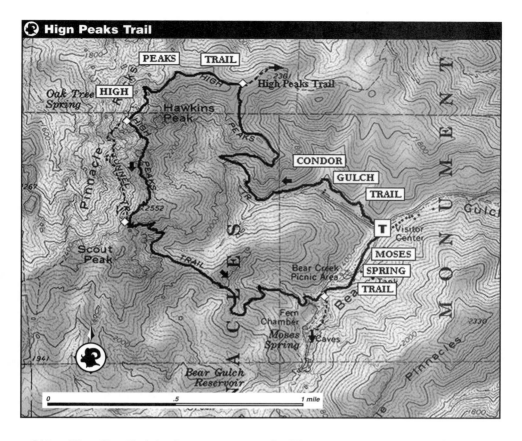

Hign Peaks Trail

G13 at King City. Park in the nature center parking lot, 5 miles past the turnoff. The trailhead is across the road. While it is also possible to approach the Pinnacles (but not this hike) from the west through Soledad, there is no connection on Hwy. 146. There is an entrance fee of $5, which is valid for 7 days.

Description: From the trailhead (0.0/1650´), you begin climbing on the Condor Gulch Trail through large gray pines and deciduous blue oaks, quickly passing above a maintenance station. As you ascend, coast live oaks can be spotted in the riparian valley below. Toyon soon appears by the path, a shrub easily identified by its stiff, toothed, elliptical leaves and bright red berries, which first appear in December. At the first switchback, a rounded squat formation dubbed

the Hippopotamus sits across the small gully. Looking like a stack of chips, Casino Rock is visible to the north. The trail then leads to an overlook where a small runnel of water gurgles down in season.

From the overlook, you leave the gulch behind and wrap around the ridge above you. Where the trail winds through open chaparral dominated by chamise, good views east of deeply furrowed San Benito Valley open up.

Views to the north appear as you intersect High Peaks Trail (1.7/2290´)—go left. This is a good place to start looking for California condors. Since 2003, the park has taken part in the California Condor Recovery Program. Nearly two dozen juvenile condors have been released here in recent years; the park is currently home to more than a dozen of these majestic—

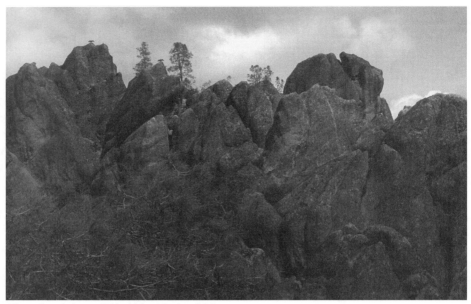

The volcanic jags of Pinnacles National Monument

and enormous—endangered birds. Also keep an eye out for prairie falcons. Every year from January through June, roughly a dozen pairs of these raptors nest in the cliffs of the Pinnacles and can often be seen swooping between the peaks. They are readily identified by their pointed wings, narrow tails, quick wingbeats, and distinctive cries.

Curving through massive boulders and outcrops, the trail then offers up views of the Balconies, a large, deeply sliced outcrop visible northwest. Reaching a junction with Tunnel Trail (2.3/2480'), continue straight on High Peaks Trail to begin an exciting section where bolted iron railings provide handholds for steep stairways, whose steps are mere scoops in the rock. Passage is tight beneath Condor Crags and descending those scoops is challenging; you soon reach a junction on the opposite side (3.0/2470') where an outhouse is conveniently situated.

Keeping left on High Peaks Trail, you begin the steep switchbacking descent to Bear Gulch. You pass the aptly named Anvil along a brief level section, before

continuing down past large manzanitas to the junction with Rim Trail (4.5/1600'). Descend left past Discovery Wall among handsome coast live oaks, and then go left again at the Moses Spring Trail junction (4.8/1550') to quickly reach Bear Gulch Picnic area. Cross the road and follow the easy path back to the visitors center.

Nearest Visitors Center: Pinnacles Visitors Center, located in Pinnacles Campground, (831) 389-4485, is open daily 9 AM–5 PM.

Nearest Campground: Pinnacles Campground is located on Hwy. 146 near the park's eastern boundary; the fees are $23 per tent site for up to six people and $36 for RV sites with hook-ups. Reservations are recommended for spring weekends; contact the visitors center or visit www.recreation.gov.

Additional Information: www.nps.gov/pinn

HIKE 9

Fremont Peak

The Invisible Canyon

Highlights	Superlative view of the entire Monterey Bay
Distance	1.0 mile
Total Elevation Gain/Loss	350'/350'
Hiking Time	1 hour
Optional Map	USGS 7.5-min. *San Juan Bautista*
Best Times	After winter storms
Agency	Fremont Peak State Park
Difficulty	★

Atop Fremont Peak on March 6, 1846, John C. Frémont defiantly raised the first American flag in California. Three days later, as he sat surrounded by Spanish forces threatening to attack, his flagpole blew down. Taking this as a bad omen, Frémont departed and left behind this unrivaled panorama of Monterey Bay.

The Hike is a quick and easy ascent of Fremont Peak (3169'), a prominent summit located due east from the center of Monterey Bay. Unparalleled views are the reason to come here, making it critical to correctly time your visit. The air is cleanest and the grass greenest immediately following winter storms, but air quality rapidly declines without rain and will usually begin to deteriorate within 24 hours. Prepare for chilly and windy conditions during the winter months. Fog can completely obliterate the view during the summer. Crowds are minimal, especially in the winter. Water is available in the nearby campground.

To Reach the Trailhead: Take Hwy. 156 east of Hwy. 101 for 3 miles to San Juan Bautista and head south on the Alameda (Hwy. G1). Approaching from the east, the turnoff is 9 miles past the junction of Hwys. 156 and 25. Immediately bear left on San Juan Canyon Rd. (Hwy. G1) at the complex four-way intersection and pro-

ceed 11 miles to the upper parking lot at road's end. There is a nominal day-use fee.

Description: From the trailhead, proceed up the paved road signed AUTHORIZED VEHICLES ONLY. A single-track dirt trail quickly splits off across from a few, stout Coulter pines, passing through coyote brush punctuated by some valley oaks and small madrones. It wraps around the western slope where the antenna complex comes into view. A series of short switchbacks lead you to the rocky summit.

Savoring the view, ignore the antennas as you behold the curving expanse of Monterey Bay. Its southern arm is formed by the Monterey peninsula, visible beyond the city of Salinas. Its northern end contains south-facing Santa Cruz on its shores. Two main rivers drain into Monterey Bay: the longer Salinas River on the south, which flows 190 miles northwest through the broad Salinas Valley, and the Pajaro River on the north, which flows by Watsonville before entering the bay near its center. Between the two is Elkhorn Slough, a tidal embayment extending 7 miles inland, whose mouth is marked by the enormous 500-foot-high boiler stacks of the Moss Landing Power Plant. The slough is a haven for birdlife—the North American record for the most birds seen

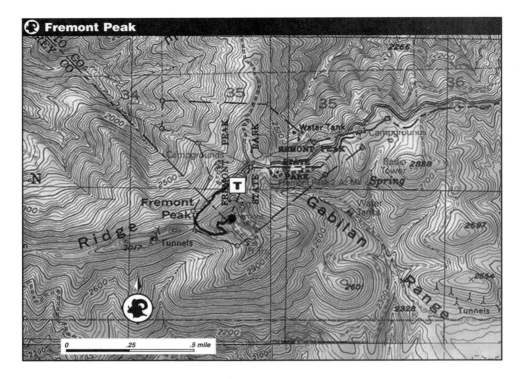

from a single location in one day (116) was set here in 1982. The broad alluvial plain around Monterey Bay is rich agricultural land and annually produces the country's largest crop of artichokes.

Immediately offshore of Elkhorn Slough is the beginning of Monterey Canyon, California's deepest submarine canyon. Twisting slightly southwest, it reaches a depth of 6000 feet less than 15 miles from the shore, almost twice the elevation of Fremont Peak, which is 16 miles from the shore. To create so deep a submarine canyon requires erosive power far greater than that provided by the current rivers that flow into Monterey Bay. To explain its origin, theory holds that in the recent geologic past (up to 5 million years ago) a large amount of California drained through present-day Monterey Bay unhindered by any Coast Ranges, carving a deep offshore canyon over the course of millions of years. As the San Andreas Fault system moved Monterey Bay north, the rising Coast Ranges limited its drainage basin to its current watershed. Cold water upwelling from March through September funnels nutrient-rich waters up Monterey Canyon, providing sustenance for the incredible diversity of sea life that makes Monterey Bay world-famous.

Nearest Visitors Center: There is not a staffed visitors center. Call (831) 623-4255 for general information. An astronomical observatory near the summit offers public programs; call (831) 623-2465 or visit www.fpoa.net.

Nearest Campground: Fremont Peak State Park Campground (20 sites, $7–$10, price varies depending on season), is open March 1–November 30.

Additional Information: www.parks.ca.gov

HIKE 10

Coit Lake

Mountains of Deception

Highlights	Ridges, lakes, and remote adventure on the edge of the Bay Area
Distance	12.4 miles round-trip
Total Elevation Gain/Loss	3800′/3800′
Hiking Time	6–10 hours
Optional Maps	*Henry W. Coe State Park Trail and Camping Map* by Pine Ridge Association, USGS 7.5-min. *Gilroy Hot Springs*
Best Times	December through May
Agency	Henry W. Coe State Park
Difficulty	★★★★

In Henry Coe State Park, the largest state park in Northern California, the towering bulwark of Wasno Ridge guards the approach to the southern backcountry, where a furrowed land of ridges, valleys, and solitude awaits the stalwart hiker. In 1775–1776, a Spanish expedition led by Juan Bautista de Anza attempted (and failed) to find a route through this convoluted region. The Spaniards dubbed this area "Sierra del Chasco" ("Mountains of Deception"); they would be the last Europeans to visit the area for nearly a hundred years.

Today wide fire roads and clearly marked trails make navigation far easier—but the steep terrain is as taxing as ever. Wasno Ridge rises more than 1500 feet above the trailhead, a heart-pumping obstacle that keeps hiking traffic to a minimum. Beyond it lie small Kelly Lake and larger Coit Lake, the second biggest in the park, as well as extensive views across the rumpled terrain.

In September 2007, a large wildfire scorched 40,000 acres within Henry Coe, including most of the park's eastern half. Known as the Lick Fire, the conflagration reached as far west as Coit Lake, where evidence of the blaze is readily apparent today. The damage was not cataclysmic—most of the park's oak trees survived the blaze—but trails and large swaths of the landscape in the burned areas were significantly affected. Wildfires are a natural part of the park's ecosystem and the backcountry is rapidly recovering, a process on full display around Coit Lake.

The Hike begins from the Coyote Creek Trailhead on Coe's southwestern edge, steeply ascends Wasno Ridge on single-track trails, and then follows old ranch roads past Kelly Lake and over another ridge to Coit Lake. The return route follows a series of more gradual trails down the flanks of Wasno Ridge. The open terrain of oak woodland and chaparral provides excellent views throughout. Bass and crappie are abundant in both lakes for anglers. Water is usually available from Coyote Creek at the trailhead, and from several springs and ponds en route (a filter is strongly recommended). The hike can be completed year-round (Kelly and Coit lakes are reliable water sources), but the baking heat, shadeless slopes, and increasingly funky water make this a less attractive option in summer and fall.

To Reach the Trailhead: Take the Leavesley Rd. exit from Hwy. 101 in

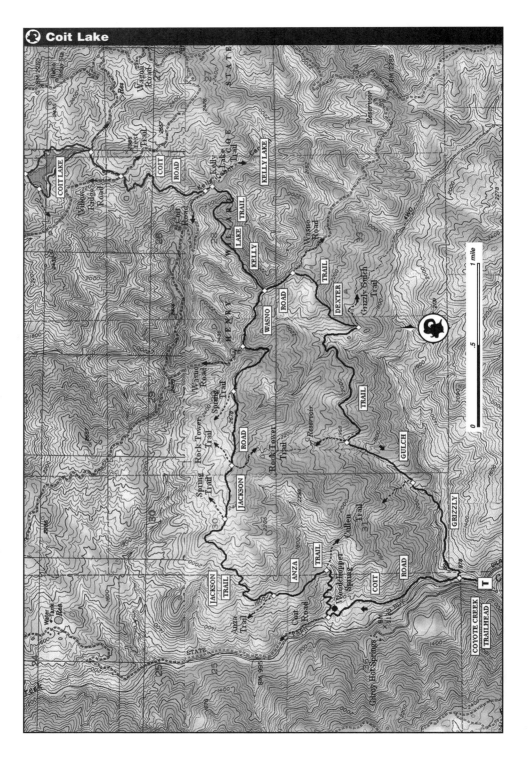

Gilroy and follow it 1.8 miles east to New Ave. Turn left, follow New Ave. 0.6 mile to Roop Rd., and turn right. Follow Roop Rd., which becomes Gilroy Hot Springs Rd. and reaches Coyote Creek County Park on the left in 3 miles. You pass Hunting Hollow Trailhead 3 miles later on the right and reach the Coyote Creek Trailhead 1.7 miles farther at a bridge.

Description: From the trailhead (0.0/940´), begin down wide Coit Rd. The route initially parallels the creek and quickly meets Grizzly Gulch Trail (your return route) on the right (0.1/960). Continue on Coit Rd. as it begins a slow climb, passes a fenced cattle-loading enclosure, and encounters large, big-berry manzanita shortly before reaching a high point. You descend briefly past valley oak and a giant rusting water tank to reach Anza Trail on the right (1.0/1090´), where an interpretive sign highlights the 1775–1776 Spanish expedition. Nearby Woodchopper Spring is a dependable water source for much of the year.

Turn uphill on Anza Trail, following the single-track path as it passes beneath bay trees and coast live oaks and switchbacks upward to reach Cullen Trail on the right (1.6/1440´). Bear left to remain on Anza Trail, which now traverses open slopes flush with spring wildflowers to reach the junction with Jackson Trail (1.9/1560´)—turn right to head toward Kelly Lake.

Views expand as you ascend Jackson Trail. Looking north, Pine Ridge and the main park entrance area (Hike 11) are visible 6 miles away—the tall and distinctive ponderosa pines that give the ridge its name can be identified on clear days. Beyond, Lick Observatory can be spotted atop Mt. Hamilton (4213´). As the trail attains the Wasno ridgeline, views reach as far south as 3171-foot Fremont Peak (Hike 9) and beyond to the Santa Lucia Range of Big Sur.

The trail passes two small ponds and reaches the junction for seasonally dribbling Elderberry Spring (3.3/2360´), widening to become Jackson Rd. Hugging the ridgeline, the route passes a four-way junction for Rock Tower Trail (3.7/2520´) shortly before attaining the ridge's highest point (2676). Jackson Rd. now begins a slow descent past hidden Spring Trail on the left (4.2/2630), then banks sharply left to reach Wasno Rd. (4.7/2420´). Turn right and briefly follow the road to Kelly Lake Trail on the left (4.9/2420´).

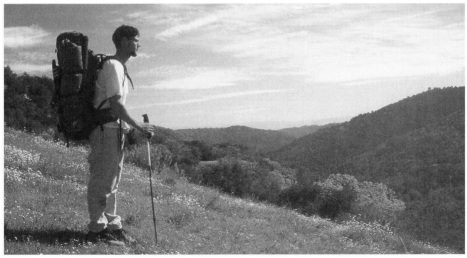

Above the Coyote Creek watershed

Follow Kelly Lake Trail as it undulates through pleasant blue oak woodlands, then plummets down shadier slopes. The lake itself remains hidden from view until the very end, when the trail deposits you on the dam enclosing the northern shore. Steep and brushy slopes make accessing the lake difficult; try the area above the lake's south end.

Continuing on to Coit Lake, the route bears left at the northern end of the dam and then turns right on wide Coit Rd. by an outhouse (5.9/1880'). Coit Rd. climbs through a lush environment of oaks, bay trees, and buckeye and then traverses across more open chaparral slopes. You crest Willow Ridge between Kelly and Coit lakes at a four-way junction with Willow Ridge Rd. (6.7/2240'). From this point, you can look east across land singed by the 2007 Lick Fire. Continue straight on Coit Rd. as it descends to Coit Lake's reedy southern shore (7.0/2080').

After savoring Coit Lake retrace your steps back to Kelly Lake Trail and its junction with Wasno Rd. (9.1/2420'). Bear left on Wasno Rd. and then quickly turn right on Dexter Trail (9.3/2420'), which descends through open blue oak woodlands and then drops steeply to reach the unsigned junction with Grizzly Gulch Trail (9.9/1940'). Turn right on Grizzly Gulch Trail, traversing a moist creek gully and contouring across shady slopes to pass Rock Tower Trail on the right (10.9/1740').

From here, Grizzly Gulch Trail descends above a narrow creek gully, where the moist environment nourishes lush valley oak, buckeye, and madrone. As you approach the canyon bottom, you pass the junction for indistinct Cullen Trail on the right (11.4/1270'). After crossing Grizzly Gulch Creek, the trail ascends and contours the slopes, passing Spike Jones Trail on the left (12.1/1060') and returning to Coit Rd. (12.3/960'). Turn left to return to the trailhead (12.4/940').

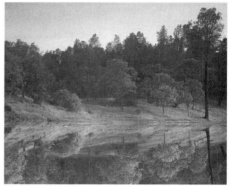

Contemplate Coe

Nearest Visitors Center: A self-service station at Hunting Hollow Trailhead is occasionally staffed on weekends. The main visitors center, (408) 779-2728, is located at the park entrance at the end of East Dunne Ave. in Morgan Hill, a long drive from this trailhead. It is open year-round 8 AM–4 PM Friday through Sunday, with later hours during busy periods in spring and summer, and is open sporadically Monday through Thursday.

Backpacking Information: A backcountry permit is required and can be obtained at the Hunting Hollow Trailhead. Camping is prohibited within a half mile of the trailhead but is permitted everywhere else along this hike. A few established sites and outhouses can be found around Coit and Kelly lakes. The park recommends leaving your vehicle at Hunting Hollow Trailhead; vandalism and theft have been reported at Coyote Creek.

Nearest Campground: Coyote Creek County Park (75 sites, $18), is located 5 miles from the trailhead on Gilroy Hot Springs Rd.; call (408) 842-7800 or visit www.parkhere.org.

Additional Information: www.coepark.org

HIKE 11

Coyote Creek

The Quiet Hills

Highlights	Deep canyons and oak woodlands in the Northern California's largest state park
Distance	12.1 miles
Total Elevation Gain/Loss	2500′/2500′
Hiking Time	6–10 hours
Agency	Henry W. Coe State Park
Optional Maps	*Henry W. Coe State Park Trail and Camping Map* by Pine Ridge Association, USGS 7.5-min. *Mt. Sizer, Mississippi Creek*
Best Times	February through May
Difficulty	★★★

Here are gentle ridgetops, steep canyons, gurgling creeks, 700 different plants, 137 species of birds, a radiant profusion of spring wildflowers, and immortal words etched on the monument to Henry W. Coe—MAY THESE QUIET HILLS BRING PEACE TO THE SOULS OF THOSE WHO ARE SEEKING.

The largest state park in Northern California, Henry W. Coe State Park encompasses 85,000 acres (more than 130 square miles) and protects a diversity of plant and animal life, including coyotes, bobcats, foxes, black-tailed deer, feral pigs, mountain lions, and abundant birdlife. Complete checklists are available at the visitors center.

In September 2007, a large wildfire scorched 40,000 acres within Henry Coe, including most of the park's eastern half. Known as the Lick Fire, the conflagration reached the northern edge of this hike; evidence of the blaze is readily apparent today in several spots. The damage was not cataclysmic—most of the park's oak trees survived the blaze—but trails and large swaths of the landscape were significantly affected in the burned areas. Wildfires are a natural part of the park's ecosystem and the backcountry is rapidly recovering, a process on full display in the areas north of Poverty Flat and Los Cruzeros trail camps.

The Hike begins from the main park entrance, cruises along diverse Pine Ridge, and then plummets more than a thousand feet to a year-round swimming hole in Coyote Creek. After winding through the Narrows, a thin creek-carved gap, the hike reaches idyllic Los Cruzeros Trail Camp along the babbling creekside. The journey returns via Poverty Flat Road, winding over the open hillsides of Jackass Peak, passing Middle Fork Coyote Creek, and then climbing steeply back up Pine Ridge. The hike can be shortened by more than 2 miles using Creekside Trail between Poverty Flat and China Hole on Creekside Trail.

To Reach the Trailhead: Take Hwy. 101 to Morgan Hill and take the East Dunne Ave. exit. Follow East Dunne Ave. east for 11 miles to the visitors center parking lot at the road's end. After leaving the residential area of Morgan Hill, the road is a narrow twisting ascent—RVs and trailers are not recommended. There is a $5 day-use fee.

Description: The hike begins across from the visitors center on single-track Corral Trail (0.0/2650′). After crossing a

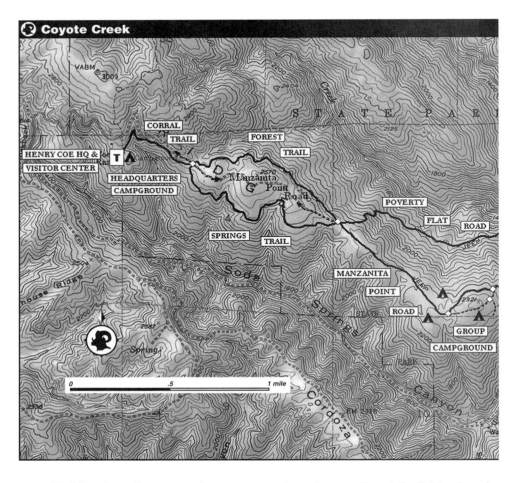

small bridge, the trail contours above precipitous slopes in a lush world of black oak, bay trees, buckeye, snowberry bushes, and coast live oak. Soon you encounter the first big-berry manzanita of the trip. Dozens of manzanita varieties exist, but few approach the massive size of these specimens; their twisting, blood-red trunks are almost treelike in girth. Chamise, toyon, and honeysuckle vines—common members of the park's chaparral community—appear alongside.

The path emerges onto open hillsides graced with large valley oaks and reaches a six-way junction at Manzanita Point Rd. (0.6/2510′). Cross the wide road, grab an interpretive brochure from the post,

and continue on Forest Trail. Numbered markers line the path and correspond to the brochure's descriptions of the park's flora. After contouring through this shady educational world, you rejoin Manzanita Point Rd. (1.8/2330′) at its junction with Springs Trail and Poverty Flat Rd.

Bear left on wide Manzanita Point Rd. and undulate along the ridgetop past valley oak and ponderosa pine. The road tours the pleasant Manzanita Group Camps and reaches the junction for China Hole and Madrone Spring trails just past Sites 6 and 7 (2.6/2260′). Turn left on China Hole Trail to begin the descent.

China Hole Trail contours below the last group sites (a spur trail splits right to

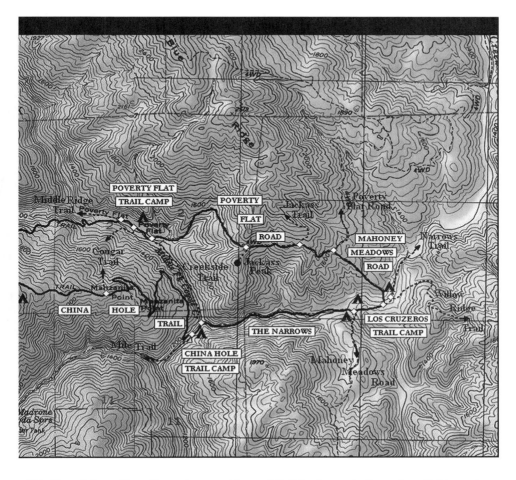

Site 9) and then dives through a corridor of massive big-berry manzanita. You next emerge in an area burned by prescribed fire (a posted sign tells the story) where thick chamise and buckbrush thrive on the regenerating hillside. Good views open up of the Coyote Creek watershed and its multiple drainages below.

The trail encounters Manzanita Point and the junction with Cougar Trail (3.7/1910′), where you continue straight on China Hole Trail to begin a series of long, descending switchbacks to the canyon bottom and the junction with Mile Trail (5.2/1150′). China Hole Trail Camp and its year-round swimming hole await a short distance upstream. In summer and

fall this stream is the only reliable water source on the hike, so fill your bottles.

Continuing, proceed upstream to quickly reach the confluence of Coyote Creek's Middle Fork (left) and East Fork (right). Here Creekside Trail splits off to connect with Poverty Flat Trail Camp via the Middle Fork, a shorter return option. To complete the full loop, bear right up the East Fork and enter the lush world of the Narrows. There is no officially maintained trail through the Narrows, but a use path is generally obvious as it closely parallels the creek. This route requires crossing the stream in several places, and, depending on season and flow, this can be a rock-hop or knee-deep ford. In times of heavy rains the Narrows may become impassable—use caution.

Profuse spring wildflowers color the ground in this canyon environment, and soon you reach wide Mahoney Meadows Rd. and the start of Los Cruzeros Trail Camp near the confluence of East Fork Coyote and Kelly creeks (6.2/1230'). Bear left on Mahoney Meadows Rd. and cross the creek near the junction with Willow Ridge Trail (6.3/1230'), located a short distance upstream.

Follow wide Mahoney Meadows Rd. as it climbs steeply through open woodlands and then turn left onto broad Poverty Flat Rd. (6.8/1620'). Remain on Poverty Flat Rd. as it ascends to reach Jackass Trail (7.0/1790') before descending to a saddle below Jackass Peak (1784'). A short side trip leads to the level summit and its near-360-degree views. Poverty Flat Rd. plummets past this point to meet Middle Fork Coyote Creek and Creekside Trail (8.2/1150') arriving from China Hole. The wide streambed of sycamores is a pleasant backdrop to nearby Poverty Flat Trail Camp, which was used as a primary staging area during the Lick Fire.

Poverty Flat Rd. meanders among the camp's five sites and junctions for Cougar and Middle Ridge trails, then begins a steady thousand-foot ascent along the flanks of Pine Ridge. Poverty Flat Rd. contours gently and ascends steeply for short, strenuous sections until an intense switch-backing climb at the end deposits you back atop Pine Ridge at the earlier junction with Manzanita Point Rd. (10.2/2330'). Return to the trailhead on the road or via Springs Trail, which travels along the margin of open oak woodland and past several dribbling springs to reach Corral Trail (11.5/2510') and the final section back to the visitors center (12.1/2650').

Nearest Visitors Center: The park visitors center, (408) 779-2728, is open year-round 8 AM–4 PM Friday through Sunday, with later hours during busy periods in spring and summer. It's open sporadically Monday through Thursday.

Backpacking Information: Backcountry camping is permitted at China Hole, Poverty Flat, and Los Cruzeros trail camps. A permit is required and must be obtained the day of your departure. All permits are first-come, first-served—no reservations are accepted. There is a permit fee of $3 per person per night and a parking fee of $5 per vehicle per night. Campfires are prohibited.

Nearest Campground: Headquarters Campground (20 sites, $12) is located below the visitors center.

Additional Information: www.coepark.org

HIKE 12

Sunol Backpack Area

Sweet Sunol

Highlights	A hidden oak woodland oasis
Distance	5.9 miles
Total Elevation Gain/Loss	1100´/1100´
Hiking Time	3–5 hours
Optional Maps	*Sunol Regional Wilderness Park Map,* USGS 7.5-min. *La Costa Valley*
Best Times	February through May
Agency	Sunol Regional Wilderness
Difficulty	★★

Shielded from view behind landmark Mission Peak, peaceful Sunol Wilderness offers escape in beautiful rolling woodlands. An idyllic backcountry camping area is located at the hike's midpoint, a tranquil spot and a wonderful way to extend your visit.

The Hike explores the multifaceted character of Sunol Wilderness, passing through majestic oak woodlands, walking open hillsides, and pausing at substantial Alameda Creek as it rushes through a scenic section dubbed "Little Yosemite." This hike can be completed year-round, but spring is the time to come as hillsides are carpeted green, wildflowers are in bloom, and temperatures are most ideal. Cows graze throughout the park, creating a pleasant manicured landscape full of cowpie minefields. Crowds around Little Yosemite can be heavy, especially on weekends, but the rest of the trails are more peaceful. Poison oak and stinging nettle are ubiquitous and unfriendly companions on this hike—be watchful. Water is available at the trailhead.

To Reach the Trailhead: Take Hwy. 680 east of Fremont to the Calaveras Rd. exit and proceed south on Calaveras Rd. for 4.3 miles to Geary Rd. Turn left on Geary Rd., reaching the visitors center parking lot and trailhead in 1.9 miles. There is a day-use fee of $5.

Description: From the trailhead (0.0/410´), head to the wooden bridge over Alameda Creek and pause to admire the babbling waters. The largest watershed in the East Bay, Alameda Creek

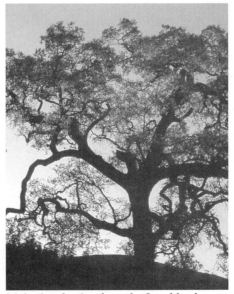

Majestic oaks rise above the Sunol landscape.

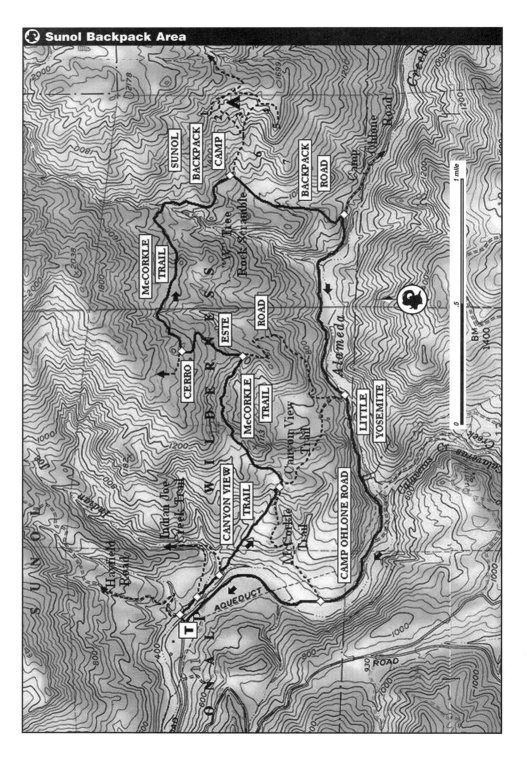

Sunol Backpack Area

drains more than 700 square miles. Here it nourishes the mottled, smooth gray trunks and twisting branches of California sycamores, which line the streambed. With their broad leaves, sycamore trees can lose up to 50 gallons of water per day and grow only where such large volumes are available.

Cross the bridge, bear right on the wide path, and continue straight on Canyon View Trail as it quickly passes junctions on the left for Hayfield Rd., Indian Joe Nature Trail, and Indian Joe Creek Trail. Canyon View Trail soon climbs away from the creek and into a drier environment populated by blue oaks, the most drought-tolerant of all oaks. Easily recognized, its leaves are shallowly lobed with smooth margins. You pass through one of numerous cattle gates to come (always leave them as you find them) and reach a four-way intersection with McCorkle Trail (0.7/700′).

Turn left on McCorkle Trail and follow the overgrown path as it climbs the ridgeline and then turns east to traverse through chaparral. This low-lying and shrubby community flourishes in arid environments and is regularly seen throughout the hike. Its common constituents include coyote brush, toyon, sticky monkeyflower, bracken fern, coffeeberry, and plenty of poison oak. Valley oak also begins to appear along this section, identified by its 2- to 4-inch deeply lobed leaves.

The trail passes beneath some huge coast live oaks and reaches the junction with wide Cerro Este Rd. (1.7/1180′). Bear left, make a steady uphill climb on Cerro Este Rd., and then bear right to return to single-track McCorkle Trail (2.1/1430′). Traversing steadily across open slopes, the route offers outstanding views of Mission Peak to the west, and south toward Calaveras Reservoir, the upper Alameda Creek watershed, and the more distant

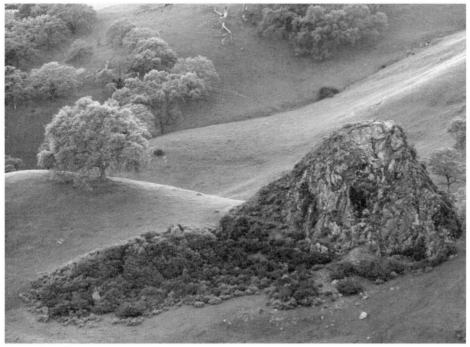

Sweet Sunol

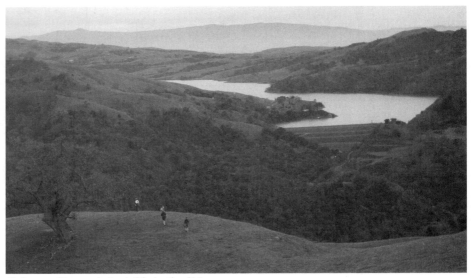

Calaveras Reservoir is visible in the distance.

peaks of the Diablo Range. The trail makes a steep, switchbacking drop into the "W" Tree Rock Scramble and then continues its traverse to reach Backpack Rd. (3.4/1150´) and the gated edge of Sunol Backpack Camp. The camp's pleasant sites and potable water (located above Site 3) make for a pleasant layover.

Continuing, follow wide Backpack Rd. as it steadily descends to Camp Ohlone Rd. (4.0/800´), where you turn right to begin your tour alongside nearby Alameda Creek. It's an easy cruise along this wide thoroughfare to Little Yosemite (4.5/450´). With a rushing river coursing through a small gorge over boulders blue and green, Little Yosemite is a pretty sight. From here, continue on level Camp Ohlone Rd. to rejoin the park road at the upper parking lot (5.5/420´). Watch for gray pine, California buckeye, and the reappearance of coast live oak and California bay along this final section. Walk the road to return to the visitors center (5.9/410´).

Nearest Visitors Center: The park visitors center, (925) 862-2601, is open 9:30 AM–4:30 PM Thursday through Sunday.

Backpacking Information: Backcountry camping is permitted only in Sunol Backpack Area. Seven campsites ($5 per person per night and a one-time reservation fee of $6) are available and can be reserved by calling the EBRPD reservation office at (888) 327-2757, 8:30 AM–4 PM Monday through Friday. It is also possible to make last-minute arrangements at the parks themselves if space is available. Fires and dogs are prohibited.

Nearest Campground: Sunol Wilderness has four drive-in campsites ($12) that can be reserved by calling (888) 327-2757 or visiting www.ebparks.org/registration. Drop-ins are accommodated if there is space, but sites are usually booked in advance during the summer.

Additional Information: www.ebparks.org/parks/sunol

HIKE 13

Coyote Hills

Bayside

Highlights	Shorebird paradise
Distance	2.5 miles
Total Elevation Gain/Loss	400´/400´
Hiking Time	1–2 hours
Optional Map	USGS 7.5-min. *San Leandro*
Best Times	December through May
Agency	Coyote Hills Regional Park
Difficulty	★

A grassy swell in the flatlands, Coyote Hills exist almost in the center of south San Francisco Bay. Protected marshlands enhance the unique perspective and offer a rich assortment of wildlife.

For thousands of years, the Ohlone Indians occupied the region around Coyote Hills, harvesting oysters, clams, mussels, cockles, and abalone from the extensive Bay mudflats; salmon, seals, seal lions, sea otters, and sturgeon from the water; and deer, elk, antelope, and rabbit from the surrounding hills. Using tule reeds from the vast marshlands, they constructed small boats for paddling in the bay. We know all this because four substantial middens still exist in Coyote Hills Regional Park. Middens—also referred to as shell mounds—are large piles of accumulated debris, the "kitchen wastes" of the Ohlone. Shells, bones, trinkets, and other discarded materials forming these large piles have shed a great deal of light on the Ohlone lifestyle.

With the arrival of the Spanish, it all came to an end. Disease and the mission system decimated the Indian population, and by the 19th century salt evaporation ponds and ranch lands began to surround Coyote Hills, all but eliminating the vast marshlands. Having passed through various owners, the ranch land that included Coyote Hills and a large remaining segment of marsh was purchased by the East Bay Regional Park District in 1967. Today it provides an excellent opportunity to imagine the bay as it was before the Europeans came.

Wildlife still abounds in this ecological oasis. At least 210 species of birds have been spotted in the park, including a variety of herons, egrets, owls, pheasants, hawks, and shorebirds. More than 30 different mammals also exist in the park, mostly small rodents hunted by foxes, weasels, and raptors.

The Hike connects several short segments of trail to form a loop, passing first along the marsh before returning via Red Hill (291´). Expansive hilltop views can only be enjoyed immediately after a winter storm has cleansed the thick South Bay air; move fast—air quality begins to deteriorate within 24 hours. The hills are velvety green from January through May, turning brown in summer and fall when the skies fill with haze. Water is available at the trailhead.

To Reach the Trailhead: Take Hwy. 84 to the east side of the Dumbarton Bridge and exit at Paseo Padre Parkway. Head north on Paseo Padre for 1 mile and turn left onto Patterson Ranch Rd., following it for 1.5 miles to the visitors center at road's end.

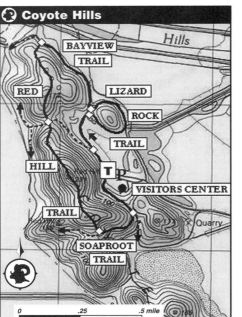

There is a $5 entrance fee per vehicle. The park opens at 8 AM and closes at sunset.

Description: From the visitors center parking lot, go through the gate and take the paved Bayview Trail, skirting the edge of the marsh partly shaded by small willow and sycamore trees. A chittering of birds and croaking of frogs keeps you company. The trail passes a few Monterey pines before reaching the junction for Lizard Rock Trail at the far end of the marsh—go right toward the red rock outcrop. This outcrop is Franciscan chert, formed from the silica-rich skeletons of microscopic sea creatures that collected on the ocean floor over millions of years. All of Coyote Hills is composed of this chert, which gains its red color from trace amounts of iron. Highly

resistant to erosion, chert has withstood the elements while the surrounding area eroded and became covered with thick layers of mud and silt washed down from the hills. In a sea of mud Coyote Hills is an isolated island of bedrock.

Stay by the marsh and loop east around the small hill before returning to Bayview Trail, passing a many-branched coast live oak along the way. Continuing on the paved path, you soon reach a junction where another paved trail splits right for the Alameda Creek Trail. Here you go left up dirt Red Hill Trail, climbing steeply to the top of the first hill before dropping down to a junction with Nike Trail, named for the NIKE missile site that was situated on these hills between 1955 and 1959 to protect the U.S. from Communist invasion. Continuing straight, the trail ascends Red Hill, high point of the park, where your best views are had. Descending Red Hill, return to the visitors center by bearing left on Soaproot Trail and left again on wide Quail Trail.

Nearest Visitors Center: Coyote Hills Visitors Center, (510) 795-9385, is open Tuesday through Sunday 9:30 AM–5 PM.

Nearest Campground: Sunol Regional Wilderness has four drive-in campsites ($12) that can be reserved by calling (888) 327-2757 or visiting www.ebparks.org/registration. Drop-ins are accommodated if there is space, but sites are usually booked in advance during the summer.

Additional Information: www. ebparks.org/parks/coyote_hills

HIKE 14

Bob Walker Ridge

Open Territory

Highlights	Remote Diablo Range wandering
Distance	5.8 miles
Total Elevation Gain/Loss	850'/850'
Hiking Time	3–4 hours
Optional Map	USGS 7.5-min. *Tassajara*
Best Times	October through May
Agency	Morgan Territory Regional Preserve
Difficulty	★★

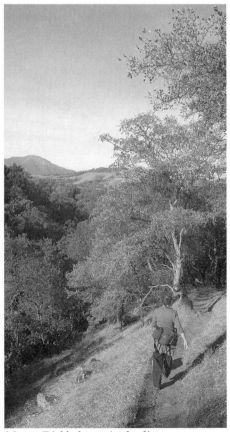

Deep in the furrows of the Diablo Range, Morgan Territory Regional Preserve protects a little-trod landscape of rolling hills, oak-studded grasslands, and quality views. On many days, your only companions will be the looming massif of nearby Mount Diablo, the nodding blooms of spring wildflowers, and the many cows that graze the grassy woodlands.

The park gets its name from Jeremiah Morgan, an early pioneer who settled here in 1857 and hunted grizzly bears in the surrounding hills. The East Bay Regional Park District acquired the first parcel here in 1976, expanding its holdings during the 1980s and early 1990s to nearly 5000 acres. Today old ranch structures belie the area's past; mountain lions, golden eagles, and a variety of other wildlife proclaim its future.

The Hike loops through the east half of the preserve, descending first along a shady creek corridor before circling around through oak woodland and open grasslands on a series of wide fire roads. The trip reaches its northernmost point below Bob Walker Ridge, where excellent views of Mount Diablo can be enjoyed from idyllic picnic spots. Water is available at the trailhead.

To Reach the Trailhead: Take Interstate 580 to the North Livermore Ave. exit, head

Mount Diablo looms in the distance as a hiker heads into Morgan Territory.

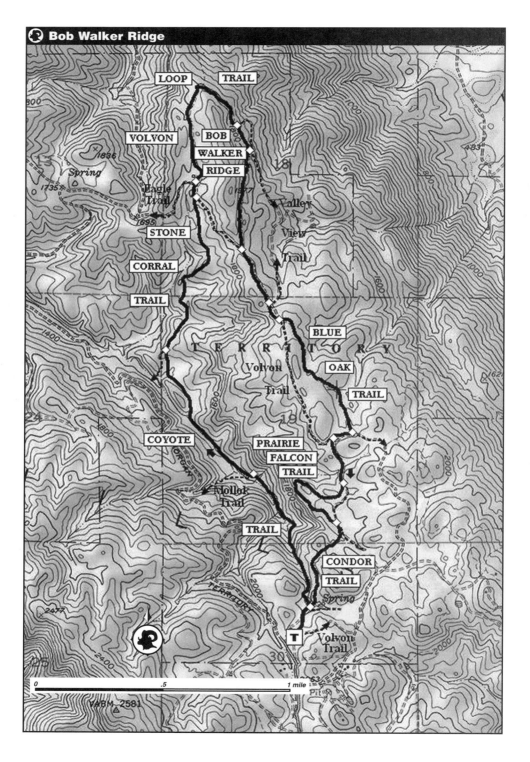

north on North Livermore Ave. for 4 miles, and turn right on Morgan Territory Rd., located 0.5 mile beyond the point where North Livermore Ave. curves west and becomes Manning Rd. Follow twisting and one-lane Morgan Territory Rd. 5.5 miles to the signed trailhead on the right.

Description: From the trailhead (0.0/2030´), look for Mt. Diablo to the north, your regular companion and landmark throughout the hike. To begin the journey, head out past the weathered ranch buildings and immediately bear left on single-track Coyote Trail. The open grassland begins its transition to woodland and you soon pass the hike's first oak on your left. Parasitic clumps of mistletoe dangle from the branches of this large valley oak; recognize the tree by its large, deeply-lobed leaves. Continue left on Coyote Trail as Condor Trail (your return route) splits off to the right (0.1/2000´).

The trail winds past a small pond and beneath twisting coast live oaks, which

can be identified by their spiny leaves that bend under at the margins. The route drops steeply into a shady ravine populated by mossy bay trees and small oaks. Maidenhair ferns line the moist north-facing slopes. During the descent, you regularly cruise along the edge of two ecosystems. The drier world of blue oaks and manzanita is visible just above, while buckeyes, black oaks, and bigleaf maples grow in the lush environment below.

The occasional switchback leads you past Mollok Trail on the left (0.9/1520´). Watch for baseball-sized buckeye seeds littering the ground as the gradient eases in the ever wider drainage. Mature blue oaks cling to the hillside above you. Recognize these drought-deciduous trees by their smaller leaves and smooth, wavy leaf margins. The mottled trunks of a few sycamore trees appear in the creekbed below as the trail curves right to leave the drainage and crosses through a gate into open fields. The trail initially runs along

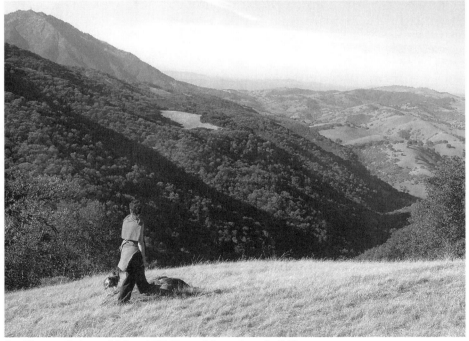

Looking north toward Mount Diablo and its eastern foothills

a barbed wire fence but quickly becomes indistinct—traverse upward toward the right side of the field to reach Stone Corral Trail near the top (1.6/1480′).

Bear right on the wide dirt road and gently rise through blue oak woodlands, soon passing through another gate. You steadily traverse upward, passing numerous sandstone outcrops, before curving left to reach the junction with Volvon Loop Trail (2.3/1780′). Follow Volvon Loop Trail, which immediately passes Eagle Trail on the left and then a small cattle pond ringed with cattails. The hike now cruises along the fields below Bob Walker Ridge; several use paths branch right to attain its rocky and tree-studded prow. A strong advocate for land protection, Bob Walker was a prolific photographer and played a major role in the expansion of Morgan Territory. He died in 1992 at the age of 40, but his 30,000 images of the East Bay region continue to inspire.

Near the end of the ridge a pleasant knoll offers exceptional views northwest of the twin summits of Mount Diablo (Hike 15). The view northeast stretches toward the Delta area, where the Sacramento and San Joaquin rivers merge in a broad wetland area. The cities of Antioch and Pittsburg line its shores. A collection of wind turbines marks the low rise of Grizzly Island near the confluence of these two mighty rivers.

Continuing, the trail wraps around the ridge, heads south, and crosses shadier, more tree-covered slopes. Intermittent views look southeast toward Los Vaqueros Reservoir. Remain on Volvon Loop Trail as Valley View Trail splits left (3.0/1770′), followed shortly by a connecting path. The trail climbs briefly, levels out in nice blue oak woodlands, and reaches another junction (3.5/1840′). Continue straight on Volvon Trail, which passes the south junction

for Valley View Trail on the left (3.8/1840′) and then quickly forks. Bear left on Blue Oak Trail, which undulates through shady and mature forest punctuated by twisting snags and other crusty specimens. Bear right on Hummingbird Trail (4.5/1960′) to quickly return to Volvon Trail, where you turn left.

The trail now encounters scrubby chaparral community, highlighted by the appearance of thick chamise, and soon reaches Prairie Falcon Trail on the right (4.8/1960′). This short side loop is a worthwhile diversion, a single-track path that winds over to a good vista downvalley before returning to Volvon Trail (5.3/1970′). Bear right and quickly right again on Condor Trail, which rises briefly before descending to the earlier junction with Coyote Trail (5.7/2000′) by the trailhead.

Nearest Visitors Center: This preserve doesn't have a visitors center. For general information, the nearest visitors center is at Black Diamond Mines Regional Park, (925) 757-2620.

Nearest Campground: Juniper Campground is located along Summit Rd. in Mount Diablo State Park. Also, you could try Junction Campground by Diablo park headquarters or Live Oak Campground on Mt. Diablo Scenic Rd./South Gate Rd (all campgrounds $15–20, depending on season). Reservations are recommended for weekends; visit www.reserveamerica.com or call (800) 444-7275.

Additional Information: www.ebparks.org/parks/morgan

HIKE 15

Mount Diablo

The Ultimate View

Highlights	Viewpoint for much of Northern California
Distance	0.7 mile
Total Elevation Gain/Loss	100´/100´
Hiking Time	1 hour
Optional Map	*Mount Diablo, Los Vaqueros, and Surrounding Parks* by Save Mount Diablo
Best Times	After storms
Agency	Mt. Diablo State Park
Difficulty	★

Dominating the landscape, Mt. Diablo offers vistas from the Sierra Nevada to the Golden Gate in an all-encompassing sweep of Northern California. There is no other view like it.

Surrounded by encroaching development and connected to no greater mountain range, Mt. Diablo is an oasis of both plant and animal life. Besides a variety of wildlife—and particularly birdlife—several plant species occur on the mountain that can be found nowhere else. Due to variations in elevation and precipitation, a variety of ecosystems are found here, and several can be explored on this short hike.

The Hike follows the Fire Interpretive Trail, an easy loop around the summit of Mt. Diablo (3849´) offering spectacular vistas in every compass direction. An interpretive brochure and informative signs enhance the experience. The optimal time to come is immediately following a spring or winter storm when the air is cleanest, the views most far-reaching, and the landscape carpeted a vibrant green. Even then, a good breeze is necessary to blow away all lingering and newly forming clouds, which can hover around the mountain. Strong easterly winds during the spring can also push the haze away. While the

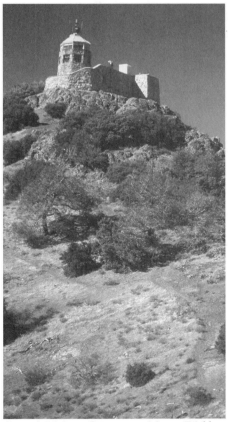

Summit Visitors Center atop Mount Diablo

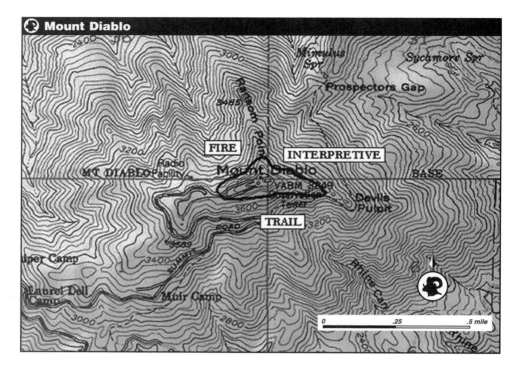

hike is open year-round, haze and heat are thick throughout summer and fall. Water is available at the trailhead.

To Reach the Trailhead: Take the Ygnacio Valley Rd. off-ramp from Hwy. 680 in Walnut Creek and proceed 3.8 miles east on Ygnacio Valley Rd. to Oak Grove Rd. Turn right on Oak Grove Rd. and then turn left onto North Gate Rd. in 1 mile. When you reach a junction with Mt. Diablo Scenic Rd. at park headquarters 8 miles later, take Summit Rd. 5 miles farther to the summit. Park in the large lot where the lanes divide near the top. It is also possible to approach from the south by taking Diablo Rd. from Hwy. 680 in Danville east for 3 miles to Mt. Diablo Scenic Rd. Turn left and proceed up the narrow, twisting road for 6 miles to the junction with Summit Rd., on which you continue 5 miles to the summit. There is a day-use fee of $6 per vehicle.

Description: Be sure to pick up an interpretive brochure at the visitors center before you start. Beginning by the picnic tables across the road from the parking lot, the first half of the hike is paved and passes through a small sample of the oak woodland plant community, offering exceptional views north of distant Mt. St. Helena (Hike 38) and northeast across the Sacramento Valley to the Sierra Buttes (Hike 76). Mt. Shasta would be visible 240 miles away were it not blocked by the curvature of the Earth. Closer to the north is nearby Eagle Peak (Hike 16). The rocks around you are greenstone and chert, the uppermost layers of what is known as an ophiolite suite, a group of rocks and minerals found close together wherever ancient seafloor is exposed.

The sea floor is composed of five layers. The bottom three form a surface that is essentially a solid piece of the Earth's crust. The upper two layers are deposited underwater on this surface. At tectonic spreading ridges, liquid basalt is squeezed out onto the sea floor, piling up in distinctively shaped pillow basalts, which compose the first of the two upper layers. These are in turn covered by sediment settling from the ocean. Primarily made up of the microscopic skeletons of tiny sea creatures, this silica-rich upper layer takes millions of years to accumulate, gradually forming thin layers mixed with small bits of sand and mud. Altered by pressure and temperature, these two upper layers eventually become greenstone and chert. The Mt. Diablo Ophiolite, as it is called, has been so heavily deformed and tilted that the sequence no longer lies flat. While its upper layers are visible at the summit, its lower layers are exposed northwest at the Lone Star Quarry, where diabase, a constituent rock of the lower sequence, is used for roadbeds and foundations. Exactly how this piece of 165-million-year-old sea floor became emplaced in the young sediments ringing Mt. Diablo remains a mystery.

As you hike into chaparral on the drier east slope of the mountain where the path becomes dirt, the peaks of Yosemite National Park (Hikes 86–89) can be identified. Let the gospel flow from atop Devil's Pulpit, a large outcropping of chert with a mildly precarious scramble to the top. Beyond it, the trail curves onto the south side of the mountain, where grassland replaces the chaparral ecosystem on this sunniest side of the summit. Coyote Hills (Hike 13) can be spotted to the southwest by the bay. The trail ends back by the parking lot.

Nearest Visitors Center: Summit Visitors Center, (925) 837-6119, constructed on the actual summit of the mountain, is open daily year-round 10 AM–4 PM with occasional extended hours during the spring and summer. For general information also call (925) 837-2525.

Nearest Campground: Juniper Campground is located along Summit Rd. Also, you could try Junction Campground by park headquarters or Live Oak Campground on Mt. Diablo Scenic Rd./South Gate Rd. (all campgrounds $15–20, depending on season). Reservations are recommended for weekends; visit www.reserveamerica.com or call (800) 444-7275.

Additional Information: www.mdia.org and www.parks.ca.gov

HIKE 16

Eagle Peak

Eagle Eye

Highlights	Flowers, oaks, and a secluded summit
Distance	4.0 miles
Total Elevation Gain/Loss	1800´/1800´
Hiking Time	3–4 hours
Optional Map	*Mount Diablo, Los Vaqueros, and Surrounding Parks* by Save Mount Diablo
Best Times	February through May
Agency	Mt. Diablo State Park
Difficulty	★★★

From a sea of rippling grassland rises Eagle Peak, a little-visited summit below the ramparts of Mt. Diablo.

The Hike climbs to the summit of Eagle Peak (2369´) from the northern boundary of Mt. Diablo State Park, ascending on Mitchell Rock Trail before returning via the Eagle Peak and Coulter Pine trails. While the hike can be done year-round, spring is the time to come as the land is carpeted green, wildflowers bloom, and temperatures are most ideal. Sections of the trail are exposed, making sun protection crucial most of the year. Ticks and poison oak are of particular concern in the brush along much of the route. Crowds are minimal. Water is available at the trailhead.

To Reach the Trailhead: Take the Ygnacio Valley Rd. off-ramp from Interstate 680 in Walnut Creek and proceed 9 miles east on Ygnacio Valley Rd. to Clayton Rd. Turn right and in 1 mile turn right again on Mitchell Canyon Rd., proceeding 2 miles to the lot at the road's end. There is a day-use fee of $6 per vehicle.

Description: From the parking lot (0.0/640´), begin by the fire gate and information sign and start up Mitchell Canyon Rd., bearing left onto Mitchell Rock Trail at the immediate junction. Stay on the wide trail as you pass two junc-

tions for Bruce Lee Trail before turning right on single-track Mitchell Rock Trail (just past the second Bruce Lee intersection). In season, abundant wildflowers liven the ground here and throughout the hike—look for California poppies, yarrow, paintbrush, lupine, irises, orange bush monkeyflower, yerba santa, blue dicks, Ithuriel's spear, and the endemic Mt. Diablo fairy lantern.

As you climb upward into thick forest, note the increasing number of pine trees. Two pines are found in this area, both producing massive cones with sharp hooks on the scales. Gray pine is the more common, abounding throughout California's foothills and easily identified by its wispy character. Its upper half, often drooping slightly to one side, tends to fork into a multitude of small branches with no clear center trunk. Its long grayish needles come in groups of three and give the tree its name. Coulter pine, on the other hand, is straight, stout, and considerably less common than gray pine, occurring only in the Coast Ranges from Mt. Diablo south. They are at the northernmost limit of their range here and can be identified by their single trunk, long stiff needles (also in groups of three), stouter appearance, and gargantuan cones. Coulter pine cones are the

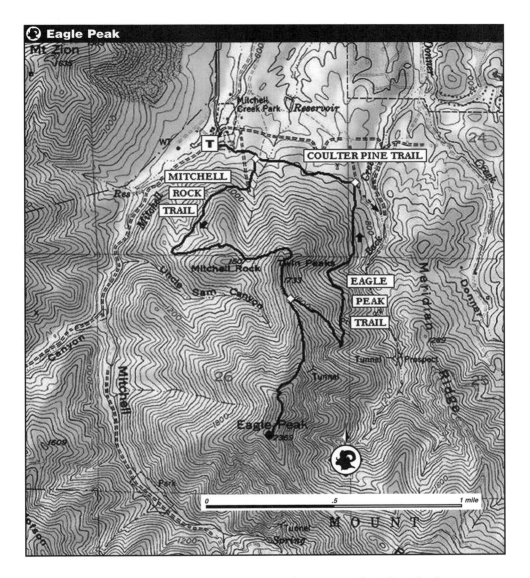

largest known, giant loaves 12–14 inches long that easily weigh several pounds.

As you climb steadily, your views north of the creeping edge of suburbia continue to improve until you reach an open rock platform (0.6/1080´). Directly across Mitchell Canyon, noisy Lone Star Quarry digs up diabase for use in road-beds and foundations. Continuing up the trail, you ascend to a small saddle below Twin Peaks. As you traverse below Twin Peaks to attain the ridge, the Sacramento River Delta appears to the north and the broad expanse of the Great Central Valley peeks out east over the hills. An eagle eye can discern the confluence of the San Joaquin and Sacramento rivers. Once on the ridgeline, views open up of the Mt. Diablo massif—both North Peak (3557´) and the summit (3849´) are visible. From Twin Peaks (1.5/ 1733´), Eagle Peak is clearly seen up the ridge.

Descending briefly, the trail passes a junction for Eagle Peak Trail (your return route) and then makes a steep, brushy, view-rich climb up the ridgeline to just below the summit, where a series of final switchbacks bring you to the top (2.3/2369′). Bear right on Eagle Peak Trail on your downhill return from the summit to take a much steeper and more direct route to the bottom than Mitchell Rock Trail. Dropping above Back Creek canyon, the trail cuts sharply back before passing over a scree gully below Twin Peaks. As you continue to descend, an increase in pines and poison oak marks the approaching junction with the Coulter Pine Trail (3.4/780′). Bear left and enjoy the gentle ramble through flowers and oaks and rippling grass that returns you to the Mitchell Rock Trail and your trailhead.

Nearest Visitors Center: Mitchell Canyon Ranger Station, located near the end of Mitchell Canyon Rd., is open 8 AM–4 PM on weekends during spring and summer, 9 AM–3 PM in fall and winter. For general information call (925) 837-2525.

Nearest Campground: There are no park campgrounds accessible from the north side of Mt. Diablo State Park, but three campgrounds are accessible from the south side: Juniper Campground, located along Summit Rd.; Junction Campground by park headquarters; and Live Oak Campground on Mt. Diablo Scenic Rd./South Gate Rd. Sites cost $15–20, depending on season. Reservations are recommended for weekends; visit www.reserveamerica.com or call (800) 444-7275.

Additional Information: www.mdia.org and www.parks.ca.gov

HIKE 17

Wildcat Peak

East Bay Escape

Highlights	East Bay escape with outstanding views of the Bay Area
Distance	7.0 miles
Total Elevation Gain/Loss	1000´/1000´
Hiking Time	3–5 hours
Optional Map	USGS 7.5-min. *Richmond*
Best Times	Year-round
Agency	Tilden Regional Park
Difficulty	★★

A surprising world hides behind the East Bay Hills. Rolling hills, soaring raptors, and superlative views of the Bay Area highlight a peaceful oasis of nature.

The Hike runs through Tilden and Wildcat Canyon regional parks, passing along Wildcat Creek before returning via San Pablo Ridge and Wildcat Peak (1280´). The excellent views from the open ridgetop are best in the morning and after storms. While the hike can be done year-round, the trails become thick with mud during the winter rainy season. As they have since European settlement of the region, cows graze on the open hillsides. People are common, especially along popular San Pablo Ridge, but quiet glades can usually be found. Water is available at the trailhead.

To Reach the Trailhead: Take the Buchanan St. off-ramp from Interstate 80 in Berkeley, and proceed east on Marin Ave. for 2 miles. Climb Marin above Marin Circle on the East Bay's steepest road,

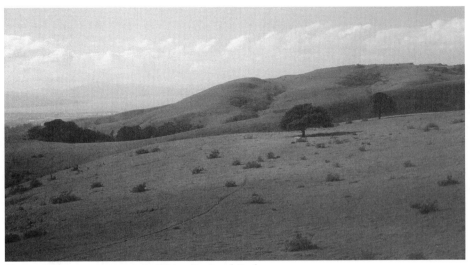

Escape to empty grasslands in Tilden Regional Park.

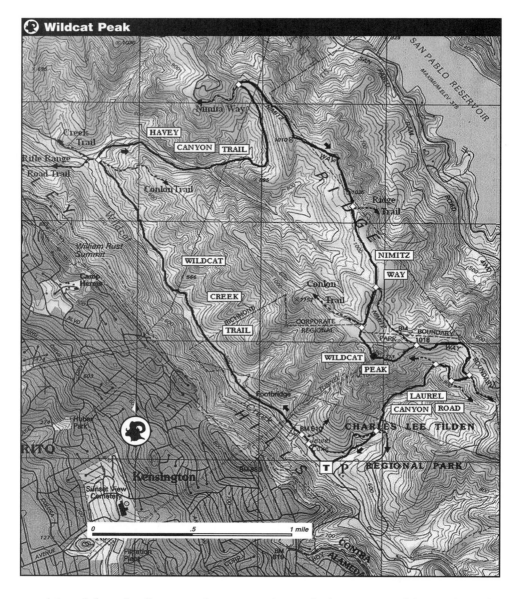

and turn left at the first stop sign onto Spruce St. Follow it to Grizzly Peak Blvd. Cross the intersection and take Canon Dr. steeply downhill to the visitors center and parking lot in Tilden Nature Center.

It is also possible to reach the trailhead by public transportation. AC Transit Bus 67 runs Monday through Friday every 30 minutes from the Berkeley BART sta-tion to the intersection of Spruce St. and Grizzly Peak Blvd. From the intersection, walk down Canon Rd. to the trailhead as described above. On weekends and holi-days, Bus 67 runs hourly from the Berkeley BART station and will drop you directly at the trailhead. Call (510) 817-1717 for cur-rent schedule and fare information or visit www.actransit.org.

Description: From the trailhead (0.0/530'), strike north from a small patch of redwood trees on wide Wildcat Creek Trail. Willow, California bay, coast live oak, coyote brush, California buckeye, poison oak, and introduced French broom line the trail as it parallels Wildcat Creek. Passing diminutive Jewel Lake, the trail soon crosses into Wildcat Regional Park. A wire fence lines the path below increasingly open hillsides. After nearly 2 miles of easy walking, you reach a gated junction for the Havey Canyon and Conlon trails (2.3/490')—on your right immediately before reaching Rifle Range Road. Go through the gate and continue straight toward Havey Canyon. The trail climbs a lush, riparian valley flush with ferns, snowberry, and some unusually massive California bay before breaking out onto open slopes dotted with coyote brush. While cows are a common sight, more exciting are the raptors often seen overhead; red-tailed hawks, easily identified by their namesake tail feathers; and northern harriers, spotted by the distinctive white patch of feathers on their rump. As the trail curves north, distant Mt. Tamalpais (Hike 32) becomes visible to the west. Soon, you go through another gate to reach paved Nimitz Way atop San Pablo Ridge (3.8/950')—bear right (south).

Views along the ridge are far-reaching, stretching from Vallejo in the north to Mt. Diablo (Hike 15) in the east. The East Bay Hills' highest peaks rise from the ridge to the south, and San Pablo Reservoir lies below you. You reach another junction near Wildcat Peak (4.8/1140')—leave the pavement and go straight up the rocky trail. After passing a few Monterey pine and Monterey cypress, you swing right along the wide path to descend the Conlon Trail. At this point, leave the trail to find a bench with incredible views of the

Golden Gate (Hike 28) and central Bay Area. From the bench, bear left on a faint, barbed-wire-lined path, and cross through the fence at a small gap to continue up to Wildcat Peak's summit (5.4/1280'). A stone platform crowns the summit and explains the purpose of the nearby Rotary Peace Grove. Savor the amazing views before dropping down to explore the grove of bushy giant sequoia, seemingly healthy despite being far removed from their native Sierra Nevada habitat.

To return to the trailhead, follow Peak Trail as it descends east from the summit, and take the single-track trail branching right to quickly reach Laurel Canyon Rd. below. Alternatively, you can continue on Peak Trail to rejoin Nimitz Way—bear right and then right again upon reaching Laurel Canyon Rd.

Laurel Canyon is within the Tilden Nature Study Area, a designated area for protection of Tilden's unique flora and fauna. A maze of trails winds through it, each marked with a symbol. Laurel Canyon Rd. is the widest and easiest route, but any number of trail combinations will return you to the trailhead (7.0/530')—just keep bearing downhill.

Nearest Visitors Center: The Environmental Education Center and Visitors Center, (510) 525-2233, located at the trailhead, is open 10 AM–5 PM Tuesday through Sunday.

Nearest Campground: There are two group campgrounds in the Tilden Nature Study Area. Reservations are required and can be made by calling (510) 636-1684.

Additional Information: www. ebparks.org/parks/tilden

HIKE 18

Little Butano Creek Canyon

Redwoods and Knobcones

Highlights	Canyon views, redwood forest, and knobcone pines
Distance	8.8 miles
Total Elevation Gain/Loss	2100´/2100´
Hiking Time	5–6 hours
Optional Maps	*Butano State Park Map*, USGS 7.5-min. *Franklin Point*
Best Times	Year-round
Agency	Butano State Park
Difficulty	★★★

Little Butano Creek slices westward in a narrow defile almost completely protected within Butano (BOO-tah-no) State Park. Less than 4 miles long yet brimming with ecological diversity, the canyon contains an isolated and diverse world representative of the entire region. Extensive stands of redwoods thrive in the park's lush environment, including 315 acres of old-growth trees.

The Hike travels on seven different trails to complete a clockwise loop around the canyon. The trip can be completed year-round, with spring and fall offering the ideal combination of good weather and light crowds. Summer is foggy and people-heavy, while winter and early spring are typically rainy, cool, and perpetually damp.

To Reach the Trailhead: Take Hwy. 1 south of Half Moon Bay for 16 miles to Pescadero Rd. and turn left. In 2.5 miles, turn right on Cloverdale Rd. and proceed 4 miles to the park entrance on the left. Approaching from the south, take Hwy. 1 north of Davenport for 14 miles and turn right on Gazos Creek Rd., located immediately north of the Beach House gas station. Follow Gazos Creek Rd. for 2 miles, turn left on Cloverdale Rd., and proceed 1 mile to the park entrance on the right.

The posted trailhead is a half mile past the entrance station by a large turnout.

Description: From the trailhead (0.0/230´), follow Mill Ox Trail across Little Butano Creek and quickly climb northeast to reach Jackson Flat Trail (0.2/430´). Redwoods, Douglas firs, tanoaks, and huckleberry bushes surround you along this early section, joined intermittently by bigleaf maples, twisting madrones, sword and wood ferns, and the soft leaves of hazel bushes. Turn right on Jackson Flat Trail and begin a gradual rising traverse along the moisture divide between a damp redwood forest (a few large old-growth trees can be spotted) and drier mixed-evergreen forest.

Bear right on Canyon Trail (1.7/800´) as Jackson Flat Trail curves left. You initially continue through thick redwood forest but the woods soon transition to canyon live oak and madrone, then abruptly transform into an entirely different ecosystem. As the trail crosses the threshold of the Santa Margarita geologic formation—a sandstone layer poor in water and organic material—it encounters species uniquely adapted to these harsh conditions. Knobcone pines, spindly conifers that sprout their namesake cones everywhere, including from their branches and trunks,

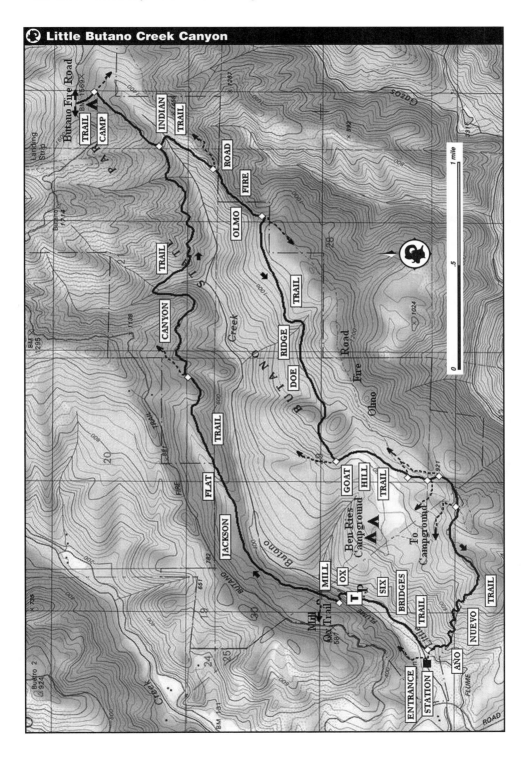

Little Butano Creek Canyon

proliferate. Knobcones survive through serotiny—their cones open only from the heat of wildfires. This strategy populates the newly charred, nutrient-rich soil with a sudden, massive influx of seeds. Other members of the drier chaparral community grow alongside: manzanita, golden chinquapin (look under the leaves), toyon, scrub oak, and chamise.

The trail winds through this open community, passing open views that reveal the depth of this diminutive canyon. The route momentarily banks left into a small tributary canyon and descends to cross a seasonally rushing creek (note the bigleaf maples and change of ecosystem as moisture again increases). Several switchbacks then return you upward to the Santa Margarita Formation and its accompanying views and flora. The path contours around several small drainages, returns to thick forest, and reaches the posted junction for the park's trail camp (3.7/1200'). (To reach the trail camp, bear left and head steeply uphill along the narrow trail for 0.5 mile to an unnamed fire road. The campsites are just uphill to your left.)

Remain on Canyon Trail as it continues briefly up the valley, crosses the headwaters of Little Butano Creek, and then curves right to start the return journey. Turn right upon reaching Olmo Fire Rd. (4.2/1240') and follow the wide trail as it winds for 0.4 mile through private property owned by Ainsley Family Tree Farm. Please stay on the road in this section and enjoy glimpses south into the adjacent Gazos Creek drainage, the only views of the hike beyond Little Butano Creek.

You slowly descend to reach single-track Doe Ridge Trail on the right (4.5/1050'), which you follow to one of the hike's most idyllic stretches—old-growth redwoods stand tall above the level and nicely contoured path. You next turn left on Goat Hill Trail (6.0/840'), which proceeds through thick Douglas fir forest recovering from recent logging. You pass a

spur trail on the left (6.5/900') leading to adjacent Olmo Fire Rd., and then another spur quickly thereafter. Goat Hill Trail continues downhill from here toward the campground and offers a more direct and less strenuous return route—just follow the park road from the campground to the trailhead.

To avoid the pavement, return to Olmo Fire Rd., turn right, and then bear left on Año Nuevo Trail (7.0/1060'). The single-track path contours briefly along a forested ridge, then banks right and heads down-canyon via a series of switchbacks. The foliage becomes thick with elderberry and blackberry, interspersed with airy views of the lower canyon. Upon reaching the bottom (8.3/220'), bear right on Six Bridges Trail and proceed along the banks of Little Butano Creek to return to the trailhead (8.8/230').

Nearest Visitors Center: The park entrance station is staffed daily in summer and most weekends in the off-season. It's open sporadically the rest of the year. Call (650) 879-2040 for general information.

Backpacking Information: Backcountry camping is permitted only at the park's designated trail camp, which features seven primitive sites at the ridgeline headwaters of Little Butano Creek. Campfires are not permitted. Open seasonally, the trail camp is first-come, first-served. Register at the park entrance station upon arrival.

Nearest Campground: Butano State Park Campground (39 sites, $25) is located near the trailhead. Reservations are recommended in summer; call (800) 444-7275 or visit www.reserveamerica.com.

Additional Information: www.parks.ca.gov

HIKE 19

Castle Rock

King of the Mountains

Highlights	Wild rocks and airy views atop the Santa Cruz Mountains
Distance	5.2 miles
Total Elevation Gain/Loss	1200´/1200´
Hiking Time	3–4 hours
Optional Maps	*Castle Rock State Park Map*, USGS 7.5-min. *Castle Rock Ridge*
Best Times	Year-round
Agency	Castle Rock State Park
Difficulty	★★

Perched on the tallest ridgeline in the Santa Cruz Mountains, Castle Rock State Park provides towering views over the San Lorenzo River and Pescadero Creek watersheds. It also harbors a geologic wonderland of sandstone boulders, a powerful draw for climbers and gawkers alike.

The Hike traverses the upper tier of the Santa Cruz Mountains, running high along the western slopes en route to a pleasantly secluded trail camp. Summer fog can obscure the hike's incredible views and winter storms can be heavy, but there

is no bad time to visit. Crowds on the trail are relatively light, but the intricate rock formations close to the park entrance usually attract large numbers of climbers on the weekends.

To Reach the Trailhead: Take Hwy. 35 south of the Hwy. 9 junction for 2.5 miles. The posted entrance and parking area are located on the west side of the road.

Description: A small forest of signs marks the trailhead at the edge of the parking lot (0.0/3070´). While the direct route proceeds straight on Saratoga Gap

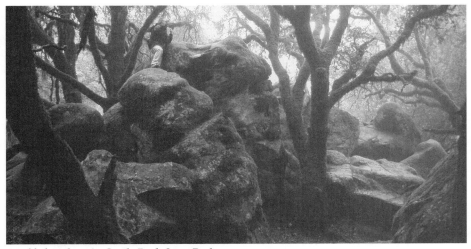

Jumbled geology in Castle Rock State Park

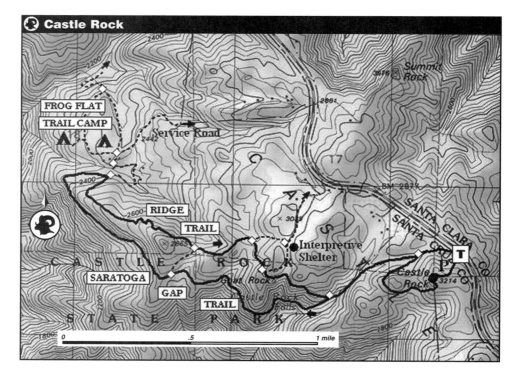

Castle Rock

FROG FLAT
TRAIL CAMP

Service Road

RIDGE

TRAIL

Interpretive
Shelter

SARATOGA

GAP

TRAIL

Goat Rock

Summit
Rock

0   .5   1 mile

Trail, you should begin your trip among the park's boulders by turning left and heading toward Castle Rock.

Heavy precipitation (45–50 inches annually) falls upon the area's unusually hard sandstone outcrops, creating conditions ideal for some bizarre chemical weathering known as *tafoni*. Rainwater seeps inside the rocks and dissolves the thin matrix of calcium carbonate that binds the individual sand grains together. When dry conditions return, the moisture trapped inside the rocks is drawn back to the surface. Its evaporation leaves behind the calcium carbonate as a hard and intricate surface residue. Without the calcium carbonate "glue" to hold them together, the interior sand grains waste away and leave small cavities behind. Over time these cavities can become intricate catacombs, their puckered walls a fascinating honeycomb of pitted rock.

You quickly reach the first wild pile of stones on the left. From here a network of

unsigned paths climbs past a variety of tafoni outcrops before reaching Castle Rock itself, an apartment-sized monolith deeply gouged by erosion. After enjoying the geology, proceed to Saratoga Gap Trail and turn left (0.5/3000′).

The trail traverses downward along the flanks of the Kings Creek drainage, one of the uppermost headwaters of the San Lorenzo River. Mixed-evergreen forest covers the slopes, dominated by the drooping evergreen branches of Douglas firs, the large spiny leaves of tanoaks, and the twisting trunks of madrones. Bigleaf maples flutter overhead and thick clumps of sword ferns sprout along the moist creekbed. A trailside understory of blackberry and poison oak discourages a departure from the soft path.

Crossing the creek, the trail reaches the junction with Ridge Trail (0.9/2730′) and the beginning of the loop. Remain on Saratoga Gap Trail as it continues briefly along the creek, joined now by a few young redwoods, and reaches an overlook for the thin cascade of Castle Rock Falls (1.1/2700′). From here Kings Creek plummets over a thousand vertical feet in less than a mile. The trail heads away from this drop and quickly passes onto drier slopes where coffeeberry, toyon, and fragrant California bay appear—plants better adapted to a world of less moisture.

Sandstone boulders protrude from the steep chaparral-cloaked slopes as you pass a connector trail on the right leading to nearby Ridge Trail (1.9/2560′) and reach the hike's first spectacular views. Looking south beyond the vast San Lorenzo River watershed on a clear day, you can see as far as the Monterey peninsula (a distance of more than 40 miles). To the west, the low ridge separating the San Lorenzo River and Pescadero Creek watersheds is apparent; the Skyline-to-the-Sea Trail follows this divide en route to Big Basin Redwoods State Park (Hike 20). Tall Bonny Doon Ridge hems the San Lorenzo River to the southwest, while Butano Ridge rises above Pescadero Creek to the west. The deep canyon of Pescadero Creek curves out-of-sight to the northwest.

Now gradually descending, you pass through chaparral thick with coyote brush and poison oak. The trail winds along sheer slopes and then turns sharply right to pass through a thick forest of tanoak and madrone and reach the junction with Ridge Trail (2.9/2400′). (To reach nearby Frog Flat Trail Camp, bear left, and then left again on the wide fire road to reach the main area in 0.2 mile.)

Turn right and follow Ridge Trail as it climbs briefly through thick forest to emerge at another incredible viewpoint of the Santa Cruz Mountains. From here, the path returns to the woods, climbs along the north side of the ridge, and reaches the connector trail to Saratoga Gap Trail (3.7/2700′). Continue on Ridge Trail as it climbs over a black oak-studded knoll and encounters a fork (4.0/2900′). A left here leads to a nearby interpretive shelter, but you should bear right to remain on Ridge Trail. You pass a return trail from the shelter (4.2/2960′) and then reach the junction for exciting Goat Rock (4.3/2920′). The rounded pinnacle of Goat Rock and its surrounding viewpoints can be accessed via numerous use trails and thrilling rock scrambles. After enjoying the most intense verticality of the hike, continue on Ridge Trail as it slowly descends along a narrow, rocky route to rejoin Saratoga Gap Trail (4.7/2730′) and the final climb back to the parking lot (5.2/3070′).

Nearest Visitors Center: This park doesn't have a visitors center, but the entrance station is occasionally staffed on busy weekends. For general information, call (408) 867-2952.

Backpacking Information: Camping is permitted at Frog Flat Trail Camp (20 sites, $10 per site) on a first-come, first-served basis. Space is always available. Water is available and campfires are permitted outside of wildfire season (typically June–November). Register at the park entrance station upon arrival.

Nearest Campground: The closest option is Big Basin Redwoods State Park, 30 to 45 minutes away on Hwy. 236. The park offers four campgrounds: Huckleberry (58 sites), Blooms Creek (54 sites), Sempervirens (32 sites), and Wastahi (27 sites). Sites cost $25 per night. Reservations are essential from Memorial Day to Labor Day and for weekends in September and October; visit www.reserveamerica.com or call (800) 444-7275.

Additional Information: www.parks.ca.gov and www.santacruzstateparks.org

HIKE 20

Berry Creek Falls

Go Big

Highlights	Continuous old-growth redwood forest and waterfalls
Distance	9.0 miles
Total Elevation Gain/Loss	3200´/3200´
Hiking Time	6–8 hours
Optional Maps	USGS 7.5-min. *Big Basin* and *Franklin Point*
Best Times	Year-round
Agency	Big Basin Redwoods State Park
Difficulty	★★★★

A continuous forest primeval, laced with gurgling streams, Big Basin State Park is a green blaze of life. Yes, the park is popular and the waterfalls are a common destination. And yes, it's worth it.

Established in 1902, Big Basin was the first state park created to protect old-growth redwood forest in the Santa Cruz Mountains. In fact, the 3800 acres initially set aside as parkland were the very first to protect coast redwoods anywhere! The park holdings have since expanded and the total park area now exceeds 19,000 acres, stretching from the Pacific Ocean at the mouth of Waddell Creek to the heart of the Santa Cruz Mountains. The old-growth redwood forest is extensive and unmatched in total area for hundreds of miles up the coast.

The Hike is a full-day adventure loop through substantial redwood forest to three waterfalls: Silver Falls, Golden Falls, and photogenic Berry Creek Falls. Fog may be present in the summer and rain might fall heavy in the winter, but there is no bad time to come here. Just be prepared for some very wet trail conditions if you arrive after a winter storm, and be ready for mud year-round. No matter what day you come, other people will be on the trail. Weekend crowds can be especially thick. A fall, winter, or spring weekday is the best

bet for some solitude. Water is available at the trailhead.

To Reach the Trailhead: Take Hwy. 236 west from one of its two junctions with Hwy. 9. Approaching from the north on Skyline Blvd. (Hwy. 35), the turnoff is 6 miles south of the junction with Hwy. 9. From this turnoff, Hwy. 236 is a one-lane twister that reaches the visitors center in 9 miles—RVs and trailers are not recommended. Approaching from the south, the turnoff from Hwy. 9 is in Boulder Creek. This more easily driven section of Hwy. 236 reaches the visitors center in 10 miles. Park in the large lot across from the visitors center. There is a day-use fee of $6.

Description: Beneath some particularly large redwoods, take broad Redwood Trail from the trailhead (0.0/990´) beyond the restrooms and across Opal Creek to your junction with the Skyline-to-the-Sea Trail. Your return trail joins from the right but you head left, passing some large Douglas firs and many tanoaks, whose toothed leaves wave everywhere. Continue toward Berry Creek Falls at the next junction and begin a steady climb out of the East Waddell Creek drainage. As you crest into the West Waddell Creek drainage (0.7/1320´), a sign warns of the strenuous hiking ahead.

As you pass a connector to Sunset Trail, your trail drops rapidly down to Kelly

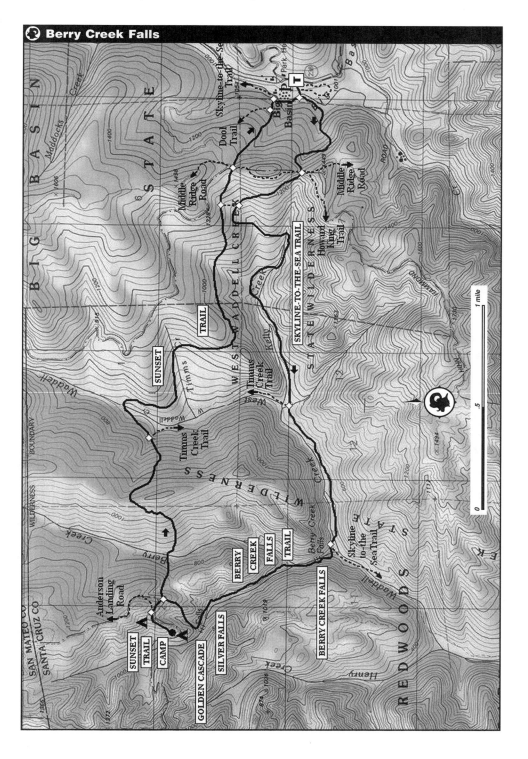

Creek. The hike passes through dense stands of large redwoods, encrusted green by the moist environment, before reaching Timms Creek Trail (2.4/560´), another shortcut to Sunset Trail. Continuing, you descend to reach the junction with Berry Creek Falls Trail (3.8/350´). Turn right toward the falls, leaving the Skyline-to-the-Sea Trail that continues to the ocean, less than 6 miles away.

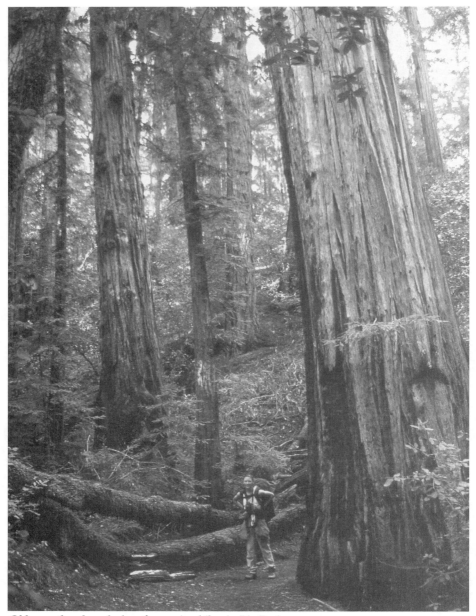

Old-growth redwoods dwarf a passing hiker in Big Basin.

Unless a recent winter storm has swollen the waters, Berry Creek Falls are thin and drop in small cascades that mist the surrounding greenery. Passing near the bottom of the waterfall, the trail then climbs left above the falls, and crosses Berry Creek. The muddy track stays close to the water and soon reaches Silver Falls, a small cascade falling over exposed sedimentary rock representative of the Santa Cruz Mountain geology.

The bedrock of the Santa Cruz Mountains is granite formed some 100 million years ago near the location of today's southern Sierra Nevada. When the San Andreas Fault became active, this piece of land began moving slowly northwest, becoming submerged beneath the sea as it went. Sand and mud settled from the ocean on this underwater surface, forming thick layers of loosely consolidated sandstone and mudstone. Within the past 4 million years, a change in the geometry of the San Andreas Fault thrust these layers above ground, folding them into the Santa Cruz Mountains and exposing the muddy layers to your boots. These loosely consolidated rocks create the huge landslide problems associated with this area today.

After climbing above Silver Falls, you soon reach Golden Falls and its series of three distinct cascades. Wooden steps and the odd switchback lead past this final waterfall to the junction with Sunset Trail (4.7/850´). Sunset Trail Camp is 0.2 mile straight uphill from here, but you turn right to begin the return journey.

Crossing Berry Creek on a solid wooden bridge, the trail then weaves slowly over a small divide between West Waddell and Berry creeks. Fleeting views of both drainages open up before the trail descends to the Timms Creek Trail junction (5.9/680´). A long undulating traverse from here along the Sunset Trail returns you to the earlier junction with the Skyline-to-the-Sea Trail. Go left on the short Redwood Trail to the trailhead.

Nearest Visitors Center: Park visitors center, (831) 338-8860, is open daily 8:30 AM–4 PM (extended hours during the summer months).

Backpacking Information: Backcountry camping in Big Basin State Park is allowed only at designated trail camps. Sunset Trail Camp is the only option on this hike, located above the waterfalls. Reservations are required and can be made by calling (831) 338-8861 Monday through Friday 10 AM–5 PM. There is a $5 reservation fee and each site costs $10 per night for up to 6 people. Campfires are prohibited and water is not available at the camp.

Nearest Campground: There are four park campgrounds: Huckleberry (58 sites), Blooms Creek (54 sites), Sempervirens (32 sites), and Wastahi (27 sites). Blooms Creek is closest to the trailhead but all are nearby. Sites cost $25 per night. Reservations are essential from Memorial Day to Labor Day and for weekends in September and October; visit www.reserveamerica.com or call (800) 444-7275.

Additional Information: www.parks.ca.gov and www.bigbasin.org

HIKE 21

Purisima Creek

Redwoods and Ridges

Highlights	A secluded redwood forest and open ridgeline
Distance	7.0 miles
Total Elevation Gain/Loss	1200′/1200′
Hiking Time	3–5 hours
Optional Map	USGS 7.5-min. *Woodside*
Best Times	Year-round
Agency	Purisima Creek Redwoods Open Space Preserve
Difficulty	★★★

Just south of Half Moon Bay, Purisima Creek slices quickly and deeply to the sea, with the northernmost redwood forest on the peninsula in its protected headwaters. So close to the urban mania yet hidden well enough to receive only light use, Purisima is a perfect place to quickly, easily, and totally get away from it all.

The rugged character of Purisima Creek canyon proved challenging to early logging efforts. While readily accessible from the coast, the sheer walls at the creek's headwaters made shipping lumber directly east to the Bay Area difficult. Despite the uncooperative topography, virtually all of the old-growth redwoods had been cut by the early 1900s, and seven different mills operated along Purisima Creek over the years. Today the forest has rebounded, with impressive second-growth redwoods now lining Purisima Creek. While no old-growth redwoods can be found along the trails, a few ancient trees are reputed to exist in the most inaccessible corners of the preserve.

The Hike follows Purisima Creek upstream through a substantial second-growth redwood forest before returning along Harkins Ridge. The open ridgetop offers excellent views of the valley, visible from mountain to sea. Fog may be thick in the summer and rains might fall heavily

in the winter, but there is no bad time to come here. While the main approach to the preserve is from Hwy. 35, this hike begins from the lower boundary, accessible only from the coast. Crowds are consequently light, although you will definitely see other people on the weekends. No water is available at the trailhead.

To Reach the Trailhead: On Hwy. 1 drive 5 miles south of the intersection with Hwy. 92 in Half Moon Bay to Verde Rd. Turn left (east) and continue straight on Purisima Creek Rd. for 0.3 mile where Verde Rd. curves right. The small parking lot is 4 miles farther at the road's deepest penetration into the valley. It is also possible to reach the trailhead on longer and twistier Higgins-Purisima Rd., which joins Hwy. 1 next to the new Half Moon Bay fire station, 1.5 miles south of the Hwy. 92 intersection.

Description: From the parking lot (0.0/420′), head up the wide path to quickly reach an information sign, where a bathroom is located and free maps are usually available. Your return trail crosses the creek on the left, but the hike continues straight on Purisima Creek Trail. As you go upstream, blackberry, hazel, thimbleberry, stinging nettle, poison oak, dogwood, deer fern, sword fern, five-finger fern, and bracken fern cover the surrounding slopes

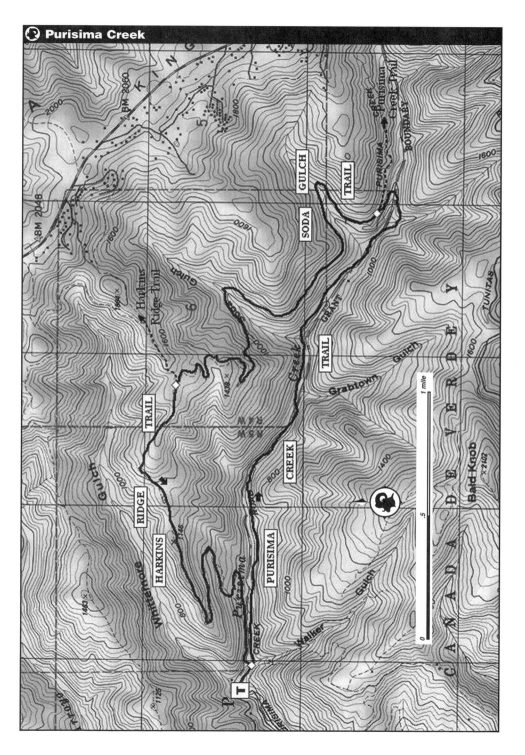

Purisima Creek

beneath the overhanging redwood trees. In addition to the redwoods, trees on this trail include the moss-coated trunks of alders, tanoaks, and bigleaf maples. Remain on Purisima Creek Trail as you pass the junctions for Borden Hatch Mills Trail and Grabtown Gulch Trail, slowly gaining elevation on the gentle gradient. When the trail switchbacks and reaches the junction with Soda Gulch Trail (2.3/1040′), go left.

Briefly joining the Bay Area Ridge Trail as you ascend on Soda Gulch Trail, the now single-track path initially winds around a small stream gully. (The Bay Area Ridge Trail is a network of paths that traverse the Bay Area's ridgelands and will eventually be approximately 550 miles long.) Look for the good-sized Douglas fir above the trail immediately before crossing the small stream, easily identified by their rougher, unfurrowed bark so distinct from that of redwoods. Continuing, a few tantalizing glimpses of upper Purisima Canyon can be had as the vegetation changes into that of the drier, sunnier upper slopes. Tanoak is still found here, but is now mixed with coast live oak and California bay. After traversing around substantial Soda Gulch, the trail suddenly bursts out into open fields of coyote brush and poison oak. Views are at their best here, as virtually the entire drainage of Purisima Creek can be seen curving west to the ocean.

Turning away from this excellent viewpoint, the trail climbs four quick switchbacks to reach the wide road of Harkins Ridge Trail (4.9/1540′). Go left to descend along the ridgetop with Higgins Creek drainage briefly visible to the north. Your views are obscured when the trail reenters thick vegetation, descending on four, long, lazy switchbacks to Purisima Creek and the earlier junction.

Nearest Visitors Center: This preserve doesn't have a visitors center. For more information call the Midpeninsula Regional Open Space District at (650) 691-1200.

Nearest Campground: Half Moon Bay State Beach Campground is closest, located just west of town in southern Half Moon Bay (52 sites, $25). Reservations are recommended for weekends; visit www.reserveamerica.com or call (800) 444-7275.

Additional Information: www. openspace.org/preserves/pr_purisima.asp

HIKE 22

Montara Mountain

Mountain Next Door

Highlights	A dominating mountain and Montara Beach
Distance	6.3 miles one-way
Total Elevation Gain/Loss	1650′/1650′
Hiking Time	4–6 hours
Optional Map	USGS 7.5-min. *Montara Mountain*
Best Times	Spring and fall
Agency	San Pedro Valley County Park
Difficulty	★★★

Montara Mountain is a solid block of granite towering over Pacifica, a landmark peak forgotten by the Bay Area. Views are tremendous. Montara Beach is an idyllic stretch of sand—hemmed by bluffs and washed by the soothing waves of the Pacific Ocean.

The Hike climbs over Montara Mountain (1813′) from San Pedro Valley County Park in Pacifica to reach Montara Beach, a one-way journey that necessitates two cars or the use of public transportation to return to the trailhead (see below for details). Alternatively, retrace your steps from the summit for an out-and-back round-trip of 5.4 miles. Fog envelops the mountain during the summer, obscuring views and making for a cold day at the beach. Winter views between storms can be spectacularly clear, but strong winds are often a problem on the exposed mountain. Bring a warm sweater and windbreaker year-round. Water is available at the trailhead.

To Reach the Trailhead: Take Hwy. 1 south from San Francisco to Linda Mar Blvd. in Pacifica and turn left (east)—the intersection is located at the southernmost stoplight in Pacifica. Proceed 1.7 miles to Oddstad Blvd. and turn right. The entrance is immediately on your left. Park in the Trout Farm Picnic Area lot to the right of the visitors center. There is a $5 day-use fee. Since the gate closes at dusk, those anticipating a post-sunset return should park outside the entrance on the street. To reach Montara Beach, take Hwy. 1 south of Linda Mar Blvd. for 4 miles and park by the northern end of the beach.

To reach the trailhead by public transportation, take BART to Daly City and SamTrans Bus 110 to the Linda Mar Shopping Center (runs every 30–60 minutes). Transfer to SamTrans Bus 14 and get off at Terra Nova Blvd. and Oddstadt Blvd. (runs every 30–60 minutes on weekdays only, no weekend service). Walk the few blocks east on Oddstadt to the park entrance. Returning to the trailhead from Montara Beach, take SamTrans Bus 294 north to the Linda Mar Shopping Center. The bus stop is at the south end of Montara Beach, located at the intersection of Hwy. 1 and 8th St. (runs every 90–120 minutes). Transfer and return as described above. Call SamTrans at (800) 660-4287 for a current schedule or visit samtrans.com.

Description: The trail begins in the Trout Farm Picnic Area lot by the restrooms (0.0/220′) and follows Montara Mountain Trail for the first half of the hike. Both poison oak and stinging nettle grow nearby and are a hazard throughout the day. Ticks are common in the brush as well—stay on the trail! The trail reaches an

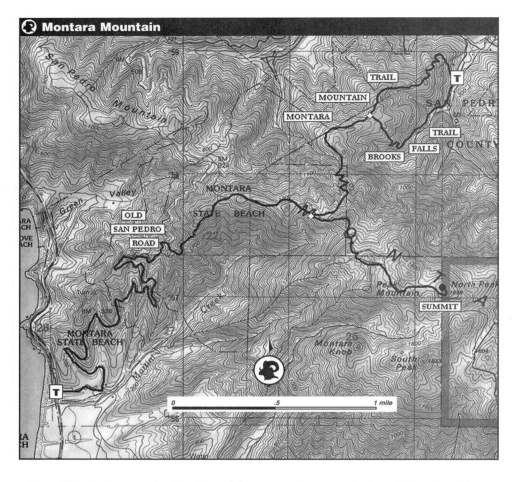

immediate fork as you begin—bear right and continue on Montara Mtn. Trail. To the left is Brooks Falls Trail, an alternate route that rejoins Montara Mtn. Trail in 0.8 mile. Crossing a road, the trail begins switchbacking through dense eucalyptus before breaking out onto increasingly open slopes.

The vegetation of Montara Mtn. is primarily coastal scrub composed of coyote brush, manzanita, and other low-lying brush highlighted with a seasonal display of wildflowers. Irises, lupine, buttercups, wild radishes, monkeyflowers, California poppies, and horse nettles are but a few of the varieties found here. Coast live oaks, California bays, and Monterey cypresses

grow in more sheltered locations. Raptors—especially red-tailed hawks—can often be seen overhead hunting for unlucky rodents. Quail, bobcats, gray foxes, and deer roam the hillsides. The rarely seen mountain lion is known to live here as well.

Passing a bench with a good view north of nearby Sweeney Ridge (Hike 23), the trail continues its steady ascent. The towers of the Golden Gate Bridge (Hike 28) and the headlands of distant Point Reyes National Seashore (Hikes 34–36) can be picked out north-northwest on clear days. The view becomes ever more expansive as the trail gets rockier on the steep upper flanks of the mountain. A steep, switchbacking climb brings you to the ridge and an intersection with the broad road leading to the summit (1.7/1460´). To head directly to Montara Beach, bear right and follow the road 0.5 mile to the junction with Old San Pedro Rd., a wide trail that drops down the southern flanks of Montara Mtn. To make the recommended trip to the summit, bear left and follow the gradual trail 1.0 mile to the top.

The rocks of Montara Mtn. are granite and can be found exposed in places along the upper sections of trail. Formed approximately 80 million years ago in Southern California, the granite has since been forced hundreds of miles north by the San Andreas Fault system. You can trace this fault as it travels underwater northwest from Mussel Rock (located just offshore north of the Pacifica Pier) and continues through the low gap between Point Reyes National Seashore and Mt. Tamalpais. Lands west of the fault, including Montara Mtn. and all of Pacifica, are currently moving north at an average rate of 1–2 inches per year. Over millennia, the exact position of the San Andreas Fault has shifted in response to various geologic forces, and the San Andreas Fault once ran along the base of Montara Mtn. on what is known today as the Pilarcitos Fault. During this period, the rocks along the fault were crushed into sediment, which easily eroded away to form San Pedro Valley after the San Andreas Fault shifted to its present course. Ancient movement along Pilarcitos Fault

brought the rocks of Montara Mtn. and landmark Pedro Point into contact with those found north of San Pedro Valley. Beyond their current proximity to each other, the two rock groups are totally unrelated.

From its junction with Montara Mtn. Trail, Old San Pedro Rd. drops west through McNee Ranch State Park on an easy gradient all the way to Hwy. 1. Prior to the construction of Hwy. 1 along Devils Slide, this was the only way to drive south of Montara Mtn. Bits of old pavement are still identifiable in the roadbed. As you descend past several confusing junctions into the Martini Creek drainage, follow the most obvious road to reach Hwy. 1 near a large yellow gate. Just across the road is the beach.

Nearest Visitors Center: San Pedro County Park Visitors Center, (650) 355-8289, is open weekends 10 AM–4 PM.

Nearest Campground: Francis Beach Campground is open year-round at the south end of Half Moon Bay State Beach, located just west of Hwy. 1 on Kelly Ave.; the turnoff is 0.3 mile south of Hwy. 92 (58 sites, $15). Reservations are recommended in summer; call (800) 444-7275 or visit www.reserveamerica.com.

Additional Information: www.eparks.net

HIKE 23

Sweeney Ridge

Discovery

Highlights	Sighting on November 4, 1769
Distance	4.8 miles round-trip
Total Elevation Gain/Loss	1000'/1000'
Hiking Time	3–4 hours
Optional Map	USGS 7.5-min. *Montara Mountain*
Best Times	September through May
Agency	Golden Gate National Recreation Area
Difficulty	★★

On November 4, 1769, Juan Crespí sighted San Francisco Bay from atop Sweeney Ridge. A member of the expedition sent north by the Spanish government to found missions at San Diego and Monterey, he had journeyed overland from San Diego through absolute terra incognita, recording a California barely imaginable today.

The Hike climbs Sweeney Ridge from Pacifica, roughly approximating the route traveled by Juan Crespí the day the expedition sighted San Francisco Bay. While easier access points exist for Sweeney Ridge, the history told below is best enjoyed by approaching from the Pacific side. Summer months are foggy in Pacifica, chilling the air and obscuring views for days on end. Weather is best in the fall, views are clearest after winter storms, and wildflowers explode from March through May. The ridge is open and exposed, making a good windbreaker worthwhile year-round. Crowds will be minimal beyond Shelldance Nursery. No water is available at the trailhead.

To Reach the Trailhead: Take Hwy. 1 south from San Francisco to the first stoplight in Pacifica, and make a U-turn to go north. In 0.3 mile turn right to Shelldance Nursery (accessible only from the northbound direction). Be ready for the sharp turn—it appears quickly and traffic moves fast around you. Proceed up the hill toward the nursery and park by the SWEENEY RIDGE sign. Approaching from the south, look for the Vallemar/Reina del Mar stoplight—the turnoff is 0.3 mile ahead.

The trailhead is also accessible by public transportation. From Daly City BART, SamTrans Bus 110 runs to Pacifica at least once per hour Monday through Saturday, with reduced hours on Sundays and holidays. Return service goes well into the evening weekdays but ends by 6 PM on weekends. Ask to be let off at Reina del Mar. Cross Hwy. 1 and walk up the road toward Shelldance Nursery (see above). Call (800) 660-4287 for a current schedule or visit samtrans.com.

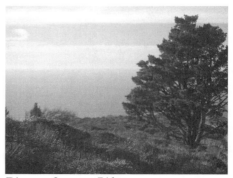

Discover Sweeney Ridge.

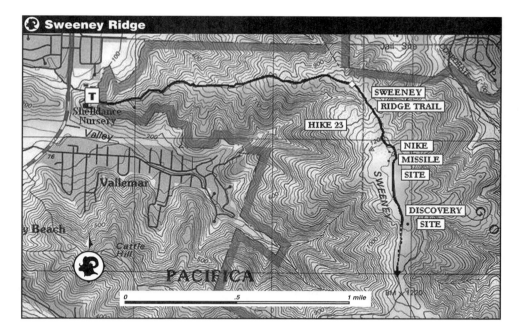

Description: Follow the dirt road adjacent to the signed trailhead (0.0/220´), cross through the gate, and climb the wide trail as it steeply ascends the ridgeline. When Father Juan Crespí was here, his journey had begun more than six months earlier.

In early 1769 a "sacred expedition," as described by Joshua Paddison in *A World Transformed: Firsthand Accounts of California Before the Gold Rush,* set forth from Baja California to establish two settlements in little-explored Alta California. To be located at San Diego and Monterey, these missions would strengthen Spain's tenuous hold on California, just as Britain and Russia had begun to eye it for their own. Initially composed of three ships and two overland parties traveling separately to a rendezvous in San Diego, the expedition rapidly dwindled to a small band of 60 men striking north from San Diego in search of Monterey Bay. Led by Captain Juan Gaspar de Portolá, 50-year-old governor of Baja California, the party included an adventurous 58-year-old missionary named Juan Crespí. After a long overland journey, the expedition reached the latitude of Monterey Bay but failed to recognize it. They continued north into the Santa Cruz Mountains.

According to Paddison, Crespí spoke of:

> a large mountain range covered with a tree very like the pine in its leaf, save that this is not over two fingers long. The heartwood is red, very handsome wood, handsomer than cedar. There are great numbers of this tree here, of all sizes of thickness, most of them exceedingly high and straight like so many candles. What a pleasure to see this blessing of timber.

Old-growth redwood forest, a forest unscarred by humankind, covered the Santa Cruz Mountains.

As the expedition proceeded along the coast just north of Waddell Creek, Crespí encountered, again according to Paddison, the native people of the area in "a large village of very well behaved good heathens, who greeted us with loud cheers and rejoiced greatly at our coming." He explained that these people gave his men "a great many large black- and white-colored tamales" and "two or three bags of the wild tobacco they use." Crespí described the scene: "One old heathen man came up smoking upon a large and well-carved Indian pipe made of hard stone. They all go naked and bare-headed, and all of them are well-featured, stout, and bearded." Between 150,000 and 250,000 native people once inhabited the area now composing California.

The expedition continued north along the coast until November 3, when, as recounted by Paddison, scouts returned to camp "firing off their guns as they arrived" and "reported that they had come upon a great estuary or very broad arm of the sea extending many leagues inland." San Francisco Bay had been discovered.

Surely excited, Crespí and the expedition began climbing Sweeney Ridge on November 4. Montara Mountain could be seen to the south with its westernmost arm dipping into the sea at Point San Pedro. To the west the jagged incisors of the Farallon Islands protruded out of the Pacific. But the towers of the Golden Gate Bridge could not be seen to the north, houses did not fill the valleys of Pacifica, and Hwy. 1 did not wind along the coast below. California's dense coastal fog and treacherous shoreline had prevented discovery of San Francisco Bay for more than two centuries. Early European explorers had failed to spot the Golden Gate through the fog, and later commercial vessels steered west of the Farallones to avoid the dangerous bottom near shore. But then Crespí was there, staring east across San Francisco Bay.

Once on the ridgetop (1.2/1030´), you go right on Sweeney Ridge Trail, passing an abandoned NIKE missile command center (1.7/1200´) from the 1950s, before reaching the Discovery Site on a paved trail (2.0/1250´). Those feeling energetic can continue 1.4 miles south along Swee-

ney Ridge to the boundary of the off-limits Peninsula Watershed.

While your current trip remains on the ridge, Crespí descended the slopes and saw:

> three or four smokes within these woods from heathen villages, of which the scouts say there are many. The soldiers report that down next to the large estuary there are many lakes and little inlets with countless fowl, ducks, geese, cranes, and others. Very large bears have been seen, and here where the camp was set up [he] saw two fresh droppings of these beasts, full of acorns.

Wetlands ringed the bay, grizzly bears roamed the hills, and between 10,000 and 20,000 native people called it home. Crespí did not see the world of Silicon Valley, the San Mateo Bridge, or the sea of asphalt. He saw a California that is today only a dream.

When you're ready, return the way you came.

Nearest Visitors Center: The Pacifica Chamber of Commerce runs an excellent visitors center in partnership with the GGNRA, (650) 355-4122, located 1 mile south of Shelldance Nursery at 225 Rockaway Beach. It's open 9 AM–5 PM Monday through Friday and 10 AM–4:30 PM on weekends.

Nearest Campground: Francis Beach Campground is open year-round at the south end of Half Moon Bay State Beach, located just west of Hwy. 1 on Kelly Ave.; the turnoff is 0.3 mile south of Hwy. 92 (58 sites, $15). Reservations are recommended in summer; call (800) 444-7275 or visit www.reserveamerica.com.

Additional Information: www.nps.gov/goga

HIKE 24

Milagra Ridge

Farallon View

Highlights	The Farallon Islands
Distance	1.5 miles round-trip
Total Elevation Gain/Loss	250′/250′
Hiking Time	1–2 hours
Optional Map	USGS 7.5-min. *San Francisco South*
Best Times	September through May
Agency	Golden Gate National Recreation Area
Difficulty	★

Thirty miles offshore, the jagged rocks of the Farallon Islands protrude from the Pacific Ocean expanse. Less than a mile from the ocean, hidden Milagra Ridge rises 700 feet above the sea, making it one of the best locations to view these remote outposts of California.

The Farallon Islands are a linear series of small rocky islets stretching 8 miles northwest from the principal island cluster. With a summit 348 feet high, the largest and most commonly sighted member of the group is Southeast Farallon, located at the far southern end of the chain. Eight miles northwest, a smaller group of rocky pillars known as the North Farallones jut from the water, ranging in elevation from 78 to 112 feet. Between the two groups is the lonely pinnacle of Middle Farallon, a single rock 50-feet wide standing 22 feet above the sea. *Farallon,* Spanish for "rocky promontory rising from the ocean," was a generic appellation that over the course of time became exclusively associated with these islands.

The rock of the Farallon Islands is granite rifted from the southern Sierra Nevada and transported several hundred miles northwest through the actions of the San Andreas Fault. Between the islands and the mainland stretches a large shelf no more than 200 feet below the surface.

Immediately beyond the islands, the continental shelf ends and the ocean bottom plummets to over a mile deep.

On August 3, 1579, Sir Francis Drake anchored the Golden Hinde off the Farallon Islands and—with his crew—set the first European footprints on their rocky soil. During the early 19th century, New England merchants were involved in a lucrative shipping trade between Boston, the West Coast, and China. Hundreds of thousands of furs were harvested along California's coast by these traders, decimating the vast populations of fur seals then found around the Farallones. By 1834, the annual yield of fur seals had dwindled to 60 and the species was all but exterminated.

Next came the Russians. Seeking provisions for their recently established

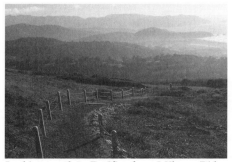

Looking south to Pacifica from Milagra Ridge

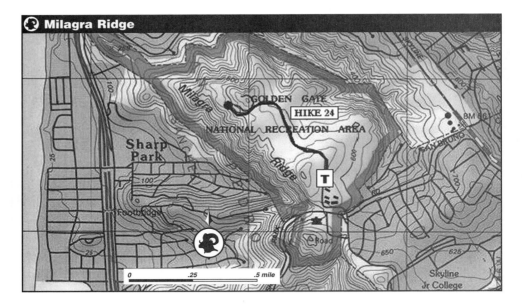

settlement of Fort Ross on the present-day Sonoma coast, they established an outpost on the islands that was permanently staffed from 1817 until the early 1830s. Sea lions, elephant seals, and other wildlife were hunted and shipped to Fort Ross. Abandoned in 1838, this remote station on the Farallon Islands marked the southernmost limit of Russian expansion in North America.

Following the discovery of gold in California, the Farallones became the site for a much-needed lighthouse. Constructed atop the summit of Southeast Farallon, the light went into operation in 1855. Over the following 117 years, the lighthouse was staffed and cared for by a long line of lighthouse keepers and their assistants. Often living with their families in a few lonely houses at the base of the peak, they were responsible for maintaining the light, foghorn, and related equipment until the lighthouse became fully automated in 1972. Today the lighthouse still perches on the narrow summit, flashing brightly at regular 15-second intervals.

During the early decades of San Francisco, a lack of poultry led to an acute egg shortage. As early as 1849, the harvesting of murre eggs from the Farallon Islands helped satisfy the demand. Double the size of a chicken egg, the common murre egg was evidently quite palatable, although the white remained transparent after frying and the yolk had a bright orange-red hue. In the mid-19th century, hundreds of thousands of murres nested on the Farallones, laying countless eggs in precarious rocky roosts, which were collected by daring men climbing on the cliffs. Egg gathering continued until 1896 when an ever-dwindling supply and increasing public pressure brought operations to a halt.

During the 20th century, Southeast Farallon was used for several military radio and radar installations. In 1909 President Theodore Roosevelt created the Farallon Reservation, a wildlife preserve protecting the North Farallones. In 1969 the southeast island group was included in the renamed Farallon National Wildlife Refuge. All of this is today a part of the vast Gulf of the Farallones National Marine Sanctuary, 948 square nautical miles of protected ocean stretching from Bodega Bay to well south of the Farallon Islands. The only remaining human inhabitants on

Southeast Farallon are a few members of the Point Reyes Bird Observatory assigned to safeguard and monitor the recovering wildlife. Since 1969, elephant seals once exterminated from the islands have returned to breed, and the diminishing murre population has rebounded from a record low of 6000 nesting birds to well over 100,000 today. Great white sharks up to 18 feet in length prey on the increasing numbers of marine mammals, and are a common underwater denizen of the Farallon Islands.

The Hike winds along the open hilltops of Milagra Ridge, offering views of Pacifica and the distant Farallon Islands. In order to see the Farallones, you will need a day with good visibility and no fog. Winter and spring provide the best opportunities, with air quality generally best immediately following storms and when strong easterly winds blow. Summer months bring fog, which almost always sits offshore, obscuring the islands. A telescope or strong pair of binoculars is useful. Crowds are generally light, especially on weekdays. No water is available at the trailhead.

To Reach the Trailhead: Take Westborough Dr. west from its exit on Interstate 280 in South San Francisco. You steeply ascend the ridge to Skyline Dr. (Hwy. 35). Cross Skyline Dr. and continue 0.5 mile to the intersection with College Dr. Turn right and go 0.2 mile past a housing complex to the gate at the road's end. Parking is limited—if there are no spaces available, the next closest parking is almost a mile away at Skyline College, located at the opposite end of College Dr. Approaching from Hwy. 1, take the Sharp Park off-ramp and drive 1.4 miles east up Sharp Park Dr. to College Dr. Turn left and continue as described above.

While reaching the trailhead by public transportation is challenging, SamTrans Bus 140 does run regularly between Pacific Manor Shopping Center in north Pacifica and Tanforan Shopping Center/San Bruno BART Station in South San Francisco, stopping at nearby Skyline College along the way. Call (800) 660-4287 for current schedule and connection information or visit samtrans.com.

Description: From the trailhead climb the stairway, passing a buried water tank. The trail winds through coyote brush and seasonal wildflowers—California poppies, paintbrush, clover, and checkerbloom are a few of the more common. The trail crests out at a vista point providing a good Farallon view. Southeast Farallon is located almost due west at 276°, and the North Farallones can be picked out on exceptionally clear days at 284°. Much of Pacifica is laid out beneath you and Montara Mtn. (Hike 22) dominates the southern skyline.

From here, the trail descends from its highest point and traverses among a maze of paths northwest along the ridgetop, providing good views north of Mt. Tamalpais (Hike 32) and northeast of upper San Bruno Mtn. (Hike 26). Passing a '50s NIKE missile launchpad, the trail terminates at an old World War II 6-inch-gun platform, where former military bunkers are buried in the hillside. Return the way you came.

Nearest Visitors Center: The Pacifica Chamber of Commerce runs an excellent visitors center in partnership with the GGNRA, (650) 355-4122, located 1 mile south of Shelldance Nursery at 225 Rockaway Beach. It's open 9 AM–5 PM Monday through Friday and 10 AM–4:30 PM on weekends.

Nearest Campground: Francis Beach Campground is open year-round at the south end of Half Moon Bay State Beach, located just west of Hwy. 1 on Kelly Ave.; the turnoff is 0.3 mile south of Hwy. 92 (58 sites, $15). Reservations are recommended in summer; call (800) 444-7275 or visit www.reserveamerica.com.

Additional Information: www.nps.gov/goga

HIKE 25

San Andreas Fault

It's Your Fault

Highlights	The San Andreas Fault and fossils on a forgotten beach
Distance	3.5 miles one-way
Total Elevation Gain/Loss	50´/50´
Hiking Time	2–3 hours
Optional Map	USGS 7.5-min. *San Francisco South*
Best Times	September through May
Agency	Golden Gate National Recreation Area
Difficulty	★

After covering 500 miles overland, the San Andreas Fault dives northwest from the bluffs of Daly City into the Pacific Ocean. North of this tectonic landmark, a beach of surprising seclusion runs for more than 3 miles below cliffs of mud, sand, and fossils.

Approximately 2 million years ago, the geography of the Bay Area differed radically. The Point Reyes Peninsula sat directly west of today's Golden Gate, partially enclosing a shallow basin between itself and the mainland. Sediments poured in from the surrounding land masses, filling the basin with thick layers of sand, mud, and gravel. In all, a deep reservoir of sediment more than a mile thick was deposited. Layers formed during periods

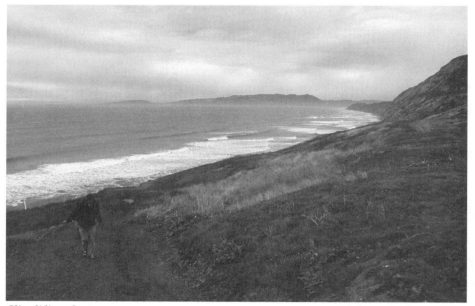

Slip sliding along

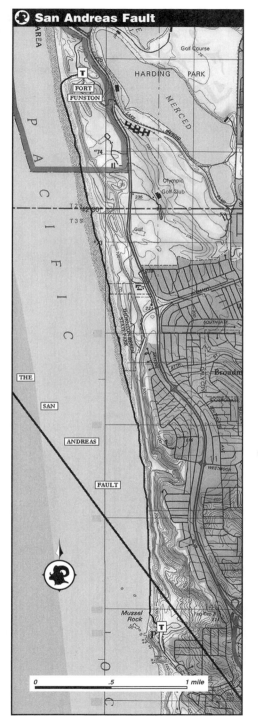

of shallow water include thick beds of fossils—crushed shells make up the bulk of the material, but entire preserved sand dollars and clams can also be found. Within the past 300,000 years, changing geometry along the San Andreas Fault lifted the entire basin and tilted its beds gently north to expose it as today's Merced Formation. A small piece of the northern basin remained attached to the southeast corner of the Point Reyes Peninsula as it was wrenched into its current position; it is now exposed in the bluffs east of Bolinas, as explained by Ted Konigsmark in *Geologic Trips*.

The Hike follows the beach north from Mussel Rock in north Pacifica to Fort Funston in San Francisco. *This trip can become dangerous during high tides, when big waves can wash to the base of the bluffs and suck people out to sea. Do not venture onto the beach if you see waves reaching the bluffs. No tide tables are posted at the trailhead—check in advance.* The hike can be made into a round-trip by returning along the beach to the trailhead. Otherwise, car arrangements must be worked out for the return to Pacifica. For those unable to do the full hike, the general flavor and experience of the locale can be had in a short 1-mile round-trip from the trailhead. While the hike can be done year-round, fog is thick in the summer and makes for a cold, low-visibility day at the beach. Crowds are light compared to other area beaches. No water is available at the trailhead.

To Reach the Trailhead: From San Francisco, follow Hwy. 1 south, take the first Pacifica exit at Manor Dr., and turn right on Palmetto Dr. Go 0.8 mile and turn left on Westline Dr. Bear left toward the Mussel Rock Transfer Station (the dump), keep left again as the road forks right to the dump, and park in the large lot at the road's end. To reach Fort Funston, take Skyline Dr. (Hwy. 35) 4 miles north from Hwy. 1 in north Pacifica—the parking lot is on the left. Approaching Fort Funston from San Francisco, follow Skyline Dr. 0.8 mile south of the Great Hwy.

Description: From the parking lot by Mussel Rock, walk through the opening in the fence and descend along roads leading down toward the beach. Looking above you to the west, notice the loose, unconsolidated slopes along the bluffs—the result of many landslides. The bluffs above the landslide area recede at a rate of up to 3 feet per year, undercutting houses that should never have been built or purchased in the first place. The edges of the landslide mark the rough boundaries of the San Andreas Fault Zone, an area approximately a half mile wide. The loose slopes mask any actual fault trace in the hillside, but it is definitely there—the great 1906 San Francisco earthquake had its epicenter immediately inland from this location.

Walking north on the beach, notice the northward tilt of the layers in the bluffs. Deposited sequentially, these layers represent a chronology of the former basin environment; they become progressively younger as you go north. Fossil beds can be identified by the white, linear exposures of crushed shells contained in a matrix of mudstone. The views north include most of the Marin coast, and Point Bonita (Hike 29) can be picked out across the Golden Gate on clear days. Fort Funston can be identified near the northern end of the bluffs as they drop in elevation. Turning south, Montara Mtn. (Hike 22) forms the skyline closest to the sea, plunging into the ocean at landmark Pedro Point.

Continuing north, you pass the deep gash that Woods Gulch makes in the bluffs. Because saturated slopes increase the risk of landslides and accelerate erosion, draining this threatened area is an attempt to slow the imminent destruction of its cliffside homes. The number of people increases as you approach the path that leads up to the viewing platform and parking lot at Fort Funston. A former military reservation developed at the turn of the century, Fort Funston is now part of the Golden Gate National Recreation Area. It's a popular site for hang gliders and parasailors between March and October, when strong west winds rise over the blufftop.

Nearest Visitors Center: The Pacifica Chamber of Commerce runs an excellent visitors center in partnership with the GGNRA, (650) 355-4122, located near the south end of Pacifica at 225 Rockaway Beach. It's open 9 AM–5 PM Monday through Friday and 10 AM–4:30 PM on weekends.

Nearest Campground: Francis Beach Campground is open year-round at the south end of Half Moon Bay State Beach, located just west of Hwy. 1 on Kelly Ave.; the turnoff is 0.3 mile south of Hwy. 92 (58 sites, $15). Reservations are recommended in summer; call (800) 444-7275 or visit www.reserveamerica.com.

San Bruno Mountain

Peak over the Peninsula

Highlights	An island of nature in a sea of humanity
Distance	4.9 miles round-trip
Total Elevation Gain/Loss	700´/700´
Hiking Time	2–3 hours
Optional Map	USGS 7.5-min. *San Francisco South*
Best Times	After storms
Agency	San Bruno Mountain State and County Park
Difficulty	★★

Four cities lap at the base of San Bruno Mountain, encircling it with the concrete bustle of the 21st century. Yet it stands, protected, an oasis of rare plant life, the hunting ground for dozens of soaring raptors, one of the premier viewpoints in the Bay Area.

Viewed from nearby freeways, San Bruno Mountain seems barren and almost lifeless. Yet this landmark ridge preserves a large native plant community akin to what once covered all the hills of San Francisco. Isolated as it is from surrounding mountain ranges, San Bruno harbors several species of plants found almost nowhere else today. At present, 14 species of rare or endangered plants exist on the mountain. In addition, four rare species of butterflies flutter over the slopes, including the endangered San Bruno elfin and Mission blue. Nonendangered rodents, prey for dozens of raptors, scurry through the thick brush.

As the tide of development reached the base of the mountain in the 1960s, efforts began to protect this unique natural feature and its native habitats. In 1978 the state purchased the core of the new park, and in 1982 the Habitat Conservation Plan was established with developers, allowing construction on some of the surrounding native habitat in exchange for funding to preserve and protect the ecosystem within the park. This unusual plan created the San Bruno Mountain Habitat Conservation Trust Fund, used to eradicate encroaching nonnative species such as eucalyptus and reestablish endangered, existing native plants.

The Hike follows the spine of San Bruno Mountain (1314´) from the central ridgetop parking lot to the eastern end above Hwy. 101, an easy hike with incredible views. The trail is entirely exposed to the elements. Wind is common and fog can envelop the mountain from May through September, so be prepared. Views are best immediately following a winter storm, hazing up rapidly in the days that follow. A camera with a telephoto lens and binoculars are best for capturing the expansive vistas. Despite the millions of people residing and working around the mountain, the trails are lightly traveled—especially on weekdays. No water is available at the trailhead.

To Reach the Trailhead: It is possible to approach from both Interstate 280 and Hwy. 101. From 101, take the Bayshore Blvd. exit and turn west on Guadalupe Canyon Pkwy., reaching the park entrance (on the north side of the road) in 1.6 miles. Approaching on I-280 from the north, take the Eastmoor Ave. exit, turn

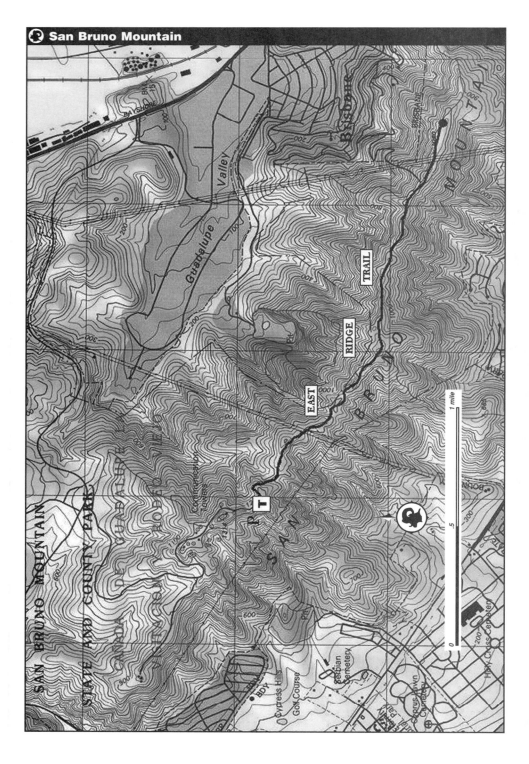

left on Sullivan Rd., then quickly left again on San Pedro Rd. to cross the freeway. As you continue on San Pedro Rd., it becomes first East Market St. and then Guadalupe Canyon Pkwy. before reaching the park entrance. Approaching on I-280 from the south, take the Mission St. exit, turn left on Junipero Serra Blvd., right on San Pedro Rd., and proceed as described above. From the parking lot at the park entrance, drive underneath Guadalupe Canyon Pkwy. and up Radio Rd. to the summit parking lot. There is a day-use fee of $5.

Description: The trail begins at the east end of the parking lot, following a disused dirt road on an undulating route to East Peak. Yarrow, wild strawberry, poison oak, and other small plants hide among the skeletal fingers of the ubiquitous coyote brush. San Francisco International Airport is less than 5 miles away and continuously fills the skies with aircraft. Raptors soar in the more immediate air. The more common include: red-tailed hawk, easily identified by its distinctive cry and orange-red tail; northern harrier, spotted by the large white patch on the rump; and American kestrel—the smallest raptor—identified by its small size, bandit black eye stripes, and constant tail twitching while in flight. While East Peak seems close throughout the hike, it takes longer to get there than you think. Where the slopes plummet down to Hwy. 101, you've arrived. Return the way you came, pondering this dramatic contrast between urban mania and Mother Nature.

Nearest Visitors Center: This park doesn't have a visitors center. For general information, call (650) 992-6770.

Nearest Campground: Francis Beach Campground is open year-round at the south end of Half Moon Bay State Beach, located just west of Hwy. 1 on Kelly Ave; the turnoff is 0.3 mile south of Hwy. 92 (58 sites, $15). Reservations are recommended in summer; call (800) 444-7275 or visit www.reserveamerica.com.

Additional Information: www.eparks.net

HIKE 27

San Francisco's Pacific Shore

Urban Wild

Highlights	The wild, scenic, historic Pacific margin of San Francisco
Distance	5.5 miles one-way
Total Elevation Gain/Loss	500´/500´
Hiking Time	5–7 hours
Optional Maps	USGS 7.5-min. *Point Bonita* and *San Francisco North*
Best Times	September through May
Agency	Golden Gate National Recreation Area
Difficulty	★★

Here is the power of the Pacific, breaking upon storied shores too rugged for development, punctuated by wild geologic exposures, immediate to the densest collection of humanity in California. Wander the urban wild of San Francisco.

The Hike follows San Francisco's Pacific shore from Ocean Beach to the Golden Gate Bridge, an all-day adventure completely accessible by public transportation. Cool ocean breezes make a warm sweater and/or windbreaker critical year-round. Avoid the summer months when fog envelops the Pacific shore, lowering the temperature and obscuring the spectacular views. A shuttle by bus or car is required to return to Ocean Beach at the end of the day. While no water is available at the trailhead, sources are plentiful along the way.

There is no safe swimming anywhere along this hike. The Pacific Ocean in San Francisco is dangerous, currents are strong, and waves can be powerful. People have been swept out to sea and drowned. Precarious cliffs are also a hazard. Respect the ocean and heed all warning signs.

To Reach the Trailhead: Head to the north end of Ocean Beach at the western edge of Golden Gate Park and park in one of the large lots adjacent to the beach. Approaching from the Golden Gate Bridge,

take Hwy. 1 south, turn right on John F. Kennedy Dr. and, when Kennedy Dr. ends, turn right again on Martin Luther King Jr. Dr. to reach the ocean. Approaching from the south on Interstate 280, take the Hwy. 1/19th Ave. exit, go north on 19th Ave. to Kennedy Dr., turn left, and proceed as described above. Approaching from the Bay Bridge, take the Fell St. exit, go west on Fell St. to Golden Gate Park, bear right on John F. Kennedy Dr., follow it through the park, and continue as described above. The northern end of this hike is in the large tourist parking lot at the southern end of the Golden Gate Bridge, located immediately east of the toll plaza.

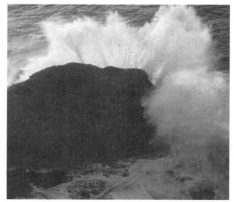

The sea breaks its back on Lands End.

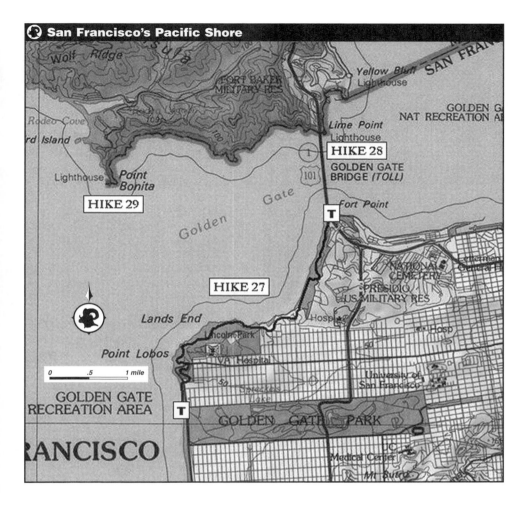

Public transportation for this hike is provided by Muni Bus 38 (service along Geary Blvd. to Point Lobos) and Bus 28 (service from the Golden Gate Bridge with a stop at Geary Blvd.). Call 511 or (415) 701-2311 for current schedule information or visit www.sfmta.com.

Description: From the parking lot at Ocean Beach, drop down a stairwell to the open sand. Four miles long, Ocean Beach is the largest beach in the Bay Area and stretches from Fort Funston to the Cliff House, visible on the rocks immediately north. The Richmond and Sunset districts east of the beach were built upon a vast field of sand dunes, which covered most

of northwest San Francisco and was once the fourth largest dune complex in California. All this sand originated between 10 and 15 thousand years ago during the last ice age when sea level was approximately 200 feet lower. San Francisco Bay was dry land, and the shoreline was roughly 20 miles west of its current location—you could have walked to the Farallon Islands! Instead of dropping its sediment in the bay as it does today, the Sacramento River flowed beyond the Golden Gate, depositing sand in a broad alluvial fan that was blown onshore by prevailing northwesterly winds to form Ocean Beach and the vast dune fields.

After enjoying Ocean Beach, walk north toward the Cliff House, head up Stairway 4, cross the Esplanade to the corner of Balboa and La Playa, and climb the stairs toward Sutro Heights. As is true throughout this hike, numerous use paths diverge in all directions as you proceed. Continue generally north through eucalyptus and Monterey cypress to reach the top of Sutro Heights, where an open area of grass and unusual trees can be found. The tall, straight-trunked trees sporting strange wandlike foliage here are monkey puzzle trees, a type of araucaria native to Chile and Argentina.

To understand the history of Sutro Heights and its surrounding landmarks requires a brief biography of Adolph Sutro. A native of Prussia, Sutro emigrated to California in 1850, and in 1869 began constructing a tunnel designed to access and ventilate the rich mines of Nevada's Comstock Lode. Completed in 1878, the Sutro Tunnel was a huge financial success, earning Sutro a tidy fortune when he sold his shares in 1879. Returning to San Francisco, he acquired vast amounts of real estate for the future structures of Sutro Heights, the Cliff House, and the Sutro Baths. At one point, he owned one-eleventh of all city land! Over the next 20 years Sutro helped build San Francisco, even serving as mayor from 1895 to 1897. After his death in 1898, the sights and wonders he created slowly fell into disrepair, leaving little but memories and the photographs so well-preserved by the National Park Service today.

Acquired by Sutro in 1881, Sutro Heights was an open blufftop with little vegetation. With the help of 11 full-time gardeners, he transformed it into an exotic plant and flower garden with a substantial greenhouse. A popular tourist destination while in operation, the structure was torn down in 1939. South from the large viewing platform, you can see the long stretch of Ocean Beach and distant Montara Mtn. (Hike 22) terminating in the ocean at Point San Pedro. Visible on clear days are

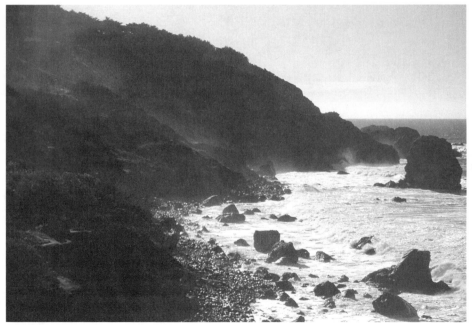

Lands End

the Farallon Islands to the west and Point Reyes to the northwest.

From Sutro Heights, head down to the Cliff House parking lot—the dirt path splits north from the paved trail by the small gazebo. Cross Point Lobos Ave. and make the quick side trip down to the Cliff House. The current Cliff House is the third structure occupying this precarious site. The first was an unassuming structure known as Seal Rock House, purchased by Sutro in 1881, that catered to San Francisco's elite. Destroyed by fire in 1894, Seal Rock House was replaced by the opulent Victorian Cliff House, an eight-story marvel styled after a French chateau, which survived the 1906 earthquake only to be destroyed by fire in 1907. Constructed in 1909 by Sutro's daughter, the third and current Cliff House is a less-exciting neo-classic building. Immediately offshore from the Cliff House sit Seal Rocks, named for the California and Steller's sea lions (once considered seals) that have historically used the rocks as a safe haven and bark boisterously into the wind. Today, Seal Rocks are much quieter as most of the sea lions seem to be congregating near Fisherman's Wharf at Pier 39.

From the Cliff House, walk back up Point Lobos Ave. and head down to the ruins of Sutro Baths. Opened to the public in 1896, the Sutro Baths complex covered more than three acres and was enclosed by 100,000 square feet of glass. In addition to one freshwater pool, 1.685 million gallons of sea water filled 6 separate saltwater swimming tanks that could be flushed in less than an hour by the incoming tides. There were 9 springboards, 7 toboggan slides, 3 trapezes, 1 high dive, 30 swinging rings, 20,000 bathing suits, 40,000 towels, 500 private dressing rooms, a 5300-seat amphitheater, 3 restaurants, natural history exhibits, art galleries, and a jungle of exotic plants. Up to 1600 bathers could swim at once, the main room had a capacity of 15,000, and more than 25,000 people could visit in a single day. Following Sutro's death, the baths slowly

fell into disrepair; they were destroyed by fire in 1966. Today the trail leads past the remaining foundation to a large concrete platform, which was the site of two-gun Battery Lobos during World War II.

The trail continues uphill north of Sutro Baths, rejoining the broad Coastal Trail via several use paths. Bear left on the Coastal Trail, the former roadbed of the Ferries and Cliff House Railroad. Continue north where a wide trail joins from the right; you will soon see the entire Golden Gate Bridge (Hike 28) through the surrounding Monterey cypress. As the large building of the Veterans Administration Hospital appears south over the bluffs above you, look left for one of the unposted trails leading down to the ocean at Lands End. A small promontory offering views of a San Francisco coastline as wild as any in California, Lands End is a side trip not to be missed.

Now heading east along the main trail, you have incredible views past off-limits Painted Rock Cliff before reaching the immaculate greens of Lincoln Golf Course. At El Camino del Mar, go left (east) down the sidewalk, bearing left at all intersections to reach the posted access for China Beach (via a hard left leading to parking above the small sandy beach). From this intersection, continue on Sea Cliff Dr. to its eastern end, where a path leads down to Baker Beach. Alternatively, you can follow the larger thoroughfare of El Camino del Mar a short distance to Bowley St., and turn left to reach the beach.

Named for a prominent San Francisco lawyer killed in the Civil War, Baker Beach was the site of San Francisco's only shark attack, a fatal incident that occurred in 1959. Walk north along the beach toward its clothing-optional section, and make the sandy, exhausting ascent up the stairway to Lincoln Blvd. Turn left and walk along Lincoln Blvd. for approximately 50 yards to a trail heading left for Battery Crosby, one of 22 coastal batteries constructed in and around the Presidio. The majority of these, including Crosby, were built and manned between 1895 and 1945 as a defense against potential invasion. From here, a maze of trails winds north on the bluffs above the ocean. While the main trail continues along Lincoln Blvd., it is possible to follow any number of the use paths—just keep heading north.

The distinctive green bluffs here are composed of serpentine, an unusual rock that produces soils inhospitable to most plants. Consequently, unique ecosystems have developed on serpentine outcrops around the state, which harbor many rare and endangered species found nowhere else. Please respect the signs and fences along this section—they are designed to protect and rehabilitate this rare San Francisco ecosystem. The heavily sheared, landslide-prone bluffs here can be closely examined by scrambling down to the secluded rocky shoreline at their base, an exciting side trip.

Continuing north past Batteries West (armed with 12 cannons and operational 1873–1898), Godfrey (3 guns, 1896–1943), Boutelle (2 guns, 1898–1917), Marcus Miller (3 guns, 1899–1920), and Cranston (2 guns, 1898–1943), the maze of trails meets at a paved path that leads underneath the Golden Gate Bridge to the large parking lot and tourist center by the toll plaza.

Nearest Visitors Center: There is not a visitors center along this hike's route. For general information, contact the Presidio Visitors Center, (415) 561-4323, which is open daily 9 AM–5 PM.

Nearest Campground: Group campgrounds in the Marin Headlands, across the Golden Gate Bridge, include Kirby Cove (4 sites, open April through October) and Battery Alexander (1 site, open year-round). The fee for each is $20. There is also an easily accessible, free, walk-in campground at Bicentennial near Battery Wallace (3 sites, maximum 2 people per site, open year-round).

Reservations are required for all campsites in the Marin Headlands and can be made up to 90 days in advance by calling the Marin Headlands Visitors Center, (415) 331-1540. Permits must be picked up at the visitors center, located 1 mile from Point Bonita on Bunker Rd. in Rodeo Valley and open daily 9:30 AM–4:30 PM.

Additional Information: www. nps.gov/goga

HIKE 28

Golden Gate Bridge

The Golden Gate

Highlights	The bridge. The view. The experience.
Distance	2.4 miles round-trip
Total Elevation Gain/Loss	60´/60´
Hiking Time	1–2 hours
Optional Map	USGS 7.5-min. *San Francisco North*
Best Times	September through May
Agency	Golden Gate National Recreation Area
Difficulty	★

SEE MAP ON PAGE 103

A graceful sweep of perfection, the Golden Gate Bridge is the defining landmark of Northern California. It is a marvel of human ingenuity that spanned an impossible gap across a violent strait, an engineering masterpiece famous the world over.

The Hike covers the length of the Golden Gate Bridge and explores its location, history, and construction. While the round-trip hike can be completed from either end, the description below begins from the south. It is usually cold and windy on the bridge with summer months bringing dense fog to the mix, obscuring the incredible views, and making the rest of the year preferable for a visit. A warm sweater and windbreaker are recommended items year-round. Tourists are thick on the bridge and the wide diversity of countries represented is entertaining. The bridge is closed to pedestrians after dark and reopens at 5 AM. Water is available at the trailhead.

To Reach the Trailhead: Take Hwy. 101 to the southern end of the bridge and park in the main tourist lot immediately east of the toll plaza. To reach the trailhead by public transportation, take Muni Bus 28 or 29. Call 511 or (415) 701-2311 for current schedule information or visit www.sfmta.com.

Description: The hike begins by the statue of Joseph Strauss, chief engineer of the Golden Gate Bridge from inception to completion. An engineer whose college graduation thesis was a bridge design for spanning the 50-mile-wide Bering Strait between Alaska and Russia, Strauss was a man of intense vision, purpose, and ingenuity. By the time construction began in early 1933, he had completed more than 400 bridges around the world and was considered by many to be the only man capable of realizing such an ambitious project. It would be his final and greatest work.

From here, head to the bridge itself, passing the rotunda gift shop to get to the east sidewalk near a barrage of signs and regulations. As you begin walking across the bridge, contemplate the fury beneath your feet. The Sacramento River drains more than 59,000 square miles (40 percent of the entire state), pouring into shallow San Francisco Bay from the northeast. The bay has only one outlet—the Golden Gate—a narrow 1-mile-wide channel to the sea that is affected twice daily by the changing tides. During incoming tides, the rising waters pour into the bay and impound the freshwater brought in by the Sacramento River. As the tides reverse, an unbelievable volume of water rushes out the narrow entrance. Every 12 hours, the bay disgorges one-sixth of its entire volume through the Golden Gate at a rate of roughly 2.3 million gallons per second. Moving at a speed of between 4.5 and 7.5 knots, the average flow is seven times that of the Mississippi River! Add to that powerful winds capable of reaching 60 miles per hour and the fury of nature here is readily apparent.

Savor the views as you walk toward the south tower. Southeast, Coit Tower and downtown San Francisco are apparent, connected to the East Bay via the Bay Bridge. Looking east across the bay, the summit of Mt. Diablo (Hike 15) can be seen crowning the East Bay Hills, and downtown Berkeley is visible beyond nearby Alcatraz Island. Northeast is substantial Angel Island and the Tiburon peninsula. While views west are somewhat obscured by the far railings, the jagged spit of Point Bonita (Hike 29) juts from the north. Fort Point is directly beneath you, a pre-Civil War fort built during the 1850s to safeguard America's newfound western possession. In designing the bridge, Strauss recognized that preservation of this important historical landmark was imperative; he built the distinctive rainbow arches above to frame it visually. The many emergency phones along the sidewalk are to help prevent potential suicides—to date more than 1000 people have leapt to their deaths from the bridge.

Reaching the south tower, look up its fluted form. Tapering as it rises to its peak of 746 feet above sea level, this tower proved to be one of the greatest engineering challenges of the bridge. Its concrete foundation pier sits more than 1100 feet offshore on a sloping underwater ledge between 60 and 80 feet deep, fully in the brunt of waves and tidal current. To build it required construction of a precarious trestle from shore to site, building fenders around the pier site, blasting a foundation hole to a level depth of 100 feet below sea level, extending the fenders from surface to bottom, and then dewatering (pumping out the water) the entire thing. The trestle and fenders were destroyed by waves during early construction and had to be rebuilt prior to pouring the concrete. The north pier foundation proved less difficult; it was built close to shore on a flat, shallow ledge located a mere 20 feet below the surface.

The massive steel towers sit on top of these concrete piers, each constructed of 43 million pounds of steel designed to support 85 million pounds of dead weight. Surprisingly, they are not solid, constructed instead of hollow cells 42" square by 35′ high, which allow each tower to move lat-

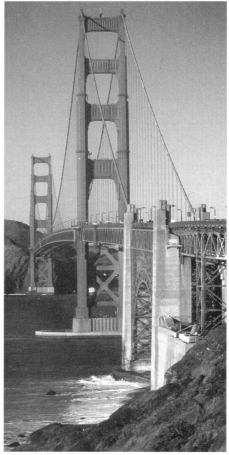

The Golden Gate Bridge

erally up to 13" and to bend 18" toward the channel and 22" toward the shore, as the cables expand and contract with the temperature. In driving the 600,000 rivets required to put each tower together, workers had to scramble inside and through the honeycombed boxes. Remarkably, the entire south tower was constructed in a scant 101 days.

The distance between the two towers is 4200 feet and as you walk it, admire the catenary curve of the two main bridge cables. These huge cables measure 36.5" in diameter, are 7650´ long, and each weigh 7125 tons. They attach to the earth at four, massive, concrete anchors buried 12 stories deep in the ground and capable of each withstanding 63 million pounds of pull. Essentially spun in place, each cable is composed of 27,000 strands of thin wire, which were individually strung from anchorage to tower to tower to anchorage and back again. Approximately 80,000 miles of this pencil-thin wire were used, enough to wrap around the equator three times.

The Golden Gate Bridge is a suspension bridge. That is, the roadway is suspended from cables supported by towers. Once the cables were complete, construction of the 90-foot-wide roadway began. Strauss was farsighted enough to build a bridge six lanes wide, a width considered somewhat excessive at the time—the traffic around you today probably would have surprised him. Construction began from both towers simultaneously and the roadway was joined in November 1936. Paving the roadway followed; it resulted in the main fatalities of the construction process. An innovative safety net had been rigged beneath the expanding and precarious roadway, saving fallen men from plummeting to their death. (Those so saved by the net formed a small "Halfway

to Hell" club.) Unfortunately, in February 1937 a platform supporting a work crew detached, ripping through the net and killing 10 men. An earlier crane accident had claimed the bridge's first victim, making a final count of 11 fatalities. Yet, construction proceeded and on May 27, 1937, the $35 million bridge opened to the public amid great fanfare. Joseph Strauss died the following year.

Continue to the viewing platform at the north end of the bridge and admire this masterpiece before returning.

Nearest Visitors Center: The Golden Gate Bridge Gift Center on the southeast side of the toll plaza is open daily 8:30 AM–6:30 PM, with extended hours during the summer.

Nearest Campground: On the north side of the Golden Gate, the Marin Headlands provide group campgrounds in Kirby Cove (4 sites, open April through October) and at Battery Alexander (1 site, open year-round). The fee for each is $20. There is also an easily accessible, free, walk-in campground at Bicentennial near Battery Wallace (3 sites, maximum 2 people per site, and open year-round).

Reservations are required for all campsites in the Marin Headlands and can be made up to 90 days in advance by calling the Marin Headlands Visitors Center, (415) 331-1540. Permits must be picked up at the visitors center, located 1 mile from Point Bonita on Bunker Rd. in Rodeo Valley and open daily 9:30 AM–4:30 PM.

Additional Information: www.goldengatebridge.org

HIKE 29

Point Bonita Lighthouse

Que Bonita

Highlights	The jaws of the Golden Gate and the legacy of "wickies" and "surfmen"
Distance	1.0 mile round-trip
Total Elevation Gain/Loss	50´/50´
Hiking Time	1 hour
Optional Map	USGS 7.5-min. *Point Bonita*
Best Times	September through May
Agency	Golden Gate National Recreation Area
Difficulty	★

SEE MAP ON PAGE 103

Take a short stroll to the farthest edge of the Bay Area. Perched on a naked fin of rock jabbing into the ocean, Point Bonita Lighthouse is a lonely sentinel with extraordinary views.

The Hike follows an easy paved path through a tunnel and over a unique suspension bridge to the lighthouse. Unfortunately, the lighthouse path is only open Saturday through Monday from 12:30 to 3:30 PM; otherwise, it is closed at the tunnel. While the hike to the tunnel is pleasant, it cannot rival the full lighthouse experience. Prepare for wind—lots of wind—as Point Bonita is always blustery. Timing is important—fog blankets the point for days on end during the summer months, making the rest of the year better for a visit. The lighthouse may be closed if wave and weather conditions are too severe.

To Reach the Trailhead: Take Hwy. 101 to the Alexander Ave. exit, the first off-ramp north of the Golden Gate Bridge. Following signs to the Marin Headlands, quickly turn left to pass through the one-lane tunnel. A mile past the tunnel turn left onto McCullough Rd., follow it uphill, and then turn right onto spectacular Conzelman Rd., which becomes a narrow

one-lane road that drops precipitously to a T-junction by a YMCA. Go left and park in the posted Point Bonita lot.

Public transportation to nearby Battery Alexander is available from San Francisco on Sundays and holidays aboard Muni Bus 76, which departs once an hour from downtown. For current schedule information, visit www.sfmta.com.

Description: From the parking area, follow the paved path below a stand of Monterey cypress. Dropping toward the tunnel, you reach an informative placard detailing the story of the Point Bonita Lifesaving Station and the "surfmen" who manned it. According to a 1908 *San Francisco Chronicle* article describing the surfmen, "Every man enlisted in this daring work must have had at least three years of experience as a sailor. He must be an expert boatman and physically perfect. He is not allowed to drink while in uniform, and to be caught intoxicated means immediate dismissal. As a matter of course he must be courageous. The discipline is very strict."

As you approach the tunnel, the first views north open up and Point Reyes and Bolinas are visible beyond the pounding

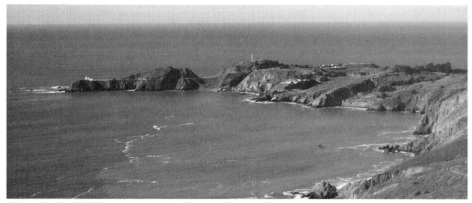

Point Bonita Lighthouse perches on the tip of a jagged peninsula.

surf. The shark fin of rock through which the tunnel passes is composed of pillow basalt, a rock highly resistant to erosion. It is formed on the ocean bottom when liquid magma is extruded from the sea floor. As the molten rock encounters seawater, its outer shell is instantly cooled to form a distinctive pillow shape. Liquid magma remains inside, however, and as it is squeezed out again another pillow is formed on top, creating large stacks of these distinctive formations.

Before you enter the tunnel, notice the odd, large-leafed plants clinging to cracks in the rock. These are feral cabbages, escaped from the gardens of past lighthouse keepers and now uniquely adapted to survive the hostile environment of Point Bonita. On the other side of the tunnel, railings protect you from the drop to the rocks below. When you reach the suspension bridge, please observe the five-person limit.

When Point Bonita Lighthouse opened in 1855, it was the third lighthouse constructed on the West Coast, built in response to the more than 300 ships that had run aground near the Golden Gate during the Gold Rush period. The original Fresnel lens, constructed in France, was capable of bending 70% of radiant light onto a horizontal plane. Its original light was the flame on an oil-fed wick, tended by resident lighthouse keepers known as "wick-ies." Incredibly, the same lens is still in use today, sending a beam of light visible for 18 miles. In 1980 the lighthouse was the last in the U.S. to become automated, and today a single 1000-watt bulb provides the light. The lighthouse building is open to the public but the light itself is off-limits.

Nearest Visitors Center: Marin Headlands Visitors Center, (415) 331-1540, located 1 mile from Point Bonita on Bunker Rd. in Rodeo Valley, is open daily 9:30 AM–4:30 PM.

Nearest Campground: Group campgrounds in the Marin Headlands include Kirby Cove (4 sites, open April through October) and Battery Alexander (1 site, open year-round). The fee for each is $20. There is also an easily accessible, free, walk-in campground at Bicentennial near Battery Wallace (3 sites, maximum 2 people per site, open year-round). Reservations are required for all campsites in the Marin Headlands and can be made up to 90 days in advance by calling the visitors center. Permits must be picked up at the visitors center during open hours.

Additional Information: www.nps.gov/goga

HIKE 30

Gerbode Valley

The Nature of Things

Highlights	Wildflowers, wildlife, and wild land—so close, yet so far away
Distance	6.1 miles
Total Elevation Gain/Loss	1500′/1500′
Hiking Time	3–5 hours
Optional Maps	Tom Harrison's *Mt. Tam*, USGS 7.5-min. *Point Bonita*
Best Times	September through May
Agency	Marin Headlands, Golden Gate National Recreation Area
Difficulty	★★

It is as it was. Rolling hills cleft by valleys, split by ridges, battered by the sea; a land of sweeping vistas, vibrant life, and dramatic geology in a natural world protected from the bustle of the Bay Area. The Marin Headlands await.

The Hike loops around broad Gerbode Valley in the central Headlands, offering far-reaching views of sea, slopes, and city from the heart of this protected landscape. The clear skies and abundant wildflowers of spring are optimal for a visit, though the sunny days of fall and crystalline air of winter are also pleasant. Summer brings fog and windy conditions. The area's immediate proximity to San Francisco draws regular crowds and you'll likely encounter dozens of hikers and mountain bikers, especially on weekends. No water is available at the trailhead.

To Reach the Trailhead: From the south, take Hwy. 101 to the Alexander Ave. exit (the first off-ramp north of the Golden Gate Bridge) and follow signs toward the Marin Headlands, turning left to pass through the one-lane tunnel and then continuing straight on Bunker Rd. for approximately 2 miles to the visitors center. Bear right toward Fort Cronkhite, reaching the trailhead on the right in a quarter mile.

Approaching from the north, take the last Sausalito exit immediately before the Golden Gate Bridge, turn left at the stop sign, bear right up steep Conzelman Rd., and continue on Conzelman Rd. for 3 miles to the intersection by Battery Alexander. Turn right, continue 0.5 mile to the visitors center, and turn left toward Fort Cronkhite.

Description: From the trailhead (0.0/20′), begin on broad Miwok Trail as it passes through open grassland punctuated by coyote brush, blackberry brambles, and a seasonal display of lupine, poppies, paintbrush, checkerbloom, irises, and other wildflowers. As you proceed, watch for quail and jackrabbits in the brush, black-tailed deer and the elusive bobcat in open clearings, and red-tailed hawks and other raptors overhead.

The trail briefly enters a small riparian alley filled with willows, stinging nettle, wild cucumber vines, horsetail, elderberry, dogwood, bracken fern, vetch, and other moisture-loving plants, a marked contrast to the surrounding dry slopes. You pass a feeder trail on the right from nearby Bunker Road (0.4/20′) and then quickly reach Bobcat Trail (your return route) on the right (0.5/30′). Remain on Miwok Trail as it turns toward the valley slopes

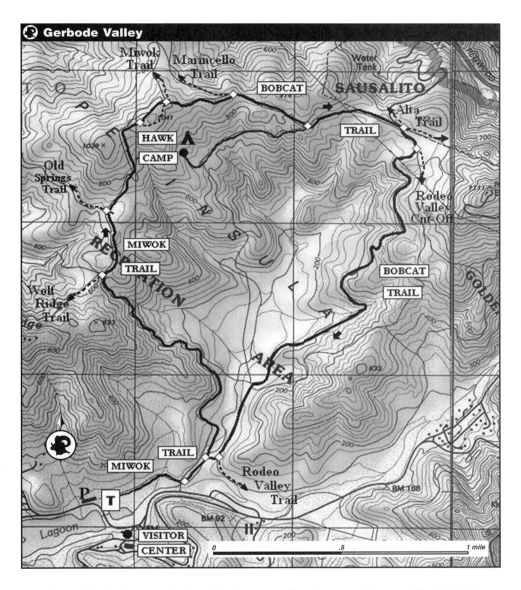

and steadily climbs toward the ridgeline. Enjoy views north into adjacent Tennessee Valley as you pass Wolf Ridge Trail on the left (1.6/600´) and briefly undulate along the ridge. Downtown San Francisco peeks over the hills to the south and the long spine of Mt. Tamalpais slowly rises to the north. Miwok Trail narrows to single-track shortly before reaching Old Springs Trail (1.9/640´).

Continue straight on Miwok Trail as it climbs steeply toward the FAA facilities atop Hill 1041, offering stratospheric views across the Bay Area. To the south are the Golden Gate Bridge, downtown San Francisco, antenna-lined San Bruno Mountain (Hike 26), and distant Montara Mountain (Hike 22). To the east are Mt. Diablo (Hike 15), the Bay Bridge, Oakland, Berkeley, and the entire East Bay hills. To the north

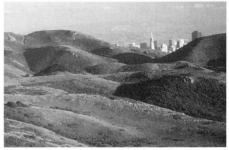
So close, so far away—San Francisco peeks over the hills of the Marin Headlands.

Mt. Tamalpais (2571) dominates above Mill Valley, the Tiburon peninsula, and Angel Island. To the west is the vast Pacific Ocean, pimpled with the Farallon Islands on clear days. The trail splits and rejoins around the fenced-off FAA facilities, which remind you that INTERRUPTION OF SERVICE MAY RESULT IN THE LOSS OF HUMAN LIFE.

Past the FAA hilltop, continue straight on Bobcat Trail as Miwok Trail splits left to descend into Tennessee Valley (2.5/1000′). Descending briefly, Bobcat Trail quickly reaches the junction with Marincello Trail (2.8/900′). This is an appropriate point to marvel at the protected world of Gerbode Valley, a world almost lost to development.

Imagine 30,000 people living in the valley below, with hundreds of homes lining Wolf Ridge and 19 high-rise buildings towering over schools, churches, shopping centers, and light industry. During the 1960s, it almost happened. A master development plan for a town named Marincello was drawn up for the privately owned valley and an access road (Marincello Trail) was built to facilitate construction. Financial and bureaucratic delays slowed the project, however, and a key court decision in the late '60s ultimately stopped it altogether. The Nature Conservancy later purchased the land for $6.5 million and bequeathed it to the National Park Service, forever protecting it for public enjoyment.

Bear right on Bobcat Trail, soon passing the junction for Hawk Camp (3.1/780′) on the right. A small copse of trees marks the

camp location a half mile away. Continuing, Bobcat Trail dips beneath power lines and passes junctions on the left for Alta Trail (3.6/730′) and Rodeo Valley Cut-Off Trail (3.7/720′). As you begin the slow downward traverse back toward the trailhead, note the different vegetation in the adjacent north-facing gullies—bay, hazel, coast live oak, elderberry, and the occasional Douglas fir flourish in these moist pockets. Bobcat Trail passes Rodeo Valley Trail on the left (5.5/50′) shortly before reaching the earlier junction with Miwok Trail (5.6/30′) and the final return stretch to the trailhead (6.1/20′).

Nearest Visitors Center: Marin Headlands Visitors Center, (415) 331-1540, is open daily 9:30 AM–4:30 PM.
Backpacking Information: Backcountry camping is allowed at Hawk Camp (3 sites, free). Each site accommodates a maximum of four people. An outhouse and picnic tables are provided, but water is not available. Reservations can be made up to 90 days in advance by calling the visitors center; unreserved sites are available at the visitors center on a first-come, first-served basis.
Nearest Campground: Group campgrounds in the Marin Headlands include Kirby Cove (4 sites, open April through October) and Battery Alexander (1 site, open year-round). The fee for each is $20. There is also an easily accessible, free, walk-in campground at Bicentennial near Battery Wallace (3 sites, maximum 2 people per site, open year-round). Reservations are required for all campsites in the Marin Headlands and can be made up to 90 days in advance by calling the visitors center. Permits must be picked up at the visitors center during open hours.
Additional Information: www.nps.gov/goga

HIKE 31

Ring Mountain

Ring It In

Highlights	Bay-sweeping views and cathedral oaks
Distance	3.2 miles
Total Elevation Gain/Loss	600´/600´
Hiking Time	2–3 hours
Optional Map	USGS 7.5-min. *San Quentin*
Best Times	Year-round
Agency	RingMountain Open Space Preserve, Marin County Open Space District
Difficulty	★★

Ring Mountain bulges upward from the shores of San Francisco Bay, a bald hillock offering exceptional 360-degree views of the northern Bay Area. A few ancient live oaks line the ridges, twisting in gnarled and fantastic form. Add in some unusual rock outcrops and you've got a full array of natural highlights.

The Hike loops to the summit of 602-foot Ring Mountain from the north, winding upward to meet a series of fire roads near the top. After a visit to hulking Turtle Rock and the nearby summit, you loop downward past several enormous live oaks. The hike can be completed year-round, though wet conditions make for muddy walking at times. The far-reaching views are the primary attraction; aim for a fog-free day. No water is available at the trailhead.

To Reach the Trailhead: Take Hwy. 101 to the Paradise Dr. exit and follow Paradise Dr. east for 1.5 miles to the signed trailhead on the south side of the road. Park by the roadside.

Description: From the trailhead (0.0/10´), the wide path strikes out past coyote brush, toyon, and young bay trees. You quickly reach a junction, where you

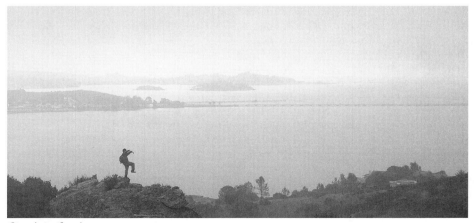

Step into the ring.

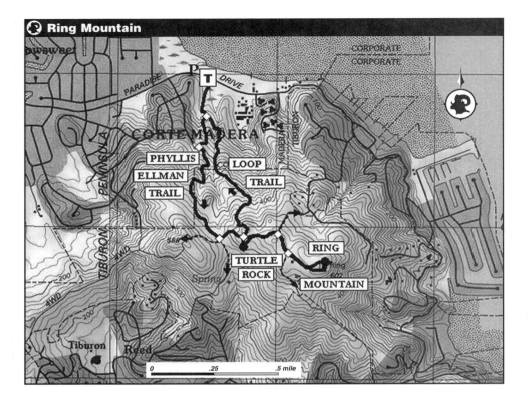

bear right on Phyllis Ellman Trail (you'll return from the left on Loop Trail). The single-track trail winds upward past blackberry vines and abundant rock outcrops, evidence of the site's unusual geology.

As a tectonic plate is forced beneath an adjacent continent—or *subducted*—it descends 10–30 miles into the earth's mantle, where temperatures are hot enough to melt all rocks. However, since the diving plate is cool and warms slowly, not all of it may melt. Instead, portions are altered into new rock-forms by extreme pressure, reemerging much later to indicate the site of the former subduction zone. Subduction occurred along the coast of California for approximately 150 million years, until the San Andreas Fault became active roughly 20 million years ago. On Ring Mountain, these telltale rocks include blueschist, a vibrantly dark-blue stone; and waxy-green serpentine, California's state rock.

Views steadily expand as you ascend, peering north toward the San Rafael Bridge and San Quentin Prison on its western end. Two unnamed side paths soon split off to the right—remain left to begin traversing up the hillside. The route switchbacks above a small ravine, where your return route on Loop Trail is visible on the opposite side.

The trail soon forks again. Stay right on the posted trail to quickly crest at a copse of ancient live oaks (0.6/340´). From here, the trail widens and becomes steeper as it ascends the grassy flanks to Ring Mountain Fire Rd. (0.9/460´). Views now open south toward the spires of San Francisco and the central San Francisco Bay. Bear left, passing Loop Trail on your left (1.0/520´) and hulking Turtle Rock—a popular bouldering spot—on your right. Less technical climbers can easily scramble atop its shell from behind.

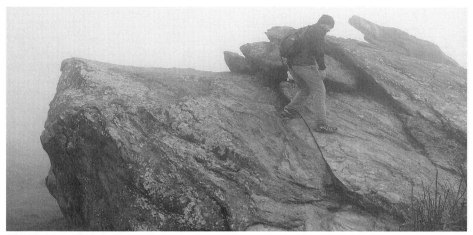

The Turtle suffers no fools.

The trail crests and drops briefly to Taylor Fire Rd. (1.2/540′). Turn right on the asphalt path, then quickly bear left on an unpaved road that wanders over to Ring Mountain's highest point on the east end of the broad hilltop (1.4/602′). A small grove of wind-sculpted bay trees marks the spot. From here, enjoy some of the hike's most expansive views. Paradise Cay and the swanky shoreline homes of Tiburon lie below you to the southeast. The Oakland-Berkeley hills line the eastern horizon; the pyramidal summit of Mt. Diablo (Hike 15) peeks over the top on clear days. To the west, the flanks and summit of Mt. Tamalpais (Hike 32) loom, while the rolling hills of the Marin Headlands (Hike 30) hide just out of sight to the southwest. San Francisco pincushions the sky farther south.

Retrace your steps to the earlier junction with Loop Trail (1.8/520′) and turn right to begin your downward journey. The single-track trail steadily drops down a small ridgeline intermittently shaded by bay trees. You pass another incredible coast live oak along the way (2.8/420′) whose elephant leg branches extend far down the hillside. Enjoy continuous views north as you descend past numerous use paths crisscrossing the hillside; the main path is obvious and marked by a series of numbered interpretive posts. As you approach the preserve boundary, the trail curves left into the adjacent gully, crosses its ephemeral rivulet, and reaches the earlier junction with Phyllis Ellman Trail (3.1/60′). Turn right to return to the trailhead.

Nearest Visitors Center: This preserve doesn't have a visitors center. Call the main Marin County Open Space District office at (415) 499-6387 for general information.

Nearest Campground: Nearby Mount Tamalpais State Park has Pantoll Campground, located by Pantoll Ranger Station (16 first-come, first-served sites that require a short 100-yard walk-in and usually fill by late afternoon). Also Steep Ravine Environmental Campground, located on a marine terrace 1 mile south of Stinson Beach on Hwy. 1, has 10 rustic cabins ($75/night) and 7 primitive campsites ($15). Reservations are essential months in advance; call (800) 444-7275 or visit www.reserveamerica.com.

Additional Information: www.co.marin.ca.us/depts/PK/main

HIKE 32

Mount Tamalpais

Tam

Highlights	A summit challenge with premier views of the Bay Area
Distance	6.8 miles
Total Elevation Gain/Loss	1900'/1900'
Hiking Time	4–6 hours
Optional Map	USGS 7.5-min. *San Rafael*
Best Times	Year-round
Agency	Mt. Tamalpais State Park, Marin Municipal Water District
Difficulty	★★★

Visible throughout the Bay Area, the long spine of Mt. Tamalpais constantly beckons the hiker with a few recreational hours to spare. Read on for an excellent taste of all the mountain has to offer.

The Hike climbs steeply from Mountain Home Inn on Panoramic Hwy. directly to the summit of Mt. Tamalpais (2571'), before looping around the mountain's eastern flanks to return to the trailhead. With a maze of trails crisscrossing the mountain, the hike utilizes the following ones in this order: Gravity Car Grade, Old Railroad Grade, Vic Haun, Temelpa, Verna Dunshee, Eldridge Grade, Wheeler, and Hoo-Koo-E-Koo. The hike can be done year-round, with spring and fall offering the most idyllic weather. The stunning views are clearest following winter storms. Summer fog can be thick in the area, but even then views tend to remain dramatic. Water is available at the trailhead.

To Reach the Trailhead: From Hwy. 101 in Marin City, take Hwy. 1 northwest toward Stinson Beach and bear right on Panoramic Hwy. at the posted Y-junction. Remain on Panoramic Hwy. for 5 miles following the ridgetop, and park in the lot across from Mountain Home Inn (at the edge of Mt. Tamalpais State Park). If the lot is full, go down the small paved road across the highway and park at the side where it turns to dirt.

Public transportation is available on West Marin Stagecoach Route 61, which makes four runs daily to Bolinas from Marin City, stopping at Mountain Home Inn along the way (415-499-6099, www.marintransit.org).

Description: From the trailhead (0.0/930'), Muir Woods' deep watershed is visible southwest below you and the summit towers due north above you. The trail begins across the highway on a small paved road that immediately brings you to a fork by a watershed boundary sign—bear right. Now on a dirt road, the trail soon crosses a gate. Beyond the gate, Douglas fir, madrone, coast live oak, toyon, and tanoak all appear along the broad trail, as do abundant second-growth redwood trees. Tantalizing views

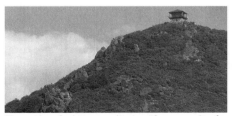

Exceptional views await atop the summit of Mt. Tamalpais.

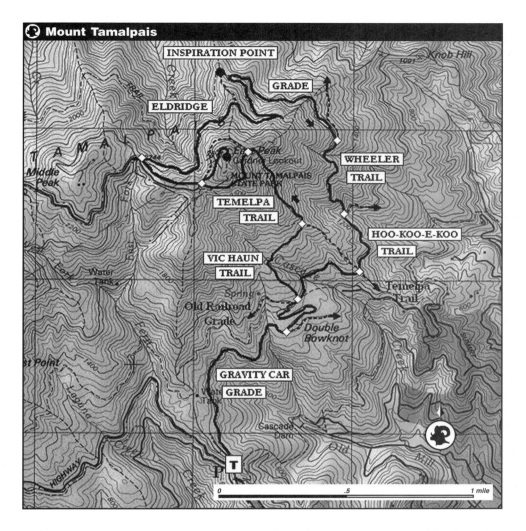

of San Francisco and the Bay Area open up intermittently as you proceed, soon reaching an area where several wide roads intersect (0.8/1100´)—continue left toward East Peak on Old Railroad Grade.

For the next 0.3 mile, you are walking on the old roadbed used by steam trains of the Mount Tamalpais and Muir Woods Railway between 1896 and 1930. While in operation, "the crookedest railroad in the world" journeyed 8.25 miles from Mill Valley to the summit on an estimated 281 curves. After making two of those curves, the roadbed reaches a posted junction with the wide Hoo-Koo-E-Koo Trail (1.1/1200´), which heads east while Old Railroad Grade curves back west. Between these two wide paths, directly at the junction, the unposted single-track Vic Haun Trail strikes almost directly uphill—take it!

Vic Haun Trail immediately begins climbing through a tunnel of manzanita and small redwoods before breaking out onto more open slopes with increasingly excellent views south. Large chinquapin bushes appear occasionally by the trail before it traverses east, crossing a small stream thick with California bay. When you

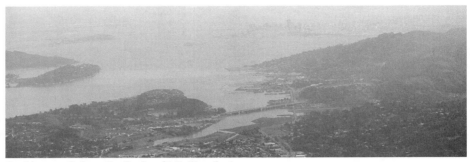

Looking south from the flanks of Mt. Tamalpais

reach the Temelpa Trail, your path continues steeply upward via numerous switchbacks to the paved Verna Dunshee Trail, which encircles the summit (2.3/2320´). Go either left or right; either way gets you to the parking lot at the crowded summit. The fire lookout above you marks the top and is easily accessible by a popular and partially boardwalked trail.

The summit and spine of Mt. Tam are composed of an unusual erosion-resistant tourmaline, formed by a reaction when sandstone becomes permeated with boron-rich water. Exposures are plentiful as you make the final push to the lookout. From the top you can see the heart of the Bay Area.

Back down at the parking lot, walk a short distance down the main paved road to find the posted gate for Eldridge Grade on the right. Drop down the wide rocky trail, noting the change in vegetation. California bay and madrone are common, joined by California nutmeg trees with pointy firlike needles. Winding below the summit, the trail reaches an obvious spur on the left due north from the peak. This is a steep, single-track shortcut to Inspiration Point that bypasses a long switchback on Eldridge Grade. From Inspiration Point (4.0/1880´), continue descending east on Eldridge Grade until you reach a posted junction (4.6/1580´) at a large switchback—continue straight on single-track Wheeler Trail.

Wheeler Trail is steep, descending rapidly through thick, young redwood forest and huckleberry bushes to reach the wide Hoo-Koo-E-Koo Trail (5.0/1110´). Turn right and stay on Hoo-Koo-E-Koo Trail until you rejoin the Old Railroad Grade (5.7/1200´). Retrace your earlier steps to the trailhead (6.8/930´).

Nearest Visitors Center: Summit Visitors Center, located by the summit parking lot, is open approximately 10 AM–5:30 PM on summer weekends and noon–4 PM on winter weekends. Also try Pantoll Ranger Station, (415) 388-2070, located 2.8 miles west of the trailhead on Panoramic Hwy.; it's open approximately 8:30 AM–7 PM daily in summer, with reduced hours (usually weekends only) in winter.

Nearest Campground: Pantoll Campground is located by Pantoll Ranger Station; it has 16 first-come, first-served sites that require a short 100-yard walk-in and usually fill by late afternoon. Also Steep Ravine Environmental Campground, located on a marine terrace 1 mile south of Stinson Beach on Hwy. 1, which has 10 rustic cabins ($75 per night) and 7 primitive campsites ($15). Reservations are essential months in advance; call (800) 444-7275 or visit www.reserveamerica.com.

Additional Information: www.parks.ca.gov

HIKE 33

Bolinas Lagoon Preserve

The Birds

Highlights	Developing avian awareness at a major heronry
Distance	2.3 miles
Total Elevation Gain/Loss	700'/700'
Hiking Time	2–3 hours
Optional Map	USGS 7.5-min. *Bolinas*
Best Times	Weekends April through July
Agency	Audubon Canyon Ranch
Difficulty	★★

With more than 100 pairs of great egrets, great blue herons, and snowy egrets nesting in a perfectly visible tree-top community, Audubon Canyon Ranch is a terrific draw. Add Bolinas Lagoon, a shallow mudflat alive with more than 60 species of birds, and an impressive oak forest, and the allure becomes difficult to resist. Together these two landmarks form the 1000-acre Bolinas Lagoon Preserve.

In the preserve, three small canyons cut down to the edge of a large, shallow mudflat and protect a rich array of life regenerating from past human influences. Logged to build 19th-century San Francisco and once used for dairy ranching, the landscape is recovering well. More than 90 species of birds can be sighted here, amphibians crawl its moist creek-beds, and steelhead trout once again swim its streams. The herons and egrets arrive by March, choose mates after elaborate courtship rituals, and then raise their young for 12 weeks in the heronry.

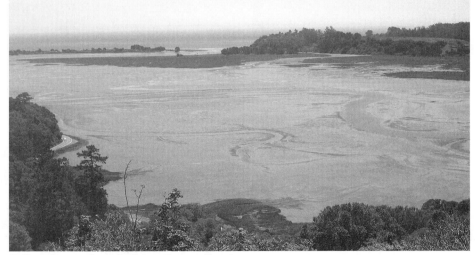

Bolinas Lagoon from Audubon Canyon Ranch

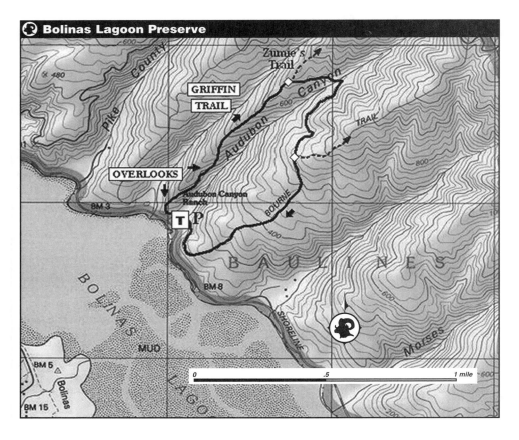

Located in the upper canopy of a few redwood trees in lower Picher Canyon, the
site provides shelter and ready access to
the fish and crustaceans found in Bolinas
Lagoon. From mid-June through mid-July
volunteers keep careful track of the nesting pairs, follow the development of the
chicks, and then watch the entire community gradually disperse.

The Hike is a circuit around Picher Canyon on Griffin Trail, passing the overlooks
of Bolinas Lagoon and the heronry early
on. Telescopes are provided and friendly
docents enrich the experience, making this
one of the best sites in California to learn
about birds. The preserve is only open to
the public from mid-March until mid-July
on Saturdays, Sundays, and holidays from
10 AM until 4 PM (open Tuesday–Friday by
appointment). While April and May are

the most eventful months in the heronry,
a powerful telephoto lens is necessary to
capture the scene on film. Crowds tend to
concentrate at the overlooks, leaving the
trails surprisingly empty. Water is available at the trailhead.

To Reach the Trailhead: Drive 3 miles
north of Stinson Beach on Hwy. 1—the
posted turnoff has an open sign hanging
if you've come at the right time. Volunteers usually greet you and tell you where
to park. While there is no entrance fee,
donations are strongly encouraged and
help support Audubon Canyon Ranch, a
private nonprofit managing this and two
other nature preserves in Marin and Sonoma counties.

Reaching the trailhead by public transportation is challenging but possible. West
Marin Stagecoach Bus 62 goes to Audubon

Canyon Ranch daily, leaving Marin City in the morning and returning midafternoon. Call (415) 526-3239 for current schedule information or visit www.marintransit.org.

Description: Pick up a free map of the preserve from the visitors center before walking briefly back down the entrance road to the start of Griffin Trail (0.0/10′). The wide trail immediately starts climbing through California buckeye, live oak, and California bay to reach the first overlook. Depending on tides, Bolinas Lagoon may be filled with shallow water or exposed as fractal-patterned mudflats. Birdlife is always abundant, and the preserve's interpretive panels and telescopes are lots of fun.

Past the lagoon overlook, the trail forks—bear right toward the next overlook. Climbing through dense foliage, you soon reach another fork—bear right again and climb the short spur to Henderson Overlook (0.3/200′). Note the sign: QUIET—BIRDS NESTING. White splotches in the green canopy, enlarged and defined by powerful telescopes here, compose the heronry below you to the east. Learn all you can of these beautiful birds before returning to the main trail.

Back on Griffin Trail, you ascend the ridge. Look for redwood trees providing excellent examples of basal sprouting. Once cut, a redwood tree immediately sprouts a series of saplings from its root system, forming a roughly concentric circle around the stump known as a "fairy ring." Some rings here include more than a dozen trees. Where Zumie's Loop splits left at the junction near the top (0.8/720′), keep right on the Griffin Trail. After cresting out, the trail swings right and crosses the lush creek gully; then it continues on a level traverse through a dense alder thicket. The path gradually descends through a thick forest of redwood and Douglas fir to an open ridgetop before beginning its steep descent to the trailhead.

Views of Stinson Beach, Bolinas Lagoon, and Olema Valley open up as you descend. The San Andreas Fault underlies these landmarks, and fault movement in the Olema Valley during the 1906 earthquake was more than 12 feet in places. One earth fissure reportedly swallowed an entire cow—except for the legs left protruding upward from the ground! The trail descends the ridgeline steeply to the visitors center, passing beneath some very impressive coast live oaks at the end.

Nearest Visitors Center: Audubon Canyon Ranch visitors center and bookstore, (415) 868-9244, located among the old ranch buildings, is open when the preserve is open.

Nearest Campground: Privately owned Olema Ranch Campground (200 sites, $30–35) is located in Olema on Hwy. 1. Also try the campground in Samuel P. Taylor State Park (60 sites, $20–25, depending on season), located 6 miles east of Hwy. 1 on Sir Francis Drake Blvd. Reservations are recommended for Samuel P. Taylor April through October; call (800) 444-7275 or visit www.reserveamerica.com. Also try Pantoll Campground, located by Pantoll Ranger Station, in Mt. Tamalpais State Park; it has 16 first-come, first-served sites that require a short 100-yard walk-in and usually fill by late afternoon ($15).

Additional Information: www.egret.org

HIKE 34

Alamere Falls

Sea Spray

Highlights	Mind-bending geology, ocean vistas, and a beachside waterfall
Distance	8.5 miles round-trip
Total Elevation Gain/Loss	900´/900´
Hiking Time	5–7 hours
Optional Maps	USGS 7.5-min. *Bolinas* and *Double Point, Point Reyes National Seashore and West Marin Parklands* by Wilderness Press
Best Times	September through May
Agency	Point Reyes National Seashore
Difficulty	★★

Alamere Falls is an accessible yet re-mote destination, where a small stream tumbles directly over coastal bluffs onto a sandy beach. The oceanside cliffs, Double Point view, and inviting freshwater lakes along the trail are all expressions of the unique geology of southern Point Reyes National Seashore.

The Hike follows the Coast Trail from Palomarin Trailhead to Alamere Falls, a fairly long dayhike that can be extended to an overnight trip by continuing 1.5 miles past Alamere Falls to Wildcat Camp. Fog is common in the summer months and should be avoided. Swimming and fish-ing are possible in freshwater Bass Lake halfway to the falls, but ocean frolicking is not recommended due to the strong rip currents, undertow, and frigid water. This is not an isolated hike, especially on the weekends, and you can expect to see other people on the trail and at the waterfall. Poison oak, stinging nettle, and ticks are common hazards in the brush. No water is available at the trailhead and there are no reliable sources before Alamere Falls.

To Reach the Trailhead: Take Hwy. 1 north from Stinson Beach for 4.4 miles to the northern edge of Bolinas Lagoon and turn left onto Olema-Bolinas Rd. The turn-

off is not posted so keep your eye out. In 1.3 miles the road reaches a T-junction—go left, continuing on Olema-Bolinas Rd. for another 0.6 mile before turning right again on Mesa Rd. Follow Mesa Rd. 5 miles to the parking lot at the road's end, passing a Coast Guard radar station and the Point Reyes Bird Observatory along the way. The last 1.5 miles are unpaved.

Description: From the trailhead (0.0/280´), the wide path immediately enters a thick eucalyptus grove where wild cucumber vines twine and a few enormous trees dominate—one huge Hy-dralike specimen is by far the largest euca-lyptus on any hike described in this book. Good views south open up next as the trail winds along open blufftops, and the Farallon Islands are visible southwest on

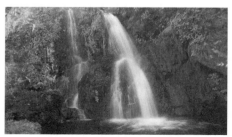

Upper Alamere Falls

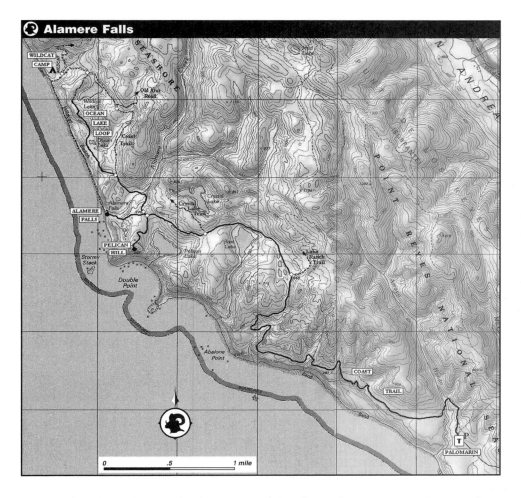

Alamere Falls

a clear day. The trail turns inland, crossing two small creek gullies choked with brush, horsetail, watercress, monkeyflower, and ferns before resuming ocean views. At the third significant creek gully, the trail continues inland, climbing over a small divide to the Lake Ranch Trail (2.2/570´) junction. Continuing ahead on the Coast Trail, you meander through a dense forest of Douglas fir, the conifer common throughout this hike. The trail passes several swampy ponds full of lily pads before Bass Lake comes into view. Gradually descending along its northern shore, the path leads to a short spur trail and an open space excellent for a break on hot days. Beyond the

lake, the trail soon passes a junction for unexciting Crystal Lake before traversing above beautiful Pelican Lake. Point Reyes and the long curving arc of beach and coastal bluffs appear north.

Descending, you reach a spur junction on your left (4.0/290´) immediately after views north are hidden by coastal bluffs. This small trail leads 0.3 mile to the top of Pelican Hill (380´) and the north end of Double Point, a spectacular, recommended side trip. Besides far-reaching views south and north from the summit, the inaccessible cove beach below is often filled with hundreds of hauled-out seals. This is also a good vantage point to contemplate the geologic forces that created this landscape.

The rock of this area is called the Monterey shale, a sequence of sedimentary layers up to 8000 feet thick that were deposited on top of the granite bedrock of Point Reyes National Seashore over the past 20 million years. In the region around Double Point, this shale has become involved in a huge landslide nearly 4 miles long and at least a mile wide. As this huge block of land slips slowly toward the sea, as explained by Alan Galloway in *Geology of the Point Reyes Peninsula*, depressions are formed that fill with freshwater lakes such as Pelican and Bass lakes.

Immediately past the junction for Pelican Hill, another unposted spur trail splits left. This overgrown and brushy path leads down to Alamere Falls, unseen until the very end, where some scrambling is required to reach the stream and its series of cascades. Some more challenging scrambling will take you down to the beach via a rocky chute. The bluffs are impressive, and the tilted, exposed layers of Monterey shale are spectacular south of the falls.

From here, it is possible to hike 1.3 miles north along the sands of Wildcat Beach to Wildcat Camp. Note, however, that sections of the beach can be impassable during high tides and heavy surf, and that there is *no exit* from the beach between the falls and camp. The narrow beach section immediately north of the falls is a good indication of the route's feasibility—if waves are reaching the cliff base, do not proceed.

To continue inland, return to Coast Trail and head north into the watershed of Alamere Creek. Contouring around the creek, Coast Trail next reaches the junction with Ocean Lake Loop (4.2/240´). While both trails lead equidistantly to camp, bear left on more scenic Ocean Lake Loop Trail (perhaps returning on Coast Trail for variety).

The single-track trail drops gently to bank around marshy Ocean Lake and then climbs abruptly to a bench with great views

of Wildcat Beach. You next descend past brush-lined Wildcat Lake and reach Coast Trail joining from the right (5.3/220´). Bear left to quickly reach the blufftop views from Wildcat Camp (5.5/70´).

Nearest Visitors Center: Bear Valley Visitors Center, (415) 464-5100, located on Bear Valley Rd. just west of Olema, 8 miles north of the turnoff for the Olema-Bolinas Rd., is open 9 AM–5 PM weekdays and 8 AM–5 PM weekends and holidays.

Backpacking Information: Backcountry camping at Wildcat Camp is by permit only. Seven sites are available, including three group sites. Reservations are essential and can be made up to three months in advance by calling (415) 663-8054 between 9 AM and 2 PM Monday through Friday. Call as early as possible for weekend reservations. Permits cost $15–$40 per night, depending on group size, and must be picked up at the Bear Valley Visitors Center prior to leaving on your trip. After-hours pickup is allowed—permits are placed in a wooden box by the information board in front of the visitors center. If sites are available, walk-in registration is possible for same-day departures. Wood fires are prohibited.

Nearest Campground: There are no drive-in campgrounds within Point Reyes National Seashore. The closest campgrounds are Pantoll Campground in Mt. Tamalpais State Park, located by Pantoll Ranger Station (16 first-come, first-served sites that require a short 100-yard walk-in and usually fill by late afternoon, $15), and privately owned Olema Ranch Campground (200 sites, $30–35), located in Olema on Hwy. 1.

Additional Information: www.nps.gov/pore

HIKE 35

Sky and Coast Trails

Sky High and Ocean Bound

Highlights	Old-growth ridgeline and wave-swept coastline
Distance	10.8 miles
Total Elevation Gain/Loss	1800′/1800′
Hiking Time	5–7 hours
Optional Maps	Tom Harrison's *Point Reyes National Seashore*, USGS 7.5-min. *Double Point, Point Reyes National Seashore and West Marin Parklands* by Wilderness Press
Best Times	September through May
Agency	Point Reyes National Seashore
Difficulty	★★★

This loop hike explores the full spectrum of Point Reyes National Seashore, from the lush forest atop its highest ridges to the sculpted promontories above its salty shore. Along the way, you'll tag the peninsula's tallest point, stand atop a wave-tunneled bluff, and savor abundant views of the cerulean sea.

The Hike directly ascends 1407-foot Mt. Wittenberg from Bear Valley Visitors Center and then descends Sky Trail to the ocean, winding through verdant mixed-evergreen forest and past open viewpoints en route to the coast. The journey then heads south on Coast Trail to striking Arch Rock, returning inland beneath the majestic trees of Bear Valley Trail.

To Reach the Trailhead: Take Hwy. 1 to Olema and head west on Bear Valley Rd.; the turnoff is located immediately north of the intersection of Hwy. 1 and Sir Francis Drake Blvd. In 0.5 mile, turn left to reach the Bear Valley Visitors Center and trailhead parking.

Public transportation is available Monday through Saturday on West Marin Stagecoach Route 68, which makes 4–5 runs daily to Inverness from San Rafael, stopping at Bear Valley Visitors Center along the way (call 415-499-6099 or visit www.marintransit.org).

Description: From the trailhead (0.0/80′), follow Bear Valley Trail past Rift Zone and Woodpecker trails to reach Mt. Wittenberg Trail by a stand of coast live oaks and a massive bay tree (0.2/80′). Bear right and ascend Mt. Wittenberg Trail beneath the arcing branches of fragrant bay trees. The shady woodlands slowly

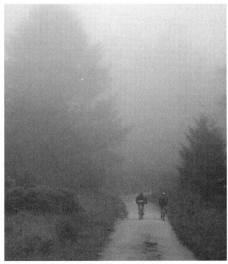

A foggy day on Sky Trail

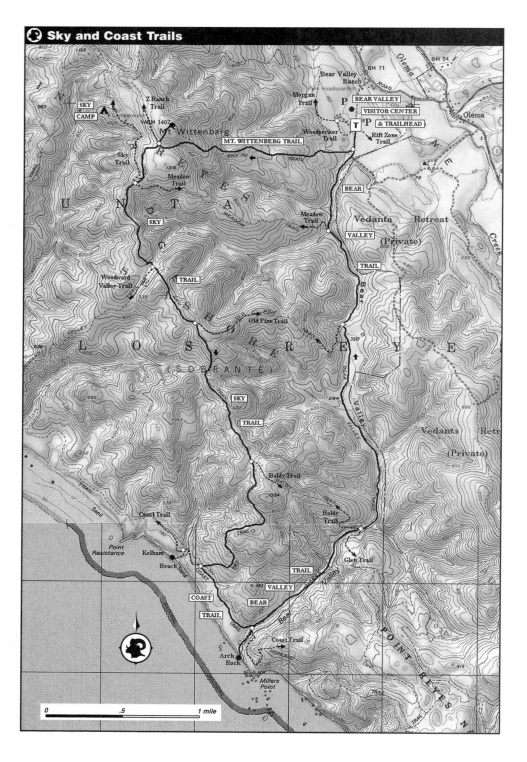

Sky and Coast Trails

transition into a mixed-evergreen forest of Douglas fir, hazel bushes, sword ferns, interspersed with the occasional buckeye and tanoak tree.

The trail rises steadily, passing intermittent glimpses of Bolinas Ridge across Olema Valley. You eventually reach a clearing ringed by coast live oaks and dotted with coyote brush—you are now halfway up the hill. The trail narrows, climbs three steep switchbacks, and levels briefly to contour around a small drainage. Upon cresting Inverness Ridge, you are rewarded with northwest views toward Limantour Beach, Drakes Estero, and Point Reyes itself. Z Ranch Trail and the spur to Wittenberg's summit lie just ahead (2.0/1260′).

This spot marks the boundary of the 1995 Vision Fire, a human-caused conflagration that scorched 12,000 acres of the seashore. Its effects can be seen in the regular size and age of the young, regenerating Douglas firs in the area, as well as the burned trunks of nearby fire survivors. From here it's a short 0.4 mile round-trip to the top of Mt. Wittenberg (1407′), the highest point in Point Reyes National Seashore. The summit is ringed by young Douglas firs but a few tantalizing glimpses peek south to Olema Valley and beyond to the long spine of Mt. Tamalpais.

Continue on Mt. Wittenberg Trail as it curves down past a shrubby undergrowth of yerba santa and bracken fern and reaches the junction with Sky and Meadow trails (2.4/1120). Sky Camp is 0.6 mile away to the north but your continuing journey heads left, following Sky Trail into the woods. Douglas firs tower overhead and strain moisture from the fog, keeping the environment green year-round. Moss-bearded branches and tree-bound ferns droop above abundant elderberry, huckleberry, blackberry tangles, and sword ferns. In September, the huckleberry bushes dangle with abundant—and deliciously edible—blue-black berries.

Sky Trail passes Woodward Valley Trail on the right (3.1/890′), climbs briefly to pass Old Pine Trail on the left (3.4/1020′), and then gently descends. The surrounding environment transitions to low-lying coastal scrub as you crest a small rise

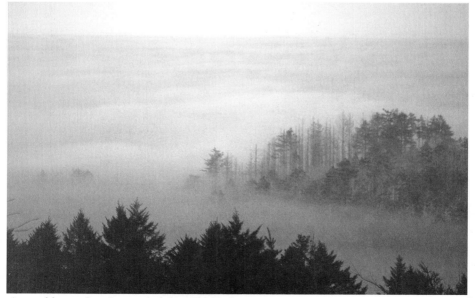

A sea of fog washes the terrain below Sky Trail.

and reach the junction with Baldy Trail (4.8/870′). Continue your descent on Sky Trail toward the increasingly visible ocean. The route passes a few burnt snags—more remnants of the Vision Fire—and makes a final drop via two switchbacks to reach Coast Trail (6.3/130′).

A right turn leads in 0.2 mile to an enormous eucalyptus by the access point for Kelham Beach, a remote strand of cliffs and sandy solitude. The continuing hike heads left (south) on wide Coast Trail, which quickly leads to Bear Valley Trail and the nearby promontory of Arch Rock (6.8/110′). Take the time to visit the open blufftop of Arch Rock and its excellent views, which stretch north along adjacent Kelham Beach to Point Resistance and beyond. On the south side of Arch Rock, a well-worn but precarious path descends into the mini-gorge of Coast Creek. At low tide, you can walk north through the arch to access Kelham Beach. To the south, a small pocket beach stretches a short distance to Millers Point.

You now leave the ocean behind and head inland on wide and well-traveled Bear Valley Trail, which quickly returns to thick woods alongside alder-choked Coast Creek. The curving branches of massive bay trees shade your journey past Glen and Baldy trails (7.7/180′) and onward to Divide Meadow (9.2/320′). Ringed by coast live oaks, the meadow sits on the divide between the Olema Valley and Coast Creek watersheds and is the only low-elevation gap through Inverness Ridge. A hunting lodge owned by the Pacific Union Hunting Club of San Francisco once sat in the northwest corner; it served as a backcountry base for pursuing bears and mountain lions from the 1890s until the Great Depression. The lodge has long since been removed; two huge introduced Monterey pines and a few patches of exotic pink flowers are all that remain.

Continuing on Bear Valley Trail, you enter one of the seashore's most majestic forests. California bay, alders, and tanoak thrive. Mighty Douglas firs rise

above, each unique in form and character. On your way out, you pass Meadow Trail (10.0/150′) and Mt. Wittenberg Trail just before returning to the trailhead (10.8/80′).

Nearest Visitors Center: Bear Valley Visitors Center, (415) 464-5100 is located on Bear Valley Rd. just west of Olema and open 9 AM–5 PM weekdays, 8 AM–5 PM weekends and holidays.

Backpacking Information: Backcountry camping at Sky Camp is by permit only. Twelve sites are available, including one group site. Reservations are essential and can be made up to three months in advance by calling (415) 663-8054 between 9 AM and 2 PM, Monday through Friday. Call as early as possible for weekend reservations. Permits cost $15–$40 per night, depending on group size, and must be picked up at the Bear Valley Visitors Center prior to leaving on your trip. After-hours pickup is allowed—permits are placed in a wooden box by the information board in front of the visitors center. If sites are available, walk-in registration is possible for same-day departures. Wood fires are prohibited.

Nearest Campground: There are no drive-in campgrounds within Point Reyes National Seashore. The closest campgrounds are Pantoll Campground in Mt. Tamalpais State Park, located by Pantoll Ranger Station (16 first-come, first-served sites that require a short 100-yard walk-in and usually fill by late afternoon), and privately owned Olema Ranch Campground (200 sites, $30–35), located in Olema on Hwy. 1.

Additional Information: www.nps.gov/pore

HIKE 36

Tomales Point

Cold Tomales

Highlights	A herd of tule elk and prairie blufftops above pounding surf
Distance	9.0 miles round-trip
Total Elevation Gain/Loss	1300'/1300'
Hiking Time	4–5 hours
Optional Maps	USGS 7.5-min. *Tomales, Point Reyes National Seashore and West Marin Parklands* by Wilderness Press
Best Times	September through May
Agency	Point Reyes National Seashore
Difficulty	★★★

Here is a hike of sweeping coastal views along an elevated, granite peninsula, covered by an open grassland famous for its wildflowers and tule elk. The Point Reyes Peninsula is a migrant piece of land. Its deepest bedrock is granite, formed in southern California approximately 100 million years ago.

When the San Andreas Fault became active 28 million years ago, pieces of North America located west of the emergent fault began slowly migrating north at a rate of 2–3 centimeters per year, traveling hundreds of miles over the ensuing millenia. The granite of Point Reyes Peninsula was one of these pieces, and became covered by thick, waterborne sediments while submerged beneath the sea for almost 10 million years on its journey north. Roughly 4

million years ago, a slight change in the geometry of the San Andreas Fault system increased compression between the rocks on either side of the fault, pushing Point Reyes Peninsula—and most of the Coast Ranges—above sea level. Erosion then began stripping away the overlying sediment, once again exposing the erosion-resistant granite on today's Inverness Ridge and the bluffs of Point Reyes itself. Today, Tomales Point is a solid piece of granite battered by the seas into sheer cliffs of solid rock, a striking contrast to the loose slopes found most places on the California coast.

The Hike goes to land's end at Tomales Point from historic Pierce Point Ranch, a chilly trip that is almost always rainy, windy, foggy, or some combination of the three. The trail is entirely exposed

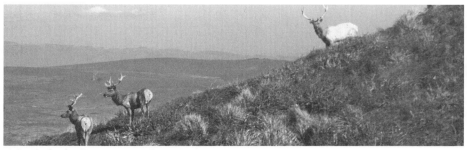

A herd of tule elk roams Tomales Point.

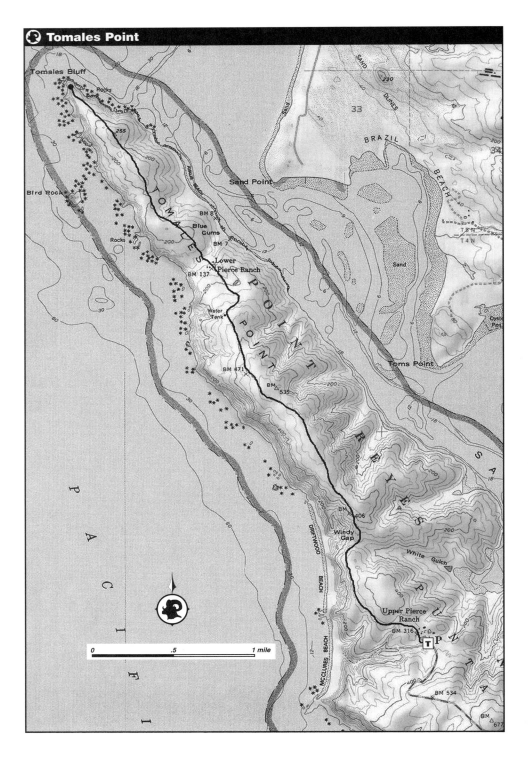

Tomales Point

Tomales Bluff

Rocks

Sand Point

Bird Rock

255

BM 8

Blue Gums

BM 7

Lower Pierce Ranch

BM 137

Rocks

Water Tank

BM 471

BM 535

T O M A L E S   P O I N T

BRAZIL BEACH

SAND DUNES

230

33

34

T5N T4N

Sand

Toms Point

Oyster

R E Y E S

BM 406

Windy Gap

White Gulch

Upper Pierce Ranch

BM 316

T   P

P   A   C   I   F   I   C

DRIFTWOOD BEACH

McCLURES BEACH

400

BM 534

BM 677

0   .5   1 mile

and offers no shelter from the elements, making a good sweater and windbreaker crucial year-round items. Fog is consistent during the summer months, obscuring views and making a visit at some other time more desirable. While you will almost surely see other people, crowds are generally light. No water is available at the trailhead or anywhere en route.

To Reach the Trailhead: Take Sir Francis Drake Blvd. west from Point Reyes Station on Hwy. 1 for 6.7 miles to the turnoff for Pierce Point Rd. Bear right on Pierce Point Rd. where Sir Francis Drake Blvd. curves left, and proceed 9 miles to the parking lot by the white buildings of historic Pierce Point Ranch.

Description: The trail begins from the west side of the parking lot by an informative sign, and for most of its length the hike follows an old lane—now a broad and friendly path—to the former site of lower Pierce Point Ranch. Passing between the still operational buildings of upper Pierce Point Ranch and a linear windbreak of Monterey cypress, the wide trail shortly breaks out into open fields of bush lupine and coyote brush where wild cucumber wraps its tendrils through the brush. Raptors—especially red-tailed hawks—are a common sight as they soar over the open fields, hunting for small prey. As you continue on the undulating route, keep an eye out for the herd of tule elk that wanders these bluffs, reintroduced in 1978 by the National Park Service. Numbering in the hundreds, these impressive creatures are a memorable and photogenic sight.

To the east the San Andreas Fault underlies Tomales Bay, a trough formed when the rocks along the fault were ground into easily eroded sediment. The fault continues northwest toward Bodega Head (Hike 37), the small peninsula immediately north of Tomales Point. Similar to Point Reyes Peninsula, Bodega Head is another piece of granite covered by sediment, separated from the mainland by the San Andreas Fault, and slowly moving northwest. Northeast, the highest peak

visible is Mt. St. Helena (Hike 38). Looking south, the long sandy stretch of Point Reyes Beach terminates at rocky Point Reyes itself.

A long undulating traverse more than 300 feet above the breaking waves eventually leads to a steady descent that ends in a grove of trees, the former site of lower Pierce Point Ranch. From here, the trail gets sandier and less distinct as it passes through fields thick with irises, climbing first before dropping down to the precipitous granite cliffs of Tomales Point itself. Bird Rock, located just offshore to the west, is a rookery for numerous seabirds and a major pupping area for harbor seals. Great white sharks are commonly sighted in the waters around Tomales Point and have attacked divers in the past. You can get close, but the ocean remains out of reach less than 30 feet below. Be respectful of the dangerous cliffs as you explore the point. Return the way you came.

Nearest Visitors Center: Bear Valley Visitors Center, (415) 464-5100, is located on Bear Valley Rd. just west of Olema and open 9 AM–5 PM weekdays, 8 AM–5 PM weekends and holidays.

Nearest Campground: There are no drive-in campgrounds within Point Reyes National Seashore. The closest campground is privately owned Olema Ranch Campground (200 sites, $30–35), located in Olema on Hwy. 1. Also try the campground in Samuel P. Taylor State Park (60 sites, $20–25, depending on season), located 6 miles east of Hwy. 1 on Sir Francis Drake Blvd. Reservations are recommended for Samuel P. Taylor April through October; call (800) 444-7275 or visit www.reserveamerica.com.

Additional Information: www.nps.gov/pore

HIKE 37

Bodega Dunes

Barefoot in the Sand

Highlights	Dune fields and barefoot beach hiking
Distance	2.2 miles
Total Elevation Gain/Loss	50´/50´
Hiking Time	1–2 hours
Optional Map	USGS 7.5-min. *Bodega Head*
Best Times	Year-round
Agency	Sonoma Coast State Beach
Difficulty	★

A chunk of granite spearheading the tectonic migration northwest, Bodega Head is backed by massive sand dunes and the longest beach on the Sonoma County coast. The fun of hiking barefoot is enhanced by distant views north up the rugged coastline.

The Hike explores the world of Bodega Dunes and the geology of Mussel Point before returning along Salmon Creek Beach. The entire hike is on loose sand that makes walking arduous but shoes unnecessary. Fog is common during the summer months, eliminating views and chilling the air. Fall offers the most consistent weather, winter the clearest views (between storms), and spring a profusion of flowering bush lupine. Crowds are heaviest in the summer months, dwindling to only the local surfers in the winter. Monarch butterflies overwinter in the park campground, making December and January an exciting time to visit. No water is available at the trailhead.

To Reach the Trailhead: Take Hwy. 1 north from the town of Bodega Bay for 6.5 miles—the posted turnoff is on the west side of the highway. Approaching from the north, the turnoff is 9 miles south of the junction of Hwys. 1 and 116. Past the entrance station, turn right on Beach Rd. and follow it to the substantial parking lot

and picnic area at the road's end. There is a day-use fee of $6.

Description: The trail begins at the gate by the parking lot entrance and immediately enters dune world. As is evident from the beginning, paths crisscross the dunes throughout this hike. The actual trail is generally obvious and parallels the beach behind the front line of dunes—please try to stay on this main trail in order to prevent erosion of the fragile environment.

The trail initially parallels a line of scrubby Monterey cypress and conspicuous flecks of white are everywhere in the sand around them. These are shell fragments, part of a midden used by the native inhabitants of the area prior to European settlement. Regularly harvesting shellfish from the ocean for food, the Coast Miwok would deposit the accumulated shell de-

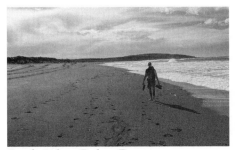

Barefoot along Bodega Dunes

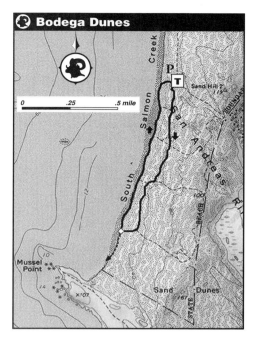

cess point is located at the posted junction for Westshore Regional Park—bear right toward the ocean.

Once on the broad beach, views of the coastline north open up dramatically. Between you and the north end of Salmon Creek Beach, the San Andreas Fault slices underground and travels just offshore before briefly touching land again 15 miles north near Fort Ross. A keen eye can pick out Goat Rock and the mouth of the Russian River 9 miles up the coast.

Continue south along the beach to its terminus at Mussel Point, which is also the northern end of Bodega Head. A surprising outcrop of granite is exposed beneath a thin layer of sandstone here. Bodega Head is the northernmost exposure of the Salinian Block, a large piece of granite bedrock torn from Southern California and thrust northwest by actions of the San Andreas Fault. Significant in size, the Salinian Block stretches from here out to the Farallon Islands and south down the entire California coast, but its granite heart is exposed in few places. At the north edge of the Salinian Block, the rocks at Mussel Point are the northernmost outcrop of granite on the California coast. Return along the beach, enjoying the views north, and reach the parking lot via the obvious wooden platform and walkway.

bris in large piles, an ancient "trash can," they also filled with discarded bones, artifacts, and tools. Built up over hundreds of years, they are now covered by drifting sand, the scattered fragments on the surface their only indication.

As you continue through the dune fields, you are gradually surrounded by a world of sand, bush lupine, and beach grass. The larger dunes here approach 150 feet in elevation, somewhat stabilized by the European beach grass planted after cattle grazing had dangerously denuded existing native vegetation. Foxes, weasels, and black-tailed deer roam the dunes. Northern harriers and red-tailed hawks scan the ground below for the mice, voles, and jackrabbits that scurry through the undergrowth.

Although several trails split left back to the campground, continue to parallel the hidden beach at all junctions. Posted Jackrabbit and Scrub Jay spur trails on your right head to the beach, providing quicker access for those unexcited about continuing through the dunes. The last beach ac-

Nearest Visitors Center: There are no visitors centers in the park. Call (707) 875-3483 for general information. Try park headquarters, located 0.7 mile north of the park turnoff on Hwy. 1. Also try the visitors center along Hwy. 1 in Jenner, which is open 10 AM–4 PM on weekends.

Nearest Campground: Bodega Dunes Campground (97 sites, $25) is located by the park entrance. Monarch butterflies congregate in the upper loop during December and January.

HIKE 38

Table Rock

Ride the Rhino

Highlights	Distant views and dead-drop cliffs
Distance	4.4 miles round-trip
Total Elevation Gain/Loss	1400´/1400´
Hiking Time	3 hours
Optional Map	USGS 7.5-min. *Detert Reservoir*
Best Times	Year-round
Agency	Robert Louis Stevenson State Park
Difficulty	★★★

Overlooking Calistoga Valley, beneath dominant Mt. St. Helena, on the lip of sheer volcanic cliffs, the view from Table Rock is something to remember.

The Hike travels to Table Rock, an unusual volcanic formation within a delightful pocket of hidden wilderness. Much of the hike is exposed, making sun protection imperative most of the year. Because the cliff edge is unprotected and a fall would be fatal, this is not a good location for children. Robert Louis Stevenson State Park is little known and has few amenities. No water is available at the trailhead.

To Reach the Trailhead: Take sinuous Hwy. 29 north from Calistoga for nearly 8 miles to the divide below Mt. St. Helena. Park in the lot east of the road exactly at the divide. Approaching from the north, take Hwy. 29 south from the junction of Hwys. 29 and 53 in Lower Lake for 26 miles to the divide.

Description: From the posted trailhead (0.0/2300´) the trail gently climbs among Douglas fir, tanoak, madrone, ponderosa pine, California bay, and black oak, while you get increasingly better views of Mt. St. Helena (4343´). In the summer of 1880, author Robert Louis Stevenson spent a month-long, cash-strapped honeymoon squatting in an old cabin on the slopes of Mt. St. Helena, penciling notes later in-

corporated into his novels. *The Silverado Squatters* and *Treasure Island* both include descriptions of the surrounding landscape.

As the trail winds briefly along northern slopes, views north down Collayomi Valley appear and Snow Mountain (7056´) can be seen capping the skyline beyond the valley's end. You'll see wispy gray

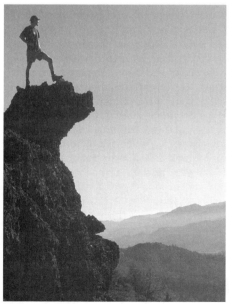

Riding the Rhino

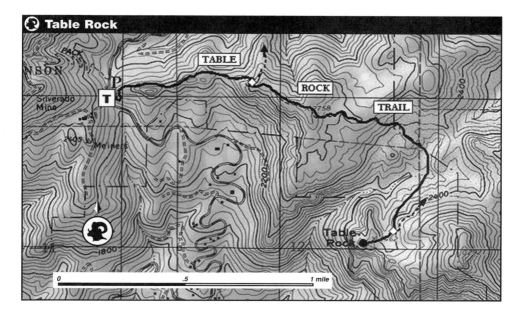

pines and get ever more distant views beyond Mt. St. Helena as the trail traverses back around to the southern exposure.

After a very brief climb, the trail reaches a junction (0.7/2550′)—go right toward Table Rock. As the trail begins to descend, tantalizing views south transform into sweeping panoramas at Devils Sofa, an exposure of large, rounded, volcanic boulders. Napa Valley's rich tapestry trends southeast toward the distant massif of Mt. Diablo (Hike 15). Looking east on a clear day, the Sierra Nevada can be seen beyond linear Blue Ridge. West, the sea is just beyond the farthest visible hills.

From here, the trail descends among thick chaparral before climbing to regain the open slopes and reach the posted junction (2.0/2350′) for nearby Table Rock, a short 0.2 mile away. Fantastical formations will delight you as you walk toward the cliff edge. Look for the Rhino (shown on the front cover). Thrill to a hair-raising view down a vertical cliff face. Contemplate the geology as you savor the view.

Over the past 28 million years, the ever-shifting geometry between the Pacific and North American tectonic plates has created a vast system of faults, associated with the greater San Andreas Fault system. These faults have ripped apart this region and formed the distinctive linear valleys and ridges visible here. Between 13 and 2.7 million years ago, some large fissures created by this activity allowed liquid magma to rise to the surface and spill across the landscape, covering it with thick layers of volcanic rock. Over time, erosion weathered the hardened basalt to form the sheer cliffs below you. Return the way you came.

Nearest Visitors Center: This park doesn't have a visitors center. For general information, call Bothe-Napa Valley State Park at (707) 942-4575.

Nearest Campground: Bothe-Napa Valley State Park Campground (50 sites, $20–25, depending on season) is located 5 miles north of St. Helena on Hwy. 29. For reservations, which are recommended in summer, call (800) 444-7275.

HIKE 39

East Austin Creek

Austin Powers

Highlights	The remote valleys of the northern Coast Range
Distance	9.1 miles
Total Elevation Gain/Loss	1150'/1150'
Hiking Time	5–7 hours
Optional Maps	*Austin Creek State Recreation Area Map,* USGS 7.5-min. *Cazadero*
Best Times	Year-round
Agency	Austin Creek State Recreation Area
Difficulty	★★★

A hidden, wild world lurks in the rumpled Coast Range just north of the Russian River. Closely packed ridges rise more than 1000 feet above narrow canyons barely 200 feet above sea level. The nearby San Andreas Fault has shaped the area, squeezing it upward, riddling it with smaller faults. Heavy rainfall then dissects the terrain, eroding the folded landscape into today's convoluted topography.

Within this tortured geography, Austin Creek State Recreation Area straddles an ecological divide between lush coastal redwood forest and drier oak woodland. Only 10 miles from the ocean, yet guarded from summer fog by several intervening ridges, the area receives significant precipitation in the winter months (more than 50 inches) yet bakes during the summer in temperatures that can approach 100°F. The results are perennial streams in lush canyons, open grasslands of twisting oaks and spring wildflowers, chaparral-cloaked southern slopes, and surprising pockets of redwood forest.

The Hike descends steeply from ridgeline to lush valley bottom, visits four mellifluous streams, and tours a wide diversity of ecosystems. This is a year-round destination. Even during the heat of summer, the park's deep valleys pro-

vide shelter from the intense sun. Winter and fall are nice, but spring is the optimal time for a visit, when wildflowers carpet the hillsides, crowds are light, and the weather is pleasant. Note that you must ford unbridged East Austin Creek at the hike's midpoint, a potential challenge during rainy spells. Water is available near the trailhead in adjacent Bullfrog Pond Campground.

To Reach the Trailhead: Take Hwy. 116 or River Rd. west from Hwy. 101 to Guerneville and turn north on Armstrong Woods Rd.; the turnoff is located 0.1 mile west of the Russian River Bridge. In 2.5 miles you reach the Armstrong Redwoods State Natural Reserve entrance and visitors center. A thrilling 2.5 miles later you reach the East Austin Creek Trailhead and parking area at Vista Point. This final 2.5 miles of road is narrow and twisting, with several steep sections (12 percent grade) and multiple 5 mile-per-hour hairpin turns. Vehicles longer than 20 feet are not permitted.

Description: From the trailhead (0.0/1400'), savor the sweeping view across the rolling terrain. Note the varied ecosystems that thrive here. Coyote brush, manzanita, and several species of oak (coast, Oregon, and black) grow on the

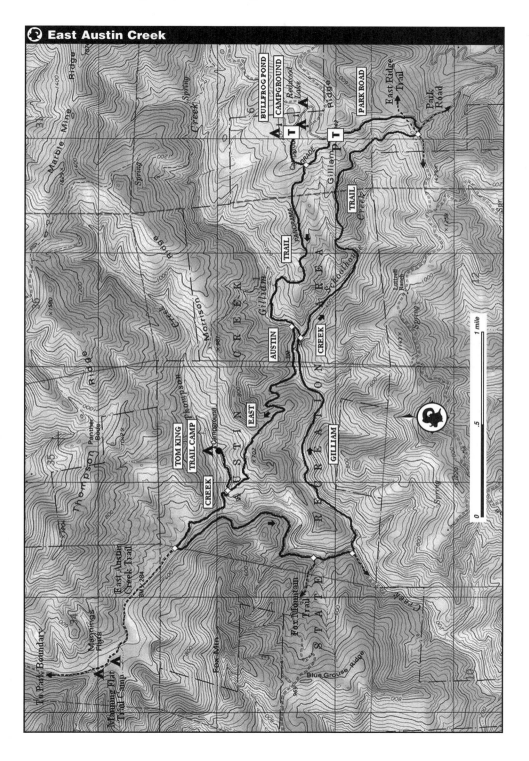

East Austin Creek

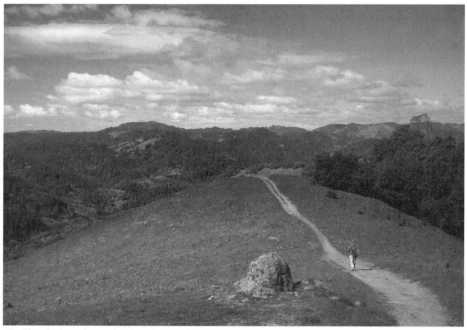

Trailhead view above the Austin Creek watershed

drier, sun-exposed west-facing slopes; bay trees, willow, buckeye, and poison oak are nourished by the moist shelter of nearby gullies; and water-loving Douglas fir and redwoods flourish on shady north and east-facing slopes. Descending on East Austin Creek Trail, you soon pass a spur trail on the right (0.2/1150´) joining from lower Bullfrog Pond Campground. The slopes are flush with seasonal wildflowers. Baby blue eyes, shooting stars, and brodiaea are particularly abundant on the descent. Also look for evidence of wild pigs; they regularly root up the hillside in search of edible roots.

Near the canyon bottom, the trail curves right and descends into a thickening mixed-evergreen forest. You briefly travel above crystalline Gilliam Creek, then reach it near a bridge and junction for the short spur trail that leads to nearby Gilliam Creek Trail (1.5/340´). Those fortunate to be here in March may witness orange-bellied newts congregating by the dozens to mate in these waters.

Cross the bridge over Gilliam Creek and continue on wide East Austin Creek Trail as it climbs briefly up a small, unnamed drainage flush with bigleaf maple, peeling madrone, and giant chain ferns (the state's largest fern). You then emerge above it all on open oak hillsides with exceptional views. The small linear valley of Thompson Creek is visible to the north and the deep drainage of East Austin Creek twists southwest toward the Russian River. The route crests near some coast live oaks (2.5/750´) and descends to the junction with Tom King Trail (2.9/450´). If you're looking for an idyllic picnic spot, turn right here and proceed a gentle 0.3 mile to the camp.

To continue, remain on East Austin Creek Trail as it switchbacks twice and crosses Thompson Creek. Old-growth redwoods appear across the stream as the wide trail parallels East Austin Creek to reach unsigned Gilliam Creek Trail (3.5/190´). Manning Flat Trail Camp lies 0.7 mile ahead, but you turn left to ford unbridged East Austin Creek and follow Gilliam Creek Trail onto shadier east-facing slopes. Climbing briefly, the trail winds well above the rushing stream and its narrow canyon before descending to pass Fox Mountain Trail on the right (4.6/290´).

Bear left at the next junction (4.8/290´) to remain on Gilliam Creek Trail and descend to the confluence of East Austin and Gilliam creeks. Ford East Austin Creek once more to immediately reach the former site of Gilliam Creek Trail Camp, located in a large grassy field near the creek. Beyond camp, the trail winds through a narrow canyon, briefly climbs a short distance above the creek, then drops to cross and recross the creek nine times over the next mile. The stream crossings are not always obvious (only a few are signed) but the trail is apparent; if you find yourself on a disappearing track, retrace your steps. At Schoolhouse Creek you encounter the unposted junction for the short connector to East Austin Creek Trail (6.5/360´) and the most direct route back to the trailhead.

This hike continues straight on Gilliam Creek Trail, which crosses the creek three more times and then climbs steeply along a small feeder creek to an open, oak-studded ridge. Manzanita, toyon, and chamise line the trail as it steadily ascends the ridgeline, levels out, and banks right to traverse the upper Schoolhouse Creek drainage (passing through several nice redwood groves en route). The trail alternately contours gently and ascends steeply to reach the junction with East Ridge Trail and the park road (8.5/1300´). Savor the beautiful vistas one last time as you bear left (north) and hike along the park road to return to the trailhead (9.1/1400´).

Nearest Visitors Center: Armstrong Redwoods Visitors Center, (707) 869-2958, is open 11 AM–3 PM daily, with longer hours in summer. Park entrance station is staffed approximately 8 AM–sunset daily in summer, weekends only in spring and fall, and sporadically in winter. For general information, call (707) 869-2015.

Backpacking Information: Backcountry camping is allowed at Manning Flat (2 sites) and Tom King trail camps (1 site) on a first-come, first-served basis. A permit is required and must be obtained from the entrance station or from an on-duty park ranger. There is a fee of $15 per site. Picnic tables, fire rings, and outhouses are provided; water is available from the adjacent creeks. Campfires are not allowed during fire season (typically late July through October).

Nearest Campground: Bullfrog Pond Campground (23 sites, $15) in adjacent Armstrong reserve. Arrive early on weekends to obtain a site at this first-come, first-served campground.

Additional Information: www.parks.ca.gov

HIKE 40

Cache Creek

Cached

Highlights	Oak woodland, bald eagles, and tule elk
Distance	3.5 miles round-trip
Total Elevation Gain/Loss	1000′/1000′
Hiking Time	3 hours
Optional Map	USGS 7.5-min. *Lower Lake*
Best Times	December through April
Agency	Bureauof Land Management Cache Creek Natural Area
Difficulty	★★

Gnarled oaks twist skyward in a rolling landscape flushed green by winter rains. Cache Creek ripples through placid pools, a herd of tule elk wanders the area, and a population of bald eagles winters here. Come for a taste of the low-lying foothills ringing the Great Central Valley.

The Hike follows Redbud Trail over a low divide to Baton Flat on the banks of Cache Creek and visits the edge of 27,245-acre Cache Creek Wilderness, one of the state's newest wilderness areas (designated October 2006). The hike is open year-round, but summer months are scorching and fall is extremely dry. Winter rains usually begin in December, coinciding with the arrival of the first bald eagles. Cache Creek can be difficult to ford after heavy storms (no bridge is provided) and the Yolo County Conservation District schedules agricultural water releases from Clear Lake during the summer with only 24-hour advance notice—these can also render the creek impassable. A herd of tule elk wanders the area, though it may be deeper in the area than this hike goes. To maximize your chances for sightings, consider an overnight trip farther along Redbud Trail. No water is available at the trailhead.

To Reach the Trailhead: Take Hwy. 20 east from the intersection of Hwys. 53 and 20 near Clear Lake for almost 7 miles. The turnoff is just west of the Cache Creek highway crossing. Approaching from the east on Hwy. 20, the turnoff is 7 miles past the junction with Walker Ridge Rd.

Description: From the lot (0.0/980′), the hike begins along a gravel road, which crosses a meadow to reach a wash gully. Veer right where the trail enters the trees and begin looking for the two types of oak that exist here: valley oak and blue oak. Blue oak is the most drought-resistant oak and can be identified by its smaller (1–3″) leaves that have wavy margins and shallow lobes. Adapting to the intense heat and dry conditions found in California at low elevations, the blue oak reinforces its leaves with cellulose, and drops them entirely in times of severe drought. Found on drier hillsides, they develop a bluish cast in the late summer and fall. Valley oak is deciduous and can be identified by its larger leaves (2–4″) that are deeply lobed. Requiring more water than blue oak, it is found along valley bottoms. Among the oak are gray pines, wispy trees that generate substantial cones.

As you slowly climb above North Fork Cache Creek, keep an eye out for elk tracks and the animals that made them. The sandstone badlands across the river con-

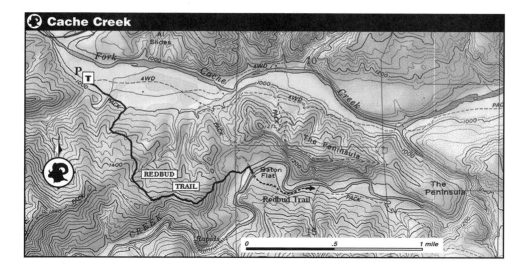

tain sediments deposited over the past 5 million years, when sea-level fluctuations submerged this low-lying region for long periods and coated it with thick layers of sand and mud. More recent tectonic compression has molded it into these rolling foothills. As you crest the ridge (1.0/1450´), the drainage of Cache Creek opens up.

Cache Creek drains Clear Lake, a large body of water formed within the past few thousand years when a large landslide dammed the headwaters of Cold Creek and blocked the westward flow of water into the Russian River drainage. Water impounding behind the new barrier filled the level valleys, creating an enormous lake. It found an outlet east in Cache Creek, draining into the Sacramento River.

As you descend toward Cache Creek, note on the opposite south slope the continued presence of gray pine but the total absence of oak. This is due to the nutrient-poor serpentine soil found there. Oaks are unable to survive in such deficient soils but gray pines continue to thrive.

A gradual, occasionally switchbacking descent brings you to the banks of Cache Creek near a delightful swimming hole at Baton Flat. A few campsites are located on both banks and the creek is fun to explore in both directions. Although this hike ends

here, Redbud Trail continues for another 4.5 miles to isolated Wilson Valley. Return the way you came.

Nearest Visitors Center: There are no visitors centers nearby. The area is managed jointly by the Bureau of Land Management in Ukiah, (707) 468-4000, and the California Department of Fish and Game in Yountville, (707) 944-5500.

Backpacking Information: Backcountry camping is permitted throughout this hike. A campfire permit is required. Cache Creek can be impassable after heavy winter storms since no bridge is provided. Campfires are allowed only in designated sites during certain times of the year, and are prohibited when fire danger becomes extreme. Call the BLM office for current information.

Nearest Campground: There's nothing close. Try Clear Lake State Park (149 sites, $15–20, depending on season) on the lake's south shore near Kelseyville.

Additional Information: www.ca.blm.gov/ukiah

HIKE 41

Gray Lodge Wildlife Area

Great Central Valley

Highlights	Valley wetlands, birdlife galore, and views of Sutter Buttes
Distance	1.0 mile
Total Elevation Gain/Loss	Negligible
Hiking Time	1–2 hours
Optional Map	USGS 7.5-min. *Pennington*
Best Times	Mid-February through late September
Agency	Gray Lodge Wildlife Area
Difficulty	★

California's greatest natural resource, the Great Central Valley produces more than a quarter of the nation's agricultural output. Before settlement, it was a world of extensive wetlands and woodlands that supported grizzly bears, elk herds, and millions upon millions of birds. Today its remaining rich diversity is compressed into small pockets of protected land, which still provide habitat for millions of resident and migrant birds. Gray Lodge Wildlife Area is one of these pockets, a wildlife delight in the shadow of Sutter Buttes.

Birdlife varies by season. The Pacific Flyway, one of North America's principal migratory routes, passes directly over much of California. Approximately 30 percent of the waterfowl population using this route winters in the Central Valley, filling available wetlands with an estimated 3 million ducks and 750,000 geese. These migrants begin to arrive in the fall, peaking in population between December and February. As they depart in the spring, shorebirds move in to feed at the mudflats and year-round residents such as herons and egrets begin their breeding season. During the hot summer months, ducklings are endearing, and many small birds arrive to feast on the plentiful insects. Animal life is also abundant—otters, beavers, coyotes, rabbits, deer, turtles, and

lizards all live in the preserve. Overhead, raptors—especially northern harriers—are a common year-round sight, and the occasional bald eagle can be spotted during the winter months.

The Hike follows an easy circuit through the refuge and offers good opportunities for viewing wildlife. Binoculars are a must. The preserve is closed to all nonhunting activities during waterfowl season (late September through early February), making spring and early fall the best times for a visit. During the unpleasantly hot summer months, visit during the early morning or evening hours when conditions are more tolerable. The preserve is a popular destination for birders but receives relatively light use overall, especially on weekdays. No water is available at the trailhead.

To Reach the Trailhead: Take Hwy. 99 north for 10 miles from the junction of Hwys. 20 and 99 in Yuba City to Pennington Rd. in the town of Live Oak. Go west on Pennington Rd. for 10 miles, turning north at the junction with North Butte Rd. The posted turnoff for the preserve is on Rutherford Rd., which reaches an outstanding bird display case near the refuge headquarters in 2 miles. The trailhead lot is just past this by the open-air information kiosk. There is a $2.50 day-use fee per

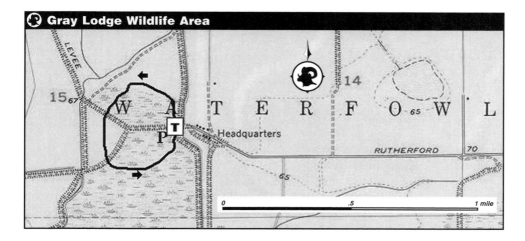

Gray Lodge Wildlife Area

person (waived for holders of a current California hunting or fishing license).

Description: While the hike can be completed in either direction, this description begins on the paved trail by the handicapped parking spaces and goes counterclockwise. The trail quickly reaches a short spur trail on the left to the first of two viewing platforms, on a small dirt hill camouflaged with reeds for more discrete viewing. The paved road continues, reaching its terminus at a large wooden platform looking north, which offers a free, high-powered telescope for your viewing pleasure. The sea of wetlands is without visible end, a limitless expanse of brown, gray, and green. Willows are the dominant tree in the area, thriving in places of abundant water supply. Grasses are thick and a wide variety can be found in the preserve, including sprangletop, smartweed, and joint grass.

Continue your loop on the unpaved trail, curving left (west) just before the second platform and offering some of the best views south of nearby Sutter Buttes. Just over 10 miles in diameter with a maximum elevation of 2117 feet, Sutter Buttes are the remains of an extinct volcano. Active in recent geologic time, their formation began with an intrusion of subsurface magma that lifted the overlying sediments from the valley floor. Between 1.6 and 1.3 million years ago Sutter Buttes underwent a period of greater activity, erupting lava directly onto the surface and forming the craggy domes of the core. Inactive today, Sutter Buttes remain a baffling mystery for geologists: It is unclear why this volcano developed as the single topographic feature of the Central Valley.

Reaching the dirt loop road of the preserve, cross it and continue on the narrow trail, passing a large thicket of bamboo adjacent to the road. Slowly looping south and then east, the trail widens again before rejoining the trailhead lot on its south side.

Nearest Visitors Center: There is no staffed visitors center. For general information call (530) 846-7500.

Nearest Campground: Colusa Sacramento River State Recreation Area Campground (14 sites, $12–15 depending on season) is located just north of Colusa by the Sacramento River.

Additional Information: ww.dfg. ca.gov/lands/wa/region2/gray lodge/index.html

HIKE 42

Fern Canyon

Coastal Greenbelt

Highlights	The lushness of a small coastal river canyon
Distance	5.0 miles round-trip
Total Elevation Gain/Loss	200´/200´
Hiking Time	2–3 hours
Optional Maps	USGS 7.5-min. *Mendocino* and *Mathison Peak*
Best Times	Year-round
Agency	Van Damme State Park
Difficulty	★

With its gurgling alley of green in a verdant canyon, Van Damme State Park provides an easy sampling of the lush ecosystem found just inland from the coast. The highlight is Fern Canyon, a small gorge 400 feet deep that shelters Little River and a lush, regenerating redwood forest. A diminutive coastal river barely 5 miles long, Little River provides critical habitat for coho salmon, steelhead, and a variety of other wildlife. Logged during the late 19th century, the forest has since rebounded to impressive dimensions with only gigantic decaying stumps to remind hikers of the past.

Logging began here on October 15, 1864, in response to the heavy demand for lumber in the burgeoning city of San Francisco. By 1865, more than three dozen schooners were hauling wood from Little River to San Francisco; activity continued unabated for the next 30 years. The redwoods were cut by burly men perched on wide planks known as "springboards," placed approximately 6 feet above the base of a tree, which allowed loggers to fell a tree at a narrower, more easily hewn point. Once cut, logs were floated downriver to be stored and milled near the river mouth. Bull teams, wagons, and a

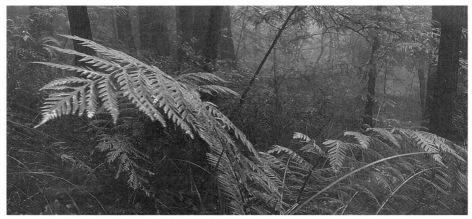

Van Damme's fern-topia is a pteridologist's delight.

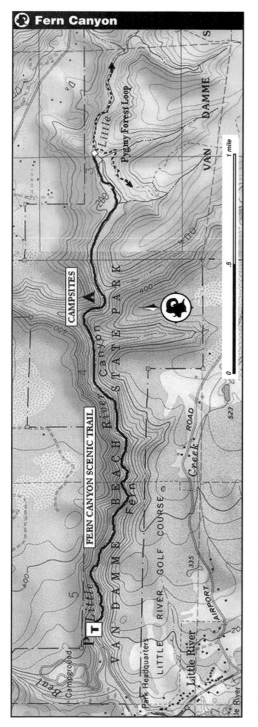

tramway moved trees from the more difficult locations, and skid roads were constructed to access ever farther up-canyon. By 1893 all profitable timber had been cut and the mills closed for good. The Jackson History Trail explores past milling operations in the park with the help of an excellent interpretive brochure, available at the visitors center or entrance station.

The Hike follows wide and level Fern Canyon Scenic Trail along Little River, an easy hike that can be extended significantly by adding the 3.5-mile Pygmy Forest loop at the hike's up-canyon terminus. The sun seldom shines in narrow Fern Canyon, making it cool and damp year-round with winter months colder and wetter than the rest. Fog does not detract from this hike—if anything, it enhances the experience—making it an excellent option for fogbound summer days. The very popular trail does not offer solitude, particularly during summer months. Water is available at the trailhead.

To Reach the Trailhead: Drive 3 miles south of Mendocino on Hwy. 1 to the park entrance. Follow the park road to its end behind the campground. There is a $6 day-use fee.

Description: From the trailhead, go through the gate and get an interpretive brochure. It explains the coho salmon life cycle with the help of metal fish markers spaced periodically along the hike. As you begin down the wide paved path, note the lush growth around you. Moss, fern, horsetail, huckleberry, stinging nettle, poison oak, thimbleberry, and the seasonal displays of tiger lilies, columbine, and irises cover the ground and cut banks. Tanoaks and Douglas firs join second-growth redwoods to form the dense canopy overhead.

The trail follows a road constructed during the 1880s to provide up-canyon logging access, which was improved by the Civilian Conservation Corps during the 1930s with the construction of several bridges. As you pass Fish 3, large redwood stumps begin to appear by the trail—look for springboard notches near the tops. Scan the river as you proceed and you may be lucky enough to spot a Pacific giant salamander. Largest of all terrestrial salamanders, they achieve lengths of up to 12 inches and can be identified by their mottled, purplish-brown backs and pale yellow underbellies. Living in moist places where they can breathe through their skins, they consume everything from insects to fish to frogs to snakes to other salamanders, lunging to grab their prey with sharp, bladelike teeth.

Once cut, a redwood tree immediately sprouts a series of genetically identical saplings from its root system, in time forming a roughly concentric circle of mature trees around the stump known as a "fairy ring." Several good examples of this basal sprouting can be spotted as you continue up-canyon—check around Fish 9. After passing 10 environmental campsites, the trail soon reaches the end of the Fern Canyon Scenic Trail in a large clearing.

Those wishing to continue their hike to the Pygmy Forest can begin the 3.5-mile loop here. Begin the loop on the trail section to the left, a single-track that delves deeper into the canyon. The return stretch is along the wide fire road to your right. Unless you are passionate about ecology,

the Pygmy Forest is not as exciting as it sounds. If you don't wish to go farther, return the way you came.

Nearest Visitors Center: Van Damme State Park Visitors Center, (707) 937-4016, is open 10 AM–4 PM daily April through October and weekends only November through March. Also try the district headquarters at (707) 937-5804.

Backpacking Information: Backcountry camping is allowed only at the 10 small but pleasant environmental campsites ($10–15, depending on season) tucked along Little River 1.75 miles from the trailhead.

Nearest Campground: Van Damme State Park Campground has 74 sites ($20–25, depending on season). Reservations are imperative from April through October, when tourists and abalone divers routinely fill the campground; visit www.reserveamerica.com or call (800)444-7275.

Additional Information: www.parks.ca.gov

HIKE 43

MacKerricher Beach

Dune World

Highlights	A vast secluded dune field
Distance	1.0 mile round-trip
Total Elevation Gain/Loss	50′/50′
Hiking Time	1–2 hours
Optional Map	USGS 7.5-min. *Inglenook*
Best Times	September through May
Agency	MacKerricher State Park
Difficulty	★

Bordered north by the vibrant ecosystem of Ten Mile River, MacKerricher State Park stretches along the coast for over 4 miles. Usually approached from the crowded south entrance, this vast enclosure of shifting sands, endangered species, foaming ocean, and windswept beach is accessed here from the secluded north end.

The Hike is a stroll along Ten Mile Dunes to the ocean via Ten Mile River and can be extended to an up to 9-mile

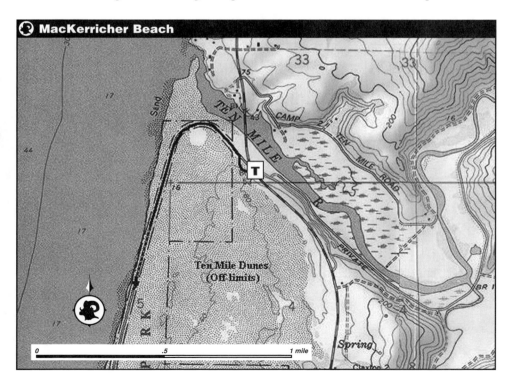

round-trip along the beach. In order to protect several threatened species, Ten Mile Dunes themselves are off-limits; yet they can be admired from the trail and the beach. Summer months bring thick fog, obscuring views and chilling the air. A windbreaker and a warm sweater are always advisable. Crowds are refreshingly light from this unposted access point. No water is available at the trailhead.

To Reach the Trailhead: Take Hwy. 1 to the Ten Mile River bridge, located 8 miles north of Cleone and 5.5 miles south of Westport. Park in the small turnout immediately south of the bridge on the west side of the road.

Description: From the trailhead, scramble briefly up the adjacent sandy slope to get a good vantage point of northern Ten Mile Dunes, and of the paved path leading down to the beach from beneath the bridge. The endangered Mendocino coast paintbrush grows in the area—be sensitive to the environment by henceforth following the paved path. Passing a sign reminding you of this, you soon reach the beach near the mouth of Ten Mile River.

Named for its distance north of the Noyo River mouth at Ft. Bragg, Ten Mile River protects 75 acres of salt marsh near its mouth, and provides habitat for spawning steelhead, salmon, and Pacific lamprey. In the dunes stretching south, the endan-

gered Menzies wallflower and Thurber's reed grass grow. The threatened western snowy plover—a plump, 6-inch-tall bird with a white chest and sandy-brown markings on its head and back—nests in the sand. The view north is excellent, unimpaired beyond the Lost Coast to Punta Delgada and the town of Shelter Cove. It is possible to walk the length of Ten Mile Beach to the park's southern entrance—an adventure that can take all day, especially if you have to walk back!

Nearest Visitors Center: Volunteers run a small visitors center at the main park entrance, (707) 964-8898. Hours vary depending on staffing, but generally it's open daily 10 AM–4 PM April through October and weekends only November through March. Also try the district headquarters at (707) 937-5804.

Nearest Campground: MacKerricher State Park Campground (142 sites, $20–25, depending on season) is located at the main, south entrance. Reservations are essential in summer; visit www.reserveamerica. com or call (800) 444-7275.

Additional Information: www. parks.ca.gov

Elder Creek

Coast Range Delight

Highlights	Coast Range old-growth, mixed-evergreen forest
Distance	3.5 miles round-trip
Total Elevation Gain/Loss	300′/300′
Hiking Time	1–2 hours
Optional Map	USGS 7.5-min. *Lincoln Ridge*
Best Times	Year-round
Agency	Northern California Coast Range Preserve
Difficulty	★

Euphonious streams of shimmering transparent clarity course beneath majestic trees here. In a land almost entirely felled by saw and ax, the little-known Coast Range Preserve protects a rare patch of pristine old-growth forest just inland from the coast.

The 7500-acre Coast Range Preserve owes its existence to Heath and Marjorie Angelo, who acquired and lived in the heart of this deep wilderness tract during the mid-20th century. Purchased by the Nature Conservancy in 1959, the preserve operates through a cooperative agreement with the Bureau of Land Management, protecting one of the best old-growth, mixed-evergreen forests left in California. The upper South Fork Eel River flows through the preserve and is joined by Elder Creek, a completely undisturbed drainage whose crystalline waters are used by the U.S. Geologic Survey as a benchmark for evaluating water quality around the state.

The Hike follows the narrow dirt road from the preserve entrance as it winds above the South Fork Eel River to reach the confluence with Elder Creek. The road continues for some distance past this point en route to a lodge at the road's end, but the views and experience do not change much. Ambitious hikers might

consider the extra 4-mile round-trip to the summit of forested Black Oak Mountain (3708′)—the posted trail junction is along the ridge where the road leaves the Elder Creek drainage. The hike can be done year-round, with cooler temperatures and rain common during the winter and fog always a possibility in the summer. The rivers swell after storms but quickly regain their remarkable clarity. While a University of California research station is located within the preserve and caretakers are often present, hikers are few and far between. The preserve is day-use only. No water is available at the trailhead.

To Reach the Trailhead: Take Branscomb Rd. 9.2 miles east from Hwy. 1—the turnoff is 1.6 miles north of Westport by lower Westport-Union Beach. The recently paved road twists and turns steeply on its way to the easily missed turnoff for Wilderness Lodge Rd. (on the north side of the road). Approaching from the east, take Hwy. 101 to Laytonville and follow Branscomb Rd. 16 miles west to the turnoff. Follow Wilderness Lodge Rd. 3.6 miles to the small visitors center at the preserve entrance. Sign the register before proceeding another 0.1 mile to park in the posted day-use lot on the right.

Description: From the trailhead (0.0/1460′), follow the narrow dirt road

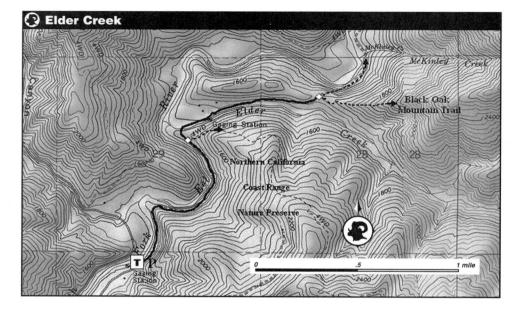

downhill a short distance and continue through the gate. The pristine nature of this preserve immediately becomes apparent as majestic redwood and Douglas fir intermingle in a tall old-growth forest along the Eel River. Tanoak, madrone, bigleaf maple, California bay, and canyon live oak fill in the middle story of the forest above an understory of huckleberry, sword fern, and moss. Wildlife here is plentiful, if reclusive. Mountain lion, black bear, river otter, bald eagle, osprey, gray fox, bobcat, mink, ring-tailed cat, Pacific giant salamander, black-tailed deer, and the rare fisher are all known to live within the preserve. Steelhead and silver salmon annually spawn here in the winter after migrating upriver more than a hundred miles from the sea.

Soon the remarkable waters of the South Fork Eel River are flowing below you. Containing 10 percent of the state's annual runoff, the Eel River is the third largest in California, and supports the second largest run of steelhead and silver salmon. Here in the preserve, less than 15 miles from the headwaters of the South Fork, the river is small and pristine. Unclouded by

the muddy runoff associated with logging and agriculture, it flows an indescribable blend of greens and grays—a wonderful piece of undisturbed California.

The road turns briefly away from the river before dropping to cross gurgling Elder Creek (1.7/1410′). A plaque commemorating it as a registered natural-history landmark can be found on the opposite bank. Oregon and black oak grow on the surrounding slopes. Continue as far as you wish along the road before returning the way you came.

Nearest Visitors Center: The rustic visitors center is not staffed. For general information, call the preserve headquarters at (707) 984-6653.

Nearest Campground: Westport-Union State Beach Campground (100 sites, $10–15, depending on season) is a view-rich but windy camping area right atop the bluffs west of Hwy. 1 and just north of Branscomb Rd.

Additional Information: http://cbc.berkeley.edu/manplan

HIKE 45

Rockefeller Forest

Humbling Humboldt

Highlights	A vast forest of redwoods enormous
Distance	11.0 miles
Total Elevation Gain/Loss	2800´/2800´
Hiking Time	5–7 hours
Optional Maps	USGS 7.5-min. *Bull Creek* and *Weott*
Best Times	Year-round
Agency	Humboldt Redwoods State Park
Difficulty	★★★★

The largest contiguous old-growth redwood forest on Earth is protected within Humboldt Redwoods State Park. Beyond amazement at individual trees, you experience an entire ecosystem that humbles all other redwood adventures in this book.

Named after the Prussian scientific explorer Alexander von Humboldt, the park began in 1921 with the purchase of 2000 acres by the Save-the-Redwoods League on the South Fork Eel River. With completion of a railroad linking Humboldt County to the Bay Area in 1914 and construction of the Redwood Hwy. in 1922, increasing tourism and logging activity magnified pressures on the diminishing old-growth redwood forests. In 1927, California created a statewide system of parks, and passed a bond measure to provide matching funds for the acquisition of state park lands. The Save-the-Redwoods League immediately began soliciting private donations and, in 1930, J. D. Rockefeller contributed a remarkable gift of $2 million to purchase 10,000 acres along Bull Creek owned by the Pacific Lumber Company. His generosity and farsightedness now protects this unrivaled redwood forest.

Humboldt Redwoods State Park today is comprised of 53,000 acres, of which 17,000 nurture old-growth redwood forest. Most of the Avenue of the Giants winds through the eastern section of the park and the entire Bull Creek watershed is now protected in its western portion. Efforts to restore park watersheds damaged by past logging are ongoing.

The Hike follows a less-traveled route through a remote corner of Rockefeller Forest on Look Prairie Road, Peavine Road, and Thornton Multi-Use Trail, before returning along the Bull Creek valley bottom. Because it climbs nearly 2000 feet from Bull Creek to traverse along a ridgetop, this is not an easy hike. That old-growth forest does not occur during the first 1000 feet of climbing also tends to limit traffic. The hike can be done year-round: Winters bring rain and guaranteed isolation; summers, tourist crowds and fog; and spring and fall, the best combination of crowds and weather. No water is available at the trailhead, and there are no reliable sources anywhere along the hike.

To Reach the Trailhead: Take Hwy. 101 to the South Fork/Honeydew exit in northern Humboldt Redwoods State Park. Head 3.5 miles west on Mattole Rd. to a small dirt lot on the right marked with a gate and sign for Look Prairie Rd.

Description: From the trailhead (0.0/220´), go through the gate and begin

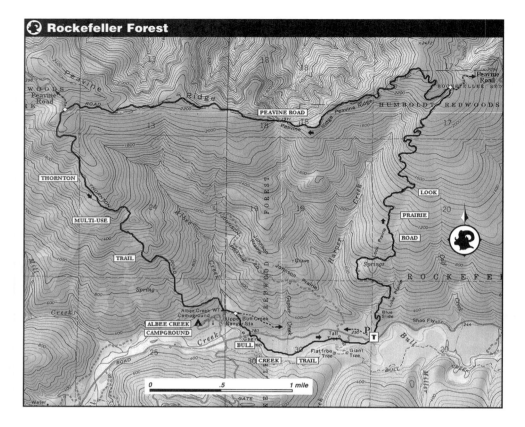

climbing. The old-growth redwoods quickly disappear as the wide service road gradually ascends through open slopes of California bay, tanoak, and second-growth Douglas fir. Obvious slumps and slides are indicative of the erosive effects that logging has had on slopes that would otherwise be held in place by redwood forest. Good views of the Bull Creek drainage open up as the trail relentlessly climbs.

Suddenly, old-growth redwood forest reappears (1.9/1400´) and stays with you for almost the entire remainder of the hike. The redwoods are huge—up to 12 feet in diameter—and many of the more massive specimens exhibit a striking resemblance to their giant sequoia cousins. Some of the largest Douglas firs you will ever see mingle with the redwoods, and gigantic madrones twist high through the understory. The Rockefeller Forest is thick, containing

the greatest density of biomass (amount of total organic material) ever measured. Estimates made at other locations in the park place the total biomass per acre at approximately 1800 tons, seven times the density of an acre of the Amazon rain forest! Near the ridgetop, you encounter the junction with Peavine Rd. (3.5/2230´)—go left.

After a brief, continued climb to the hike's greatest elevation (2500´), Peavine Rd. traverses west along the park's northern boundary. Lands north have been completely logged, harvested to the exact limit of the park's protected lands. Thankfully, these discouraging views are few and the road generally remains in undisturbed forest. After a long, gentle ramble along Peavine Rd., you reach the posted junction with single-track Thornton Multi-Use Trail (7.0/2300´)—turn left. Steadily descending the ridge that divides Mill and

Albee creeks, you soon pass a patch of incredibly thick madrones before continuing on the long descent to Albee Creek Campground (9.6/400′). From the campground, proceed down to the park road and follow Bull Creek Trail east along the broad and level stream corridor. Near the end, take the short detour across the stream to visit the Flat Iron and Giant trees. Bid farewell to two of the largest arboreal giants in the park and return to the trailhead (10.6/220′).

Nearest Visitors Center: Humboldt Redwoods Visitors Center, (707) 946-2263, located 1 mile south of Weott on the Avenue of the Giants, is open daily 9 AM–5 PM in summer; daily 10 AM–4 PM in winter.

Nearest Campground: Albee Creek Campground (40 sites, $20) is only open from mid-May through September. Burlington Campground (57 sites, $20), located near the visitors center on the Avenue of the Giants, is open year-round. Reservations are recommended during the summer.

Additional Information: www.humboldtredwoods.org

HIKE 46

Lost Coast Trail

Lost and Found

Highlights	Daunting coastal cliffs and remote beaches
Distance	16.7 miles one-way
Total Elevation Gain/Loss	3800´/3800´
Hiking Time	16–24 hours (2–3 days)
Optional Maps	USGS 7.5-min. *Hales Grove, Mistake Point,* and *Bear Harbor; California's Lost Coast* by Wilderness Press
Best Times	Spring and fall
Agency	Sinkyone Wilderness State Park
Difficulty	★★★★★

The Lost Coast can hardly be considered undiscovered. Ranching, logging, railroads, mills, and seaports have all left their mark on the land. But it is remote, too rugged for Hwy. 1, keeping all but the adventurous away.

The Lost Coast stretches from the Eel River Delta near Ferndale south to Hwy. 1, a distance of more than 70 miles. Offshore is the Mendocino Triple Junction, the point where three tectonic plates meet. North of the junction, the Juan de Fuca Plate dives beneath the Pacific Northwest, triggering the volcanoes of the Cascade Range. South, the San Andreas Fault reaches its offshore terminus, knitting the landscape with a host of faults. All this tectonic mayhem combines to cause dramatic uplift, creating cliffs that tower more than 1000 feet above the crashing sea. The dark cliffs weather to form unusual black-sand beaches, accessible only where small creeks have carved deep gullies between the bluffs. Sinkyone Wilderness State Park encompasses the southernmost section of the Lost Coast, an area of 7367 acres that protects more than 22 miles of shoreline.

Wildlife thrives in the park today. A herd of Roosevelt elk, reintroduced from Prairie Creek Redwoods State Park, wanders the coastal bluffs. Black bears and

mountain lions prowl inland. Whales and seals can be spotted offshore. Raptors of all varieties soar above. And a few stands of old-growth redwood still remain.

The Hike follows Lost Coast Trail between Orchard Camp and Usal Camp, a strenuous trek best done in three days. For being along the coast, there is virtually no level walking on this hike: The trail constantly encounters sheer creek canyons, descending quickly and ascending steeply hundreds of feet at a time. The two ends of Lost Coast Trail are far apart by road (2–3 hours' driving time) and two vehicles are required for transportation to and from the trailheads. A shuttle service is often available from local operators—contact the park or Bureau of Land Management King Range visitors center (707-986-5400, open year-round Monday–Friday 8 AM–4:30 PM and intermittently on summer weekends) for current information and rates. While the hike can be done in either direction, this description runs from north to south. Those wishing to dayhike from the north trailhead should turn around at Wheeler Camp, making a round-trip of 9.4 miles with an elevation gain/loss of roughly 1000 feet. Those interested in dayhiking from the south should climb 1000 feet to the top of the first bluff beyond Usal

Beach, a 6-mile round-trip with superlative views of the ocean and coast.

Timing is key. Fog blankets the region from June through mid-September, obscuring views and chilling the air for days on end. Heavy storms usually strike by late October and can inundate the coast with torrential rainfall well into April. From late April through May, storms are less frequent, fog is only occasional, and the lush, green terrain explodes with wildflowers. In late September and October, fog tapers off and weather is most ideal. Avoid holidays and weekends and crowds will be light. Those planning a winter visit should call ahead to verify access: Flooding and slides can close the roads for weeks at a time. Backcountry camping is allowed only at the three designated trail camps (see below). While no water is available at the trailhead, sources are plentiful along the trail.

To Reach the North Trailhead: Take the Hwy. 101 exit for Redway and Shelter Cove. From Redway, take Briceland Thorn Rd. 18 miles west toward Shelter Cove to Chemise Mtn. Rd.—turn left (south). The road rapidly turns to dirt, reaching a four-way junction in 7 miles—turn right onto the least significant road. The descent from here is steep, narrow, and not passable for trailers or RVs. While four-wheel-drive vehicles will have an easier time, low-clearance cars can make a slow descent. The Needle Rock Visitors Center is 3.5 miles from the junction. Here, dayhikers pay a $3 day-use fee per vehicle and backpackers pay their trail-camp fees. The trailhead at Orchard Camp is an additional 2.7 miles south at the road's end. After the first big rains of the season, the road is closed beyond the visitors center, making it necessary to walk this final stretch.

To Reach the South Trailhead: Take Mendocino County (Usal) Rd. 431 north from Hwy. 1. Along Hwy. 1 the unmarked and easily missed turnoff is 15.3 miles west of its junction with Hwy. 101, and approximately 3 miles north of Rockport at milepost 90.88. The one-lane dirt road

is impassable for trailers and RVs but easily handled by all other vehicles. In 6 miles you reach the area's first campsites, located in a large grassy field. Trailhead parking is 0.3 mile farther on the left, immediately before a small bridge. From here, it's a short walk to the posted trailhead at the road's end.

Description: Soon after leaving the trailhead at Orchard Camp (0.0/40´), the trail is joined by a spur trail from Railroad Camp. Then, it winds down to the coastal vista at Bear Harbor (0.4/0´), a rugged coastal access point used in the late 1800s for loading lumber. Nothing remains of prior development but pleasant campsites tucked away from the ocean. Next comes a general introduction to the Lost Coast Trail experience of repeated ascent and descent. Climbing a steep and narrow stream gully, the trail passes through luscious greenery. Large sword ferns splay everywhere, moss covers the thick trunks of alder and California bay, the large leaves of blue elderberry line the stream bank, and every possible nook and cranny bursts with life. You have time to enjoy all this because the trail is remarkably steep. After you attain the ridge, the trail traverses around Duffy's Gulch and through the first grove of old-growth redwoods before gently climbing along the blufftop. Views into

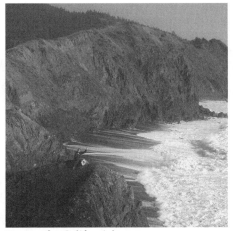

Hooray for California!

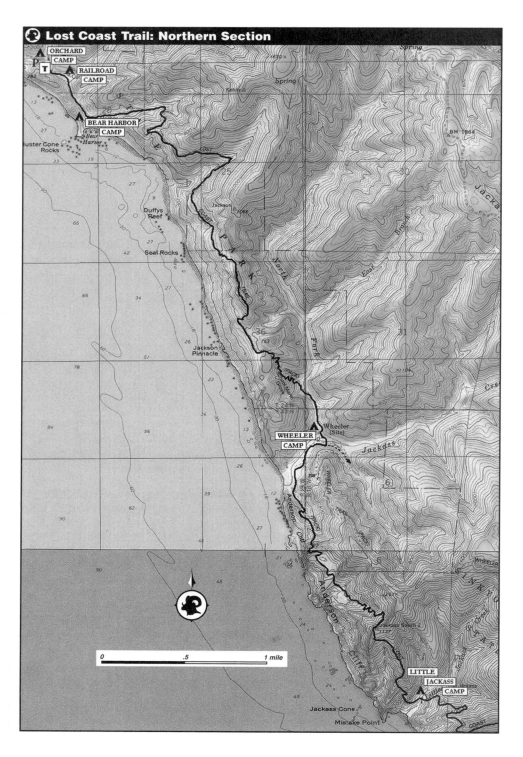

Lost Coast Trail: Northern Section

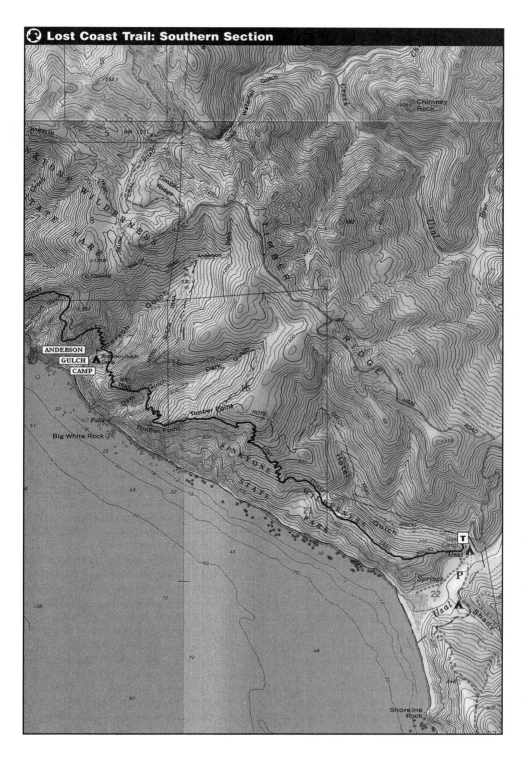

Lost Coast Trail: Southern Section

the sheer gulch of Jackass Creek open up where the trail makes its steep descent to Wheeler Camp (4.7/10´), passing through another old-growth redwood grove just before the first campsites.

Wheeler Camp was the location of a wood-processing facility from 1951 until 1960, run by the Wolf Creek Timber Company. The small company town with store, bunkhouse, and school was deliberately burned for liability reasons in 1969. Remnants of the mill include knee-high periscopelike tubes protruding from the ground, which were used to test the underground flow of toxic diesel fuel that leaked from the facility. While no fuel is known to have reached Jackass Creek, to be safe obtain your water upstream from the site. If it's raining or windy, the campsites nearest the redwood grove are nicest. If it's sunny and clear, continue along the trail to uphill sites south of the beach.

On your way to the beach, a trail diverges left as you enter the more open meadow—continue straight, winding along the edge of the beach before climbing steeply to almost 1100 feet. Keep an eye out for the small trees lining the top of the cliff. Bonsai-sized by exposure to the elements, these trees can be as old as those in the surrounding forest, with remarkably stout trunks hidden beneath their twisted foliage. Shelter Cove can be spotted north from near the cliff top, before the trail plummets down through dense tanoak forest to Little Jackass Creek Camp (9.2/20´). Sites are fewer than at Wheeler Camp, and farther from the wonderfully secluded beach.

The trail continues inland opposite the creek, quickly entering the Sally Bell Grove, an old-growth redwood stand named for a Sinkyone woman who fled here after a brutal attack on her village at Needle Rock in May 1864 by Lieutenant William Frazier and the Battalion of Mountaineers. Passing many substantial redwoods, the trail makes a very steep ascent to 800 feet before immediately dropping to Anderson Gulch Camp (11.7/250´).

Here, the campsites are small and hidden among the trees. You pass the best sites shortly after crossing the creek.

Another brief up-and-down brings you to Dark Gulch (12.3/350´), where the final and most arduous section of the hike begins. A prolonged stretch of climbing brings you to—at over 1100 feet—the highest point on this hike, almost directly above the ocean. The thick forest of tanoaks, bigleaf maples, and redwoods opens into fields of low-lying coyote brush and blackberry tangles. South, the trail can be seen winding along the bare ridgetop. Ocean views are exceptional, Usal Beach is visible, and a keen eye can identify Hwy. 1, 7 miles south of here, twisting along the coast before turning inland. It's a gradual descent from here to Usal Beach, ending with several steep switchbacks that deposit you near some nice campsites.

Nearest Visitors Center: The Needle Rock Visitors Center is staffed year-round by volunteers and open approximately 20 hours per week. Park headquarters (open intermittently, 707-986-7711) is located on Briceland Rd. in Whitethorn.

Backpacking Information: Backcountry camping is allowed only at the 3 designated trail camps—Wheeler, Little Jackass, and Anderson Gulch. There is a fee of $3 per person per night for the trail camps, payable outside the Needle Rock Visitors Center or at the Usal Camp fee station. There is no trail quota.

Nearest Campground: There are 18 walk-in campsites scattered around the Needle Rock area, including those in Bear Harbor ($10 per night October through April and $15 per night May through September).

Additional Information: www. parks.ca.gov

HIKE 47

Big Flat

Level Headed

Highlights	Endless beach, soaring cliffs, and an idyllic seaside meadow
Distance	17.0 miles round-trip
Total Elevation Gain/Loss	50´/50´
Hiking Time	9–12 hours
Optional Maps	*King Range National Conservation Area* by the BLM; USGS 7.5-min. *Shelter Cove, Shubrick Peak,* and *Honeydew; California's Lost Coast* by Wilderness Press
Best Times	Spring and fall
Agency	King Range Wilderness and National Conservation Area
Difficulty	★★★

The King Range lurches thousands of feet above from the sea, creating precipitous cliffs that back directly against black-sand beaches. Small streams carve deep ravines through the coastal bluffs, providing water and oceanside campsites for beach-walking hikers. Mountain summits lord over it all. The top of King Peak (4088´), the highest in the range, is less than 3 miles from the shore. The 42,585-acre King Range Wilderness and surrounding King Range National Conservation Area protects this rugged coastline of the northern Lost Coast, one of the most desolate stretches of sand in America.

The Hike travels along the beach to Big Flat, a rare coastside expanse of level ground awash in profuse spring wildflowers. This is not a hike for the unprepared. The loose and sloping beach is fatiguing underfoot. Strong northwest winds are common, especially in the summer, and there is little to shelter you from its onslaught. A 4.5-mile section of beach (between Gitchell Creek and Big Flat) is passable only at low tide—and is life-threatening at other times. Tide tables are posted at the trailhead; take note of when they occur. Strong storms occur regularly

from November through March and can turn the hike's many stream crossings into dangerous torrents. Water is available at the trailhead.

To Reach the Trailhead: Take the Hwy. 101 exit for Redway and Shelter Cove. From Redway, take Briceland Thorn Rd. toward Shelter Cove. In 13.2 miles you'll pass the Bureau of Land Management King Range Office on the left. Continue for another 7.1 miles to Beach Rd. and turn right toward Black Sands Beach, reaching the Black Sands Beach Trailhead and parking area in 0.9 mile.

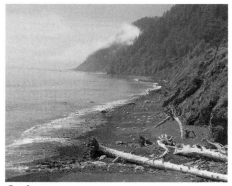

Get lost.

Big Flat: Northern Section

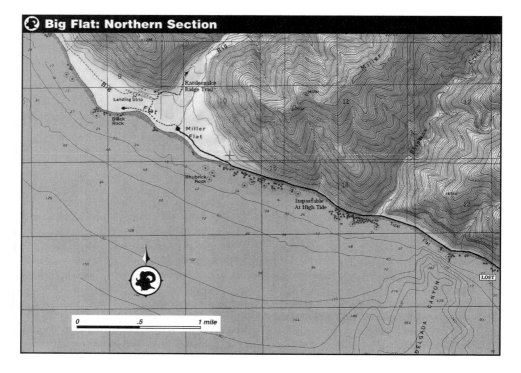

Description: A view north from the blufftop parking area (0.0/40´) reveals your approaching hike. The broad clearing of Big Flat is discernible in the distance along the shore. Inland, Horse Mountain rises as the first prominent ridgeline, followed next in the distance by Saddle Mountain. The small pyramid of 4088-foot King Peak peeks out beyond Saddle Mountain, crowning the top of Miller Ridge.

Follow the sidewalk down to the beach. Loosely consolidated layers of dark-colored sand (greywacke) and mud (shale) compose much of the mountains here, eroding to form the beach's distinctive black sand and cobbles. Heading north, you soon pass Telegraph Creek on the right (0.2/0´), followed by a rivulet emerging from below the Kaluna Cliffs. The beach narrows at this point and a giant house-sized boulder bulges from the shore. As you approach Horse Mountain Creek (1.6/0´), you encounter an elabo-

rate driftwood shelter, the first of many to come.

You pass Horse Mountain Trail (1.8/0´) just beyond Horse Mountain Creek and wander next to some low terraces. The beach narrows and offshore rocks appear as you approach Gitchell Creek (3.7/0´), which tumbles out of a 30-foot-wide gash in otherwise featureless cliffs. A huge driftwood shelter has been constructed nearby.

The next 4.5 miles of beach are impassable for several hours on either side of high tide (longer if there is significant swell). Time your passage appropriately and don't risk getting caught—there is no escape up the vertical cliffs. Past Gitchell Creek, the beach steepens and hems against sheer outcrops. Huge debris piles lie jumbled at the mouths of steep ravines. Big Flat briefly disappears from sight as you curve around a horseshoe of coastline and pass a pretty stream emerging from a lush alder grove overhead.

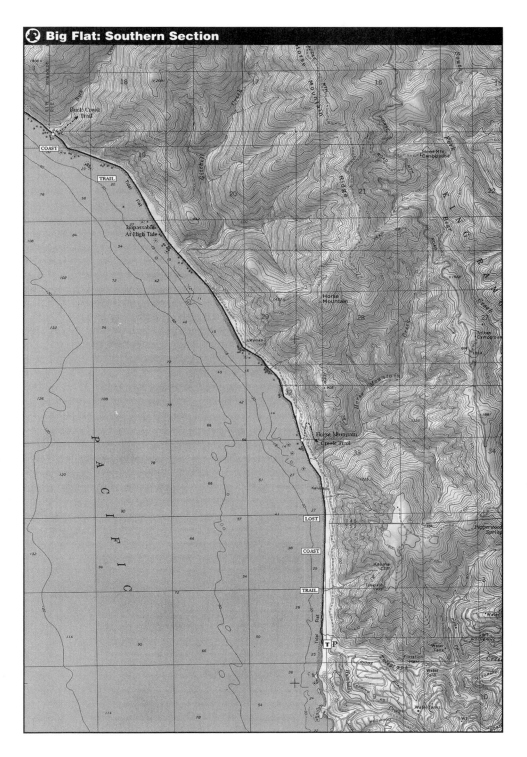

Big Flat: Southern Section

You next reach Buck Creek (5.2/0´), which pours into the surf by a wild wall of contorted rock. Numerous campsites (or rest stops) perch just inland from the shore, many with ocean views. The Buck Creek Trail heads uphill from here on its way toward Saddle Mountain, visible in the back of the valley. Past Buck Creek, the beach narrows and boulder fields extend into the tidal zone. Watch for seals hauled out on the rocks. You pass several dainty cascades, then a more significant creek that cuts a razor-thin slice in the cliff face. Next is Shipman Creek (6.6/0´), a substantial stream that emerges from a broader valley.

Beyond Shipman Creek the beach becomes rockier and strewn with cobble-stones, creating the toughest walking conditions yet. Just prior to reaching Big Flat, the cliffs shorten abruptly. There is no obvious path leading off the beach, but you should take your first available opportunity to scramble onto the easy-walking terrain above.

You emerge onto the broad outwash plain of Big Flat (8.2/20´), an open grassland interspersed with boulder piles, stunted Douglas firs, and profuse wildflowers. Burnt trees lance the surrounding slopes, mute evidence of a 2003 wildfire that scorched much of the western King Range. The trail cruises near the coastline, passing several driftwood shelters, and reaches your final stop at Big Flat Creek (8.5/20´). Retrace your steps to the trailhead.

Nearest Visitors Center: BLM King Range Office, (707) 986-5400, is open 8 AM–4:30 PM year-round Monday–Friday and intermittently on summer weekends.

Backpacking Information: Campsites are abundant at Big Flat and around the many creek mouths along the way. A backcountry permit is required, available at the trailhead or from the BLM King Range Office. A California Department of Forestry and Fire Protection permit is required for campfires, which are allowed except when a fire closure is in effect (typically late June through late October). Bear canisters are mandatory and can be rented at the BLM King Range Office for $5 per trip with a credit card deposit (violators are subject to a $150 fine). Camping is prohibited between the parking area and Telegraph Creek 0.2 mile north.

Nearest Campground: Shelter Cove Campground (105 sites, $25) is a private campground located next to the airstrip in the center of town.

Additional Information: www.blm.gov/ca/arcata

HIKE 48

King Peak

King for a Day

Highlights	The highest summit in the King Range
Distance	5.1 miles
Total Elevation Gain/Loss	1950´/1950´
Hiking Time	3–4 hours
Optional Maps	*King Range National Conservation Area* by the BLM; USGS 7.5-min. *Honeydew; California's Lost Coast* by Wilderness Press
Best Times	Spring and fall
Agency	King Range Wilderness and National Conservation Area
Difficulty	★★★

Where California bulges farthest west on the northern Lost Coast, powerful tectonic forces have crushed the King Range skyward. Touched by man and then forgotten, the mountains compose a remote topography jammed against the Pacific edge. Less than 3 miles from the sea, 4088-foot King Peak rises as the highest summit in the range, a heart-pounding destination with difficult access and superlative 360-degree views across the entire rumpled region.

Twenty-five miles northwest of King Peak, Cape Mendocino marks the westernmost point in the Lower 48. Due west from the cape, less than 10 miles from shore, three tectonic plates meet at the Mendocino Triple Junction. Land north lies along an active subduction zone where the tiny Juan de Fuca Plate dives beneath the North American continent in an underwater trench almost 2 miles deep. South, the San Andreas Fault careens offshore, slicing the land in a myriad of related faults. As the triple junction slowly migrates north, combined tectonic forces produce the most seismically active spot in the entire earthquake-prone state. The mountains are pushed upward at an as-tounding rate and major earthquakes are a frequent occurrence—a 1992 earthquake lifted the entire King Range up 3–5 feet!

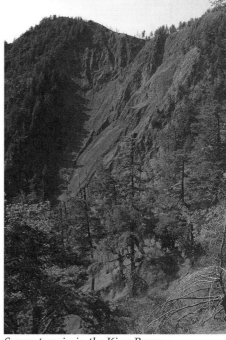

Severe terrain in the King Range

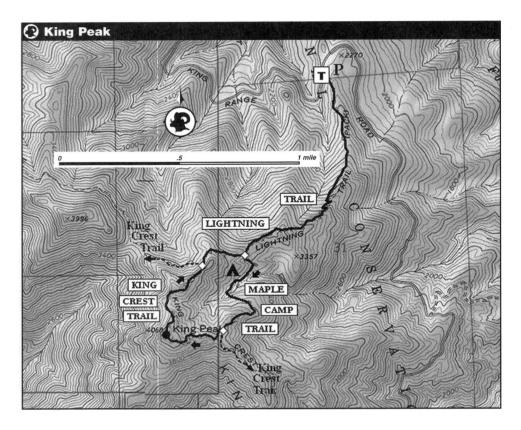

The Hike approaches King Peak from the northeast via King Range Rd., a rough and unpaved access road that necessitates a high-clearance vehicle for safe passage. The hike zigzags upward on Lightning Trail and completes a small loop near the summit to pass through pleasant Maple Camp, where a year-round stream and overnight camping area are available. The access road is closed during the rainy season (typically November through March) and the summer sun can be intense on the often shadeless slopes. These two factors make spring and fall the best times for a visit. No water is available at the trailhead; your only reliable source on this hike is at Maple Camp.

To Reach the Trailhead: Take the Hwy. 101 exit for Redway and Shelter Cove. From Redway, take Briceland Thorn Rd. toward Shelter Cove. In 13.2 miles you'll pass the Bureau of Land Management King Range Office on the left. Continue for another 4.8 miles to King Peak Rd., located at the top of a divide. Turn right and follow unpaved King Peak Rd. north, reaching Saddle Mountain Rd. on the left in 6.3 miles. Continue straight on increasingly rough King Peak Rd. for 3 miles to King Range Rd. Turn left and follow King Range Rd. 6.6 miles to the trailhead at the road's end, passing Saddle Mountain Rd. on the left 2.3 miles from the King Peak Rd. junction.

Description: From the trailhead (0.0/2220′), strike out on Lightning Trail in the shade of fluttering tanoaks, peeling madrones, and droopy Douglas firs. As you climb, the broad trail winds past several substantial Douglas firs, whose blackened trunks provide mute evidence of the 2003 wildfire that burned extensive portions of the western King Range, including much of the area visited by this hike.

Soon you encounter the trail's first switchbacks. Get used to them—you'll encounter 31 over the next 1.7 miles. You enter a burned area populated by dead madrones and young manzanita, then slowly rise close to the ridgeline beneath the shade of twisting canyon live oaks. The zigzags soon resume. Below and to the right, a seasonal creek may become audible; your best access point is just before the end of this section of switchbacks. The steep single-track trail rises steadily, traverses upslope, and soon encounters its first views northwest, which reveal the terrain of the lower Mattole watershed and Cape Mendocino area.

Then the switchbacks really begin. You rapidly gain 550 feet via 20 switchbacks, interspersed with short traverses. Large, fire-scarred Douglas firs provide company as you climb. After a final switchback, the trail makes a long gradual traverse to reach the posted junction for Maple Camp (1.7/3450′).

Turn left and follow the trail toward camp. Views quickly appear to the southeast, water becomes audible below, and the rocky path winds downward to meet a laughing brook in a stand of large, unblemished Douglas firs. A brief rise brings you to Maple Camp (2.0/3400′), where a half dozen tent sites dot the slopes like rocky nests. Bay trees and a few bigleaf maples shade the creek.

Continuing past camp, the trail runs briefly along the creekbed, crosses the brook, makes a few switchbacks, and then traverses left to enter a sun-scoured world of burnt madrone and manzanita. Views open up to the northeast, then southeast, as you ascend the loose and rocky path through scrub. Glimpses of nearby King Peak appear shortly before you reach King Crest Trail (2.4/3820′).

To the summit! Bear right and head north through the gravelly moonscape on a steady, rising traverse. A few scraggly canyon live oaks provide limited shade as you go. The route attains the ridgeline about halfway up and makes a few final

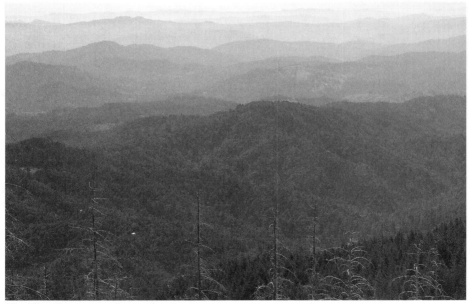

The King Range rumbles eastward.

S-turns just below the summit (2.8/4088′). A three-sided cement shelter nestles just below the top.

The view is tremendous, a 360-degree sweep. The King Range marches away to the north and south, its spine traced by King Crest Trail. The Big Flat Creek watershed pours into the ocean to the west; Shubrick Peak guards its northern flanks. Farther north, the Mattole River flows in the midst of rumpled topography; a keen eye can spot its riverbed. The deep drainage of Shipman Creek is next to the south, separated from Big Flat by Miller Ridge. The Buck Creek watershed is just beyond, separated from Shipman Creek by Fire Hill. In the southern distance you can make out the Kaluna Cliffs near Shelter Cove and the coastline of Sinkyone Wilderness (Hike 46) on the farthest horizon.

More than 10 ridges recede into the eastern distance and the high bumps of the Trinity Alps (Hike 54) dimple the northeast horizon.

Begin your return journey by following King Crest Trail north from the summit, running down the ridgeline through open manzanita and other low-lying chaparral. The trail drops slowly, offers one last view west, and then makes a brief traversing climb. Resuming the descent, the trail switchbacks eight times, enters shady oak woods, and reaches Lightning Trail (3.3/3720′). Turn right and head down Lightning Trail, enjoying another bout of switchbacks that deposits you at the earlier junction for Maple Camp (3.7/3450′). Retrace your steps to the trailhead (5.4/2220′).

Nearest Visitors Center: BLM King Range Office, (707) 986-5400, is open 8 AM–4:30 PM Monday–Friday year-round and intermittently on summer weekends.

Backpacking Information: Maple Camp is the best option and provides the hike's only reliable water source; a three-sided cement shelter just below the summit of King Peak is another (dry) option. A backcountry permit is required, available at the trailhead or from the BLM King Range Office. A California Department of Forestry and Fire Protection permit is required for campfires, which are permitted except when a fire closure is in effect (typically late June through late October). Bear canisters are mandatory and can be rented at the BLM King Range Office for $5 per trip with a credit card deposit (violators are subject to a $150 fine).

Nearest Campground: Tolkan Campground (9 sites, $8) is located on King Peak Rd., 3.5 miles north of Briceland Thorn Rd. Horse Mountain Campground (9 sites, $5) is 3 miles farther (9 sites each, $5). Neither campground has water.

Additional Information: www.blm.gov/ca/arcata

HIKE 49

Punta Gorda Lighthouse

Get Lost

Highlights	A remote, abandoned lighthouse
Distance	6.4 miles round-trip
Total Elevation Gain/Loss	100'/100'
Hiking Time	3–4 hours
Optional Maps	USGS 7.5-min. *Petrolia; King Range National Conservation Area: The Lost Coast* by the BLM; *California's Lost Coast* by Wilderness Press
Best Times	Spring and fall
Agency	King Range Wilderness and National Conservation Area
Difficulty	★★

Eleven miles north of the Mattole River mouth, Cape Mendocino marks the westernmost point in the lower 48 states. Due west from the cape, less than 10 miles from shore, three tectonic plates meet at the Mendocino Triple Junction. Land north lies along an active subduction zone where the tiny Juan de Fuca Plate dives beneath the North American continent in an underwater trench almost 2 miles deep. South, the San Andreas Fault careens offshore, slicing the land in a myriad of related faults. As the triple junction slowly migrates north, combined tectonic forces

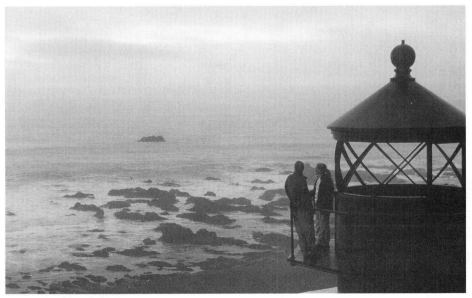

Punta Gorda Lighthouse

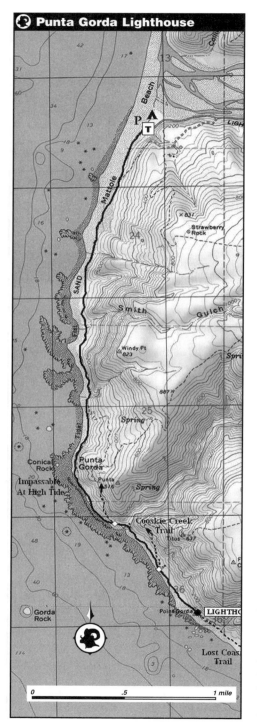

Punta Gorda Lighthouse

produce the most seismically active spot in the entire earthquake-prone state. The mountains are pushed upward at an astounding rate and major earthquakes are a frequent occurrence—a 1992 earthquake lifted the entire King Range up 3–5 feet!

Twenty-one miles south of Cape Mendocino is Punta Gorda, another bulge in the coastline sheltering remote Punta Gorda Lighthouse. Staffed for only 40 years, the lighthouse was shut down in 1951. The whole region bears traces of a 19th-century boom that busted, leaving the landscape empty and forgotten by today's world. The first oil well in California was drilled near Petrolia in 1865, and ranching and logging quickly pruned the sweeping hills and ridges. Today, the mouth of the Mattole River marks the northern limit of the King Range National Conservation Area, 60,000 acres of land protected south along the coast and inland through the heart of the King Range; 42,585 acres was set aside as designated wilderness in 2006. The seaside mountain topography catches a lot of rain, making this area the wettest in the entire state. While the mouth of the Mattole River receives an average of 50 inches per year, the surrounding ridges have recorded in excess of 200 inches— nearly 17 feet—during wet years.

The Hike follows the coastline south from Mattole River to Punta Gorda, a sandy walk that ends at the lighthouse turret. Just south of sheltering Cape Mendocino, the coastline here is reputed to have regular fog-free days during the summer months, a rarity on the North Coast. Spring and fall are the best times to come; avoid winter when storms swelling Fourmile Creek are likely to obstruct the hike. The region around Punta Gorda can be treacherous at high tides—tide tables are usually posted at the trailhead and your hike should coincide with low tide. People are few out here, and supplies are limited and very expensive. Water is available at the trailhead.

To Reach the Trailhead: You have to drive a lot of twisting roads. The easiest approach is via Ferndale, located 5 miles west of Hwy. 101 on Hwy. 211—the turn-off from 101 is at Fernbridge. In Ferndale, turn right off Main St. onto Ocean Rd., and then turn immediately left at Fifth St. to head south toward Petrolia, 30 miles away. One mile south of Petrolia, turn right on Lighthouse Rd. and follow it 5 miles to the campground and day-use parking lot at the road's end. It is also possible to get here by taking sinuous Mattole Rd. west from Humboldt Redwoods State Park to the town of Honeydew, located 25 miles (60–90 minutes) from Hwy. 101. Cross the Mattole River and continue west (down-stream) on Mattole Rd. for 15 miles to reach Lighthouse Rd. There is a $3 day-use fee for those not staying overnight at the campground.

Description: From the trailhead, go through the gate by the information sign and head south through the dunes to quickly reach a fenced-off shell midden once used by the Mattole Indians. In-terpretive signs explain its potential ar-chaeological significance and provide an excellent diagram of the tectonic forces at work in the region. Looking north, the striking point of Cape Mendocino can be seen jutting into the ocean beyond the nearby Mattole River drainage.

As you head south, follow either a trail often found running below the base of the steep bluffs or the sandy beach. Note the slopes covered with coyote brush, cow parsnip, lupine, yarrow, and mint, but be-ware the extensive poison oak. Wildlife is rich in the offshore waters and you may see harbor seals eyeing you from inside the breakers. As you slowly round Punta Gorda to reach Fourmile Creek, the light-house appears down the coast, dwarfed in scale by the landscape.

A private dwelling is located near the mouth of Fourmile Creek (2.5/0´)—please respect the property rights and the privacy of the owners here. Crossing the creek and continuing south, you soon reach the light-house, where informative placards detail the site's history. The tower itself is open and accessible from the inside via a very tight stairway ladder; it makes a great spot for lunching and relaxing. While the Lost Coast Trail continues 21 miles south along the beaches to Shelter Cove, you avoid that long sandy walk by returning the way you came.

Nearest Visitors Center: There are no visitors centers remotely close to this hike. The Bureau of Land Man-agement has an office in Arcata, (707) 825-2300, located at the north end of town, open Monday through Friday 7:45 AM–4:30 PM. There is also a visi-tors center at Thorn Junction, (707) 986-5400, located 14 miles (30–45 minutes) west of Hwy. 101 on Brice-land Rd., going toward Shelter Cove. It's open year-round 8 AM–4:30 PM Monday–Friday and intermittently on summer weekends.

Backpacking Information: Beach camping is permitted along this hike and at points farther south along the coast. Bear canisters are required and can be rented for a nominal fee at the Petrolia General Store or BLM visi-tors center at Thorn Junction (viola-tors are subject to a $150 fine). Proper human waste disposal is critical along the beaches—bury it at least 6 inches deep in the sand of the inter-tidal zone. Campfires are allowed on the beach, but a valid campfire per-mit is required (a California Depart-ment of Forestry and Fire Protection permit is valid).

Nearest Campground: Mattole Beach Campground (9 sites, $8) is located at the trailhead.

Additional Information: www. blm.gov/ca/arcata/king_range. html

HIKE 50

Trinidad Head

Hike a Head

Highlights	The North Coast and ocean views
Distance	2.0 miles
Total Elevation Gain/Loss	400´/400´
Hiking Time	1–2 hours
Optional Map	USGS 7.5-min. *Trinidad*
Best Times	Spring and fall
Agency	City of Trinidad
Difficulty	★

Beaches are few on the North Coast and the ocean cannot be seen for long stretches along Hwy. 101. Trinidad Head shelters a sandy stretch of protected coastline and offers sweeping coastal vistas from its slopes—perfect!

The Hike follows Trinidad State Beach south the short distance to Trinidad Head (362´) and makes a circuit below the summit before returning back along the beach. This is not a hike offering an isolated, wilderness experience—the small town and harbor of Trinidad are nearby—but it is an easy taste of the North Coast. Fog can be thick during the summer months, chilling the air, obscuring views, and making this a much less enjoyable hike. Be prepared for wind on Trinidad Head, and watch out for the poison oak that thrives in brush along this hike. Water is available at the trailhead.

To Reach the Trailhead: Take Hwy. 101 to the Trinidad exit and go west toward town. After crossing Patricks Point Drive, make a right at the T-junction to reach the Trinidad State Beach entrance. Park by the picnic area.

Description: From the west end of the parking lot, the trail briefly passes through Sitka spruce and shore pine before descending via several switchbacks to the beach. A short spur trail near the bottom accesses the lush gully of Mill Creek. Around the immediate point north is College Cove, another sandy beach always accessible from the parking lot, and from the main beach at low tide.

Turning south, you walk along the beach toward Trinidad Head. Keep an eye out offshore for sea lions and harbor seals. Approaching the base of Trinidad Head, you can find the start of the trail in the large parking lot surrounded by mountains of old tires. After you quickly climb 60 feet up some sandy stairs, the trail follows a paved road; bear right and walk up the road for a short distance. By several benches with good views north, the narrower, unpaved trail soon splits right from the road and begins winding through a dense corridor of coastal shrubbery. Thimbleberry, fern, sticky monkeyflower, poison oak, and impenetrable brush obscure the view but provide a good windbreak; the trail slowly traverses west around the head. Making a few switchbacks, you soon arrive at the first unobstructed views north of the jagged coastline.

The bulk of the coastline here is easily eroded sandstone and mudstone with large chunks of more resistant rocks randomly interspersed. The waves' erosive power readily strips away most material, leaving the more resistant blocks as jagged

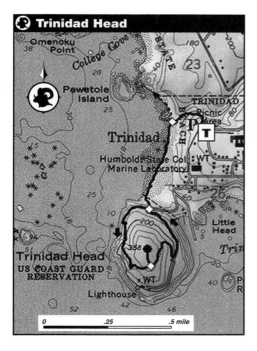

offshore rocks. The area around Trinidad is a prime example of what is known as an emergent coastline.

The trail continues its circuit, passing below a rocky rise easily accessible by an obvious spur trail. The view from on top of this small ridgelet is the best of the hike; the coastline can now be seen stretching south into the distance. Large Pilot Rock sits more than a half mile offshore south of Trinidad Head, and the city of Eureka is visible far beyond it on the distant coastline.

Resuming the circuit, you soon reach a large granite cross commemorating June 9, 1775, when Spanish explorers raised a cross here on Trinity Sunday, giving the location its name. From here, a complex of small buildings and access roads somewhat spoil the natural feel. Follow the gravel road down the east side of the head to rejoin the paved road and return to the beach.

Nearest Visitors Center: The Bureau of Land Management has an office in Arcata, (707) 825-2300, located at the north end of town and open 7:45 AM–4:30 PM Monday through Friday.

Nearest Campground: Patricks Point State Park Campground (124 sites, $20–25, depending on season) is located 5 miles north of Trinidad just west of Hwy. 101. Arrive early or reserve in advance if you plan on staying at this popular state park during the summer.

Additional Information: www.blm.gov/ca/arcata

HIKE 51

Klamath River Mouth

The Spit

Highlights	Gigantic driftwood in a dangerous place
Distance	1–2 miles round-trip
Total Elevation Gain/Loss	150′/150′
Hiking Time	1–2 hours
Optional Map	USGS 7.5-min. *Requa*
Best Times	April through October
Agency	Redwood National Park
Difficulty	★

It is a world like no other, an enormous sandy spit regularly swept clean by the fury of the ocean. Driftwood litters it, enormous stumps are buried within it, a mighty river flows behind it, and the Pacific breaks upon it.

The Hike explores the length of the broad sandbar formed at the Klamath River mouth, an easy hike that places you deep within nature's domain. *This can be a very dangerous place—especially near the mouth itself—where strong surf and high tides can completely wash across the spit and sweep the unsuspecting into the Klamath River and out to sea. Do not venture onto the sandbar if you see water washing across it.* While the hike can be done year-round, torrential winter rains are worth avoiding. The mouth of the Klamath is included within Redwood National Park but this is not an official or posted trail. Crowds will be minimal. No water is available at the trailhead.

To Reach the Trailhead: Take Hwy. 101 a half mile south of its Klamath River crossing, turn west onto Hwy. D8, and proceed 3.6 miles to a Y-junction near the

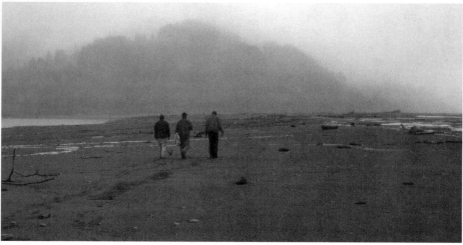

On the spit

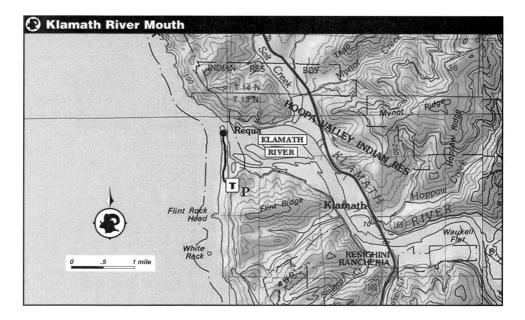

Klamath River Mouth

river level. Bear left and go 0.2 mile to the end of the pavement. Park in the small dirt lot across from the gated paved road.

Description: Be respectful of the adjacent private residence as you go through the gate and begin descending toward the beach. A few salt-pruned Sitka spruce line the upper sections, but the vegetation rapidly turns to thick brambles. Once you step onto the sandbar the world of plants has been left behind. The spit is roughly a half mile long and the washed up remains of many a gigantic redwood tree can be found along its length. Flint Rock Head (175´) can be seen protruding from the jagged coast a mile south.

Surpassed in size only by the Sacramento, the Klamath River is the second largest river in California, draining 15,500 square miles as it winds 263 miles from its headwaters in the Cascades of southern Oregon. Supporting the state's largest run of salmon and steelhead, it also provides habitat for a great diversity of life in the estuary tucked behind its mouth. Starry flounder, Pacific lamprey, American shad, and striped bass are but a few of the species that swim in the nearby waters. The wetlands just inland also attract numerous shorebirds, including godwits, willets, pintails, buffleheads, and green-winged teals. Harbor seals and sea lions can often be seen on the offshore rocks north of the river. Osprey and spotted owls nest in the surrounding forest, and bald eagles are occasionally sighted here as well.

Nearest Visitors Center: Redwood National Park Headquarters and Visitors Center, (707) 465-7306, is located in Crescent City at 2nd and K streets. Also try Kuchel Visitors Center, (707) 465-7765, located to the south in Orick. Both facilities are open 9 AM–5 PM daily in summer and 9 AM–4 PM during the off-season.

Nearest Campground: Flint Ridge Walk-In Campground (10 sites, free, no water) is located a half mile south of the trailhead on unpaved Coastal Drive.

Additional Information: www.nps.gov/redw

HIKE 52

Damnation Creek

Damnation

Highlights	Extraordinary old-growth forest and remote coastal access
Distance	4.2 miles round-trip
Total Elevation Gain/Loss	1200´/1200´
Hiking Time	3–4 hours
Optional Maps	USGS 7.5-min. *Sister Rocks* and *Childs Hill*
Best Times	April through October
Agency	Del Norte Coast Redwoods State Park
Difficulty	★★

Damnation Creek flows a scant 2 miles to the sea, yet slices a gorge more than 1000 feet deep and preserves an isolated, undisturbed old-growth forest within its sheltered walls. Its mouth provides the only coastal access point for 3 miles in either direction, a remote and rugged slice of the North Coast.

Damnation Creek lies within Del Norte Coast Redwoods State Park, one of three state parks founded during the 1920s and included today within the Redwood National and State Parks system. There are currently 856 known plant species within the parks and 202 native wildlife residents, including the threatened marbled murrelet and northern spotted owl. The parks are collectively designated a World Heritage Site and International Biosphere Preserve, testament to their unique and irreplaceable qualities. Damnation Creek is a choice example.

The Hike is a quick descent into the Damnation Creek drainage on more than 20 gentle switchbacks, passing through an awe-inspiring forest to reach a rocky and isolated beach. While fog can obscure the far-reaching coastal views, it enhances the primeval tranquility of the forest and should not dissuade you from this hike. Fog is heaviest during the summer months, with spring and fall provid-

ing the most consistent sunshine. The trail is open year-round but torrential winter rains are best not trifled with. Expect cool conditions at all times and bring a warm sweater. Crowds are relatively light but you are seldom entirely alone. No water is available at the trailhead.

To Reach the Trailhead: Take Hwy. 101 north of the Klamath River bridge for 12 miles to milepost 16.0, and park in the dirt lot on the west side of the highway. The turnout is easily missed so keep your eyes open. Approaching from the north, the trailhead is 3 miles south of the Mill Creek Campground turnoff.

Description: From the trailhead, the wide root-studded path rises briefly to its highest point (1100´); it passes through a thick ground cover of redwood sorrel and wild ginger while, overhead, enormous redwoods tower above spindly rhododendron trees. After cresting the divide the trail gradually descends, soon reaching the wide dirt road of the Coastal Trail, a former Hwy. 101 roadbed. Cross the road and continue down the posted steep, strenuous trail. As you begin the long switchbacking descent, Douglas firs become increasingly common; they are easily identified by their rough, unfurrowed bark, so distinct from that of redwoods. Fire scars are abundant in the trees along

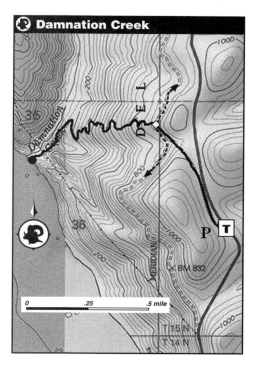

Damnation Creek

spruce has been used to build boats, airplanes, and the soundboards of concert harps, grand pianos, and violins. Victim to heavy logging, few old-growth stands remain—the trees around you are some of the largest left in California.

Thimbleberry and salmonberry twine thickly among the brush as the trail approaches the bottom. The thin trickle of Damnation Creek is heard for the first time where the trees, unable to withstand the salt-laden sea air, suddenly thin. You encounter the ocean at a small promontory, and the adventurous can explore along the coast for some distance both north and south. Then, back up you go.

the trail, and several exciting caverns can be found within their ponderous trunks.

Sitka spruce are a special highlight of this hike and begin to appear about halfway down the gorge. You can identify them by the flaky scales on their trunks and their small feathery cones. Growing in a narrow 1800-mile-long coastal belt extending from Northern California to Alaska, these majestic trees can achieve heights in excess of 300 feet, and have long been prized for their golden wood. Pound for pound stronger than steel, this

Nearest Visitors Center: Redwood National Park Headquarters and Visitors Center, (707) 465-7306, located in Crescent City at 2nd and K streets. Also try Kuchel Visitors Center, (707) 465-7765, to the south in Orick. Both facilities are open 9 AM–5 PM daily in summer and 9 AM–4 PM during the off-season.

Nearest Campground: Mill Creek Campground (145 sites, $20), located 3 miles north of the trailhead, is open May through September only. Year-round campgrounds can be found in Prairie Creek and Jedediah Smith Redwoods state parks.

Additional Information: www.nps.gov/redw

HIKE 53

Stout Grove

Rain Forest

Highlights	The lush diversity of a unique temperate rain forest
Distance	1.0 mile
Total Elevation Gain/Loss	50´/50´
Hiking Time	1 hour
Optional Map	USGS 7.5-min. *Hiouchi*
Best Times	April through October
Agency	Jedediah Smith Redwoods State Park
Difficulty	★

North America's temperate rain forest extends from northwest California to Alaska in a narrow coastal strip where rainfall is significant year-round and snow is infrequent. The coast redwood forest range extends north from Big Sur to a few miles past the Oregon border and exists in a narrow coastal belt. Jedediah Smith Redwoods State Park is one of the few places where you can experience the rare juxtaposition of these two impressive worlds.

Three members of the forest readily seen in the park are western hemlock, western red cedar, and Port Orford cedar. Common throughout the temperate rain forest, western hemlock has needles that closely resemble those of mountain hemlock—very short and continuously wrapping the ends of its drooping branches. Because germinating in the mossy green carpet on the forest floor is difficult, western hemlock use fallen trees as nurse logs. Elevated above the understory below, the trees gradually grow roots through the log and into the ground. As the log rots away, the trees are left standing in a line with their roots exposed above the surface.

Western red cedar is readily identified by the flattened sprays of delicate foliage that extend from the length of its thin branches. Cones are less than a half inch in diameter and have from four to six pairs of opposite scales. The needles are

pleasantly fragrant when crushed. Also common throughout the temperate rain forest belt, it is widely used as lumber for housing construction.

Occurring only in the Klamath Mountain region, Port Orford Cedar is a valuable lumber tree that can fetch up to $50,000 for a mature specimen. A waterborne fungus is currently decimating these trees throughout the Smith River drainage, and many unpaved U.S. Forest Service roads are closed during the rainy season to prevent further spread of the disease. They can be identified by the resemblance of their foliage to incense cedar, equally small cones (less than a half inch) with from six to ten shieldlike scales, and the deeply grooved brownish-gray bark on taller specimens. Other large trees that occur in the park are Sitka spruce (better seen on Hike 52), Douglas fir, and grand fir.

Flowing through the park is the Smith River, the only major undammed river system left in California. Roughly 300 miles of it are designated as part of the National Wild and Scenic River System—more than on any other river in the country—and its mesmerizing waters support healthy runs of salmon and steelhead throughout the winter months. In 1990 Congress created the Smith River National Recreation Area upstream from the state park to preserve land in the Smith River watershed, assur-

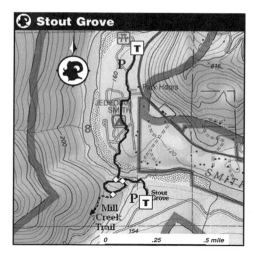

To Reach the Trailhead: Take Hwy. 199 east from Hwy. 101 (above Crescent City) for 5 miles to the park entrance. There is a day-use fee of $6. To reach the Stout Grove Trailhead from the north side, continue 2.4 miles west on Hwy. 199 past the park entrance, turn right on South Fork Rd. and then quickly right again on unpaved Howland Hill Rd./Douglas Park Dr. After you cross the two forks of the Smith, the trailhead is on your right in 2.7 miles. Trailers and RVs are not permitted on Howland Hill Rd.

Description: Wander the campground first and look for all the trees mentioned above before heading to the river crossing near Campsite 83. Then stroll through the Stout Grove, named not for the gigantic redwoods but for the Stout family who donated the 200-acre grove. An easy loop trail winds through it. As you mosey, look in the understory for salal, oxalis, western azalea, rhododendron, trillium, huckleberry, salmonberry, numerous spring wildflowers, and the nine species of ferns found within the park. Longer hikes are available for those intrigued by this short ramble—try Mill Creek Trail.

ing the long-term health of this remarkably pristine corner of California.

The state park is named for Jedediah Smith, who between 1822 and 1830 became the first Anglo-American to reach California from the east, the first to cross the Sierra Nevada, the first to travel the length of the state and, in 1828 the first to reach the Pacific Ocean overland through northwest California, camping near the future state park. During his travels he was mauled by a grizzly bear and almost lost an ear, nearly died in the Colorado River when 10 of his 19 men perished, and survived an Indian attack farther up the coast in 1828 that killed 16 of his 20-man party.

The Hike is a meandering stroll through the Stout Grove forest and the park campground on an easy, level trail. Stout Grove is across the Smith River from the campground and in summer a temporary bridge links the two. In the off-season it is necessary to drive 4 miles from the campground to the Stout Grove Trailhead. Tourist crowds are heavy during summer months, making spring and fall—with regularly occurring warm weather—the best times to visit. Winter rains can be torrential and make tent camping a dubious proposition. Expect cool, damp conditions year-round. Water is available at the trailhead.

Nearest Visitors Center: Hiouchi Information Center, located 0.2 mile west of the park entrance on Hwy. 199, is open 9 AM–5 PM daily May through September and closed in the off-season. Also Redwood National Park Headquarters and Visitors Center, (707) 465-7305, located in Crescent City at 2nd and K streets, is open 9 AM–5 PM daily in summer and 9 AM–4 PM during the off-season.

Nearest Campground: The state park campground has 90 sites ($20). Reservations are recommended in summer. Otherwise, try the national forest campgrounds east of Gasquet on Hwy. 199.

Additional Information: www. nps.gov/redw

HIKE 54

Canyon Creek Lakes

The Trinity Alps

Highlights	A serrated granite divide above lush wilderness
Distance	15.0 miles round-trip
Total Elevation Gain/Loss	3000'/3000'
Hiking Time	12–14 hours
Optional Map	USGS 7.5-min. *Mount Hilton*
Best Times	Late June through October
Agency	Trinity Alps Wilderness
Difficulty	★★★★

A land of deep canyons and jagged granite ridges, the Trinity Alps are the greatest alpine highlight of the Klamath Mountains. Impossibly alluring, they crown the thick forest of the region, a vibrant playground of lakes, rivers, and wildlife.

The Hike follows Canyon Creek Trail to Lower Canyon Creek Lake in the heart of the Trinity Alps, a very long dayhike that can easily be turned into a two- or three-day adventure. The Klamath Mountains receive heavy precipitation and, despite the relatively low elevation of this hike, snow can linger on the trail into June. Crowds funnel into this small area in unfortunate numbers during July and August, making September and even early October the best times to visit. Fishing is possible in the lakes, but Canyon Creek is too small for angling. While no water is available at the trailhead, sources are plentiful along the way.

To Reach the Trailhead: Take Hwy. 299 to Junction City, located 8.5 miles west of the intersection of Hwys. 3 and 299 in Weaverville and 6.5 miles east of East Fork Rd. and the turnoff for Helena. Turn north on Canyon Creek Rd. (Hwy. 401)—the turnoff is directly opposite the Junction City Store—and follow the increasingly narrow paved road 13.5 miles to the large parking lot at the road's end.

Description: From the trailhead (0.0/3150'), both paths leaving the parking lot quickly join to reach a posted junction for Bear Creek Trail—head left on Canyon Creek Trail. Entering the wilderness, the trail passes beneath ponderosa pines, Douglas firs, incense cedars, madrone, black oaks, bigleaf maples, dogwoods, and alders. Thimbleberry and vine maple thrive in the lush understory. Initially traversing above rushing Bear Creek, you soon descend to cross the transparent stream. A few canyon live oaks can be seen as you climb out of the gully to begin paralleling above Canyon Creek.

While Canyon Creek is often visible below through the trees, access is generally not possible. The pale granite boulders that fill the creekbed are in stark contrast to the dark metamorphic rocks of the opposite peaks, and are representative of the overall regional geology. Occupying all of northwest California, the Klamath Mountains are a complex geologic mosaic formed from a wide variety of metamorphic rocks, which accreted to the continent over the past few hundred million years. Once connected with the northern Sierra Nevada, the mountain range was intruded by magma rising through the crust in enormous subterranean bubbles between 150 and 120 million years ago.

Solidifying as granite before reaching the surface, these bubbles became exposed as erosion stripped away the overlying rock. Unlike the heavily intruded central and southern Sierra, the Klamath Mountains contain only isolated pockets of granite—the Trinity Alps is the most spectacular example. The rocks of Canyon Creek have been washed down from the granitic heart of the mountains, but here the trail still winds above a complex metamorphic assemblage. However, you soon cross the geologic divide where soaring peaks of granite become visible up-canyon.

The trail steadily climbs above Canyon Creek, becoming increasingly rocky as it navigates a few intermittent switchbacks before reaching beautiful Canyon Creek Falls (3.8/4450´) and the first easy river access. The falls mark the halfway point for the hike, and the end of the deep V-shaped river gorge of lower Canyon Creek. Above the falls, relatively recent glaciation has carved the valley into a broad U, with a delightfully flat canyon bottom. Vegetation is lush and California redbud, huckleberry

oak, and seasonal wildflowers line the trail. Leaving the vicinity of the creek, the trail switchbacks 200 feet to reach the junction with Boulder Creek Trail (6.0/5000´).

Continuing up-canyon on Canyon Creek Trail, notice the appearance of mountain hemlock and western white pine in the forest mix. As the trail begins to climb again, notice the glacial polish in evidence on nearby rocks. Red fir and aspens appear next. Soon the final push to Lower Canyon Creek Lake begins near another beautiful waterfall, this one only visible through the trees. Becoming rocky and narrow, the trail is marked by numerous small cairns as it climbs 200 feet to a rock-hop across Canyon Creek. The lake is just ahead (7.5/5606´).

With a backdrop of Wedding Cake (8569´) and more distant Thompson Peak (9002´) at the head of the canyon, the lake is scenic. It also harbors numerous specimens of Brewer spruce around the shore. The rarest spruce in the world, Brewer spruce exists only in scattered locations throughout the Klamath Mountains and is

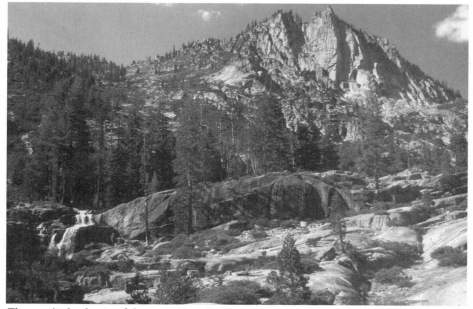

The granite landscape of the central Trinity Alps

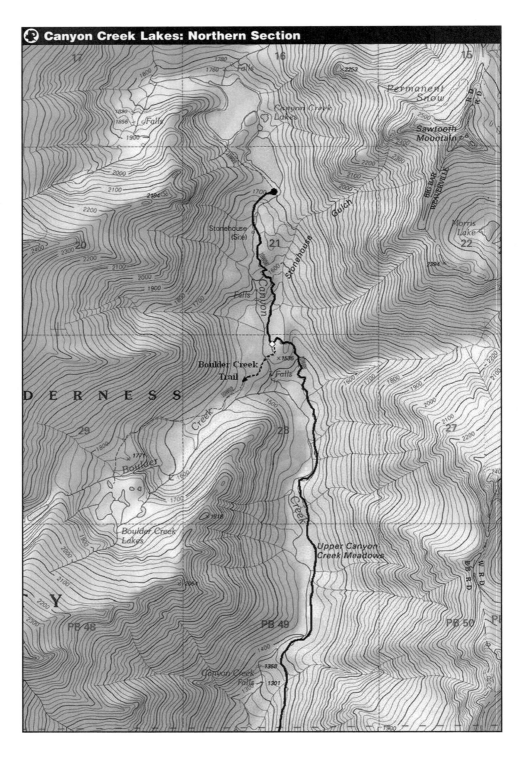

Canyon Creek Lakes: Northern Section

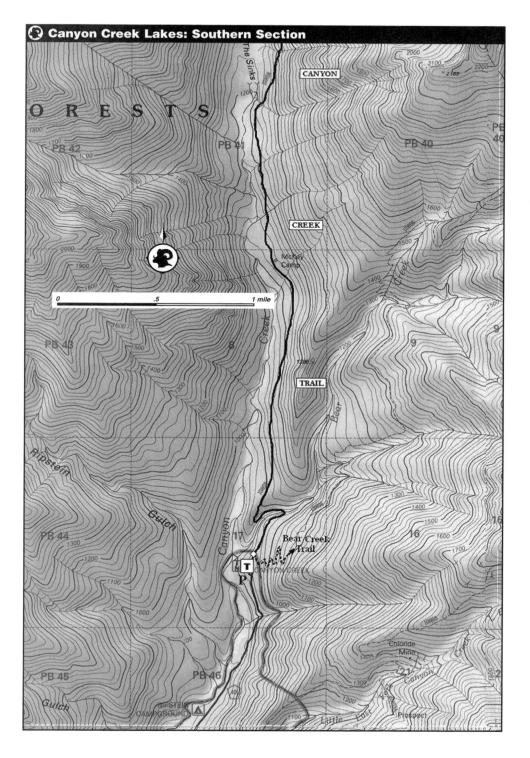

Canyon Creek Lakes: Southern Section

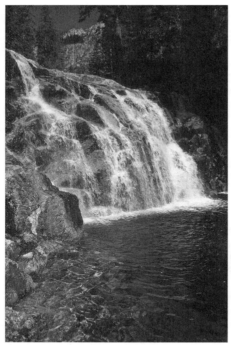

Canyon Creek Falls

easily identified by its distinctive dangling branches. Useless for lumber, and growing in generally remote locations, the tree has been little studied and its origins remain a mystery.

Several adventurous side trips are possible from the lake. Past the lake's northwest corner, more rugged Upper Canyon Creek Lake is accessible via a short brushy scramble. Tiny El Lake perches northeast nearly 800 feet above the upper lake and is reputed excellent for fishing. Thompson

Peak, the highest summit in the Trinity Alps, cannot be bagged from this approach without technical equipment. Revel in the majesty of these mountains before returning the way you came.

Nearest Visitors Center: Weaverville District Ranger Office, (530) 623-2121, located on Hwy. 299 on Weaverville's west side, is open 8 AM–4:30 PM Monday through Friday, and 8 AM–5 PM on Saturdays during summer.

Backpacking Information: A wilderness permit is required, obtainable free either outside the Weaverville District Ranger Office or at the Junction City ranger station (0.1 mile east of Canyon Creek Rd.). Campsites are abundant in the valley above Canyon Creek Falls, but only a few good sites exist around Lower Canyon Creek Lake; there are none at the upper lake. Black bears are common in the area—hang your food or bring a canister. No quota is currently in effect for this very popular trailhead.

Nearest Campground: Ripstein Campground, located on Canyon Creek Rd. 0.7 mile before the trailhead, has excellent walk-in sites (free, no water).

Additional Information: www. fs.fed.us/r5/shastatrinity

HIKE 55

Marble Rim

The Marbles

Highlights	Serene lakes, mountains of marble
Distance	17.4 miles round-trip
Total Elevation Gain/Loss	2800´/2800´
Hiking Time	10–14 hours
Optional Map	USGS 7.5-min. *Marble Mountain*
Best Times	Mid-June through October
Agency	Marble Mountain Wilderness
Difficulty	★★★★

Designated a primitive area in 1931 and established as one of California's first wilderness areas in 1953, Marble Mountain Wilderness protects nearly a quarter million acres of pristine California. You might think that the deep lakes, striking mountains, lush forest, abundant wildlife, and isolation would attract droves of hikers. But they don't.

The Hike ascends to the impressive cliffs of the Marble Mountains via serene Sky High Lakes Basin, a long dayhike best done as an easy overnight trip. Despite the low elevation, snow lingers on the trail well into June and usually returns by the end of October. This is (deservedly) the most popular hike in the wilderness, but crowds will be light relative to other alpine regions of the state. Fishing is possible in the Sky High lakes. Water is available at the trailhead until late September and sources are plentiful along the hike.

To Reach the Trailhead: Take Scott River Rd. 14.5 miles west from Fort Jones

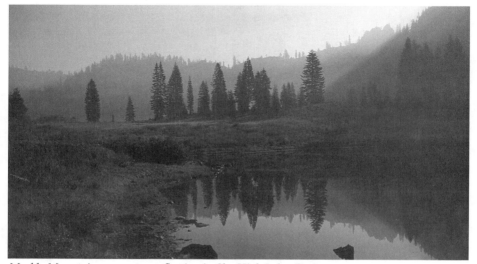

Marble Mountain moment: a reflection in Sky High Lakes Basin

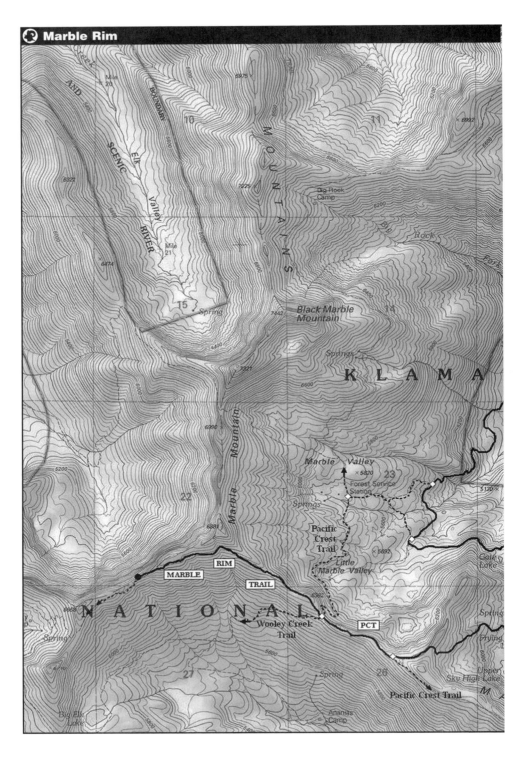

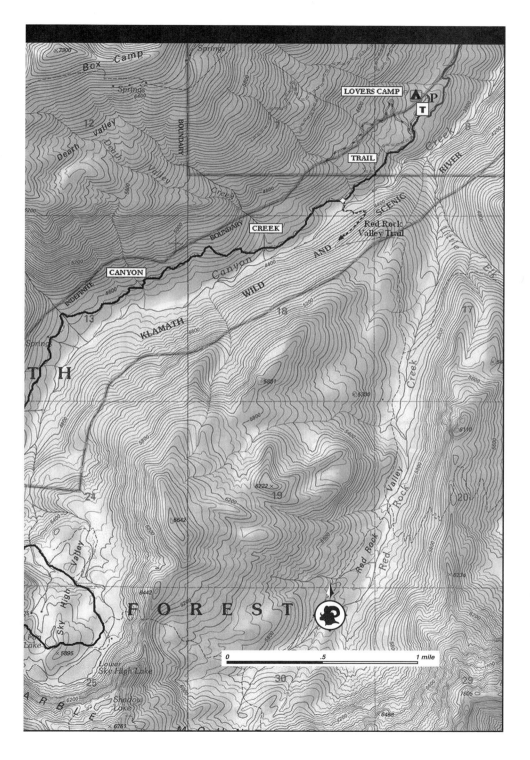

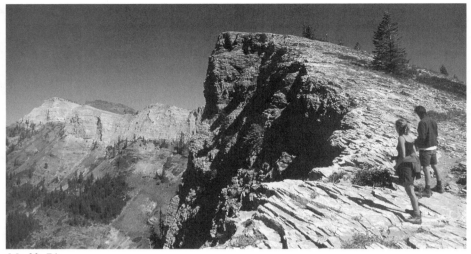

Marble Rim

on Hwy. 3 to Indian Scotty Campground and turn left (south) onto Forest Service Rd. 44N45, posted for Lovers Camp. Bear left at the immediate fork and continue on the sinuous, one-lane paved road as it climbs 7.5 miles to a large parking lot at the road's end.

Description: From the trailhead (0.0/4150´), start out on Canyon Creek Trail, passing two established campsites and entering the lush forest. Douglas firs, tanoaks, and bigleaf maples are common sights overhead, and trail markers, wild ginger, and ferns line the path. In 0.1 mile, the trail reaches a confusing intersection of unpaved roads—continue on the trail found diagonally across the road. Passing a wilderness boundary sign hammered to a Douglas fir, you soon reach a posted fork (0.7/4250´) in the level trail. The trail to Red Rock Valley heads left, but you continue right on Canyon Creek Trail toward Marble Valley.

While the hike parallels rushing Canyon Creek for several miles, it remains unseen below you for the duration. Crossing flowing Death Valley Creek, the trail then climbs briefly before dropping to cross Big Rock Fork. The logs that litter the bouldery watercourse provide evidence of the

ferocity that winter rains and flood bring to the region's otherwise small streams. Shortly thereafter, the trail abruptly turns upslope and begins climbing steeply uphill. Intermittent switchbacks eventually bring you to the junction for Marble Valley (4.1/5320´). Marble Valley provides faster and more direct access to the Marble Mountains but entirely misses Sky High Lakes Basin. If you are short on time, bear right and continue uphill to the Marble Valley Cabin (closed to the public) and the Pacific Crest Trail junction. Head south on the PCT until you reach the Marble Rim Trail. This marble-strewn route also makes an excellent return trail at the end of the day.

Bearing left toward Sky High Lakes, you climb more gradually and soon pass another junction for Marble Valley (4.4/5500´) on the right. Curving east, the trail offers the first views of the Marble Mountains to the west before making a final ascent into Sky High Lakes Basin. After you crest a final rise, diminutive and willow-choked Gate Lake welcomes you to the gently rolling basin.

Carved out by recent glaciation within the past 2 million years, the basin holds several lakes. While use paths crisscross the area, the actual trail leads first to larger Lower Sky High Lake (6.0/5775´) in the basin's southeast corner, before turning west toward tiny Frying Pan Lake, and then climbing out of the basin. The trees are diverse—white fir, red fir, mountain hemlock, western white pine, and large groves of aspen can all be found. In addition, a rare stand of subalpine fir grows here as well. A common tree throughout the Pacific Northwest, subalpine fir's range extends north to the subarctic. But in Northern California it only occurs here and in scattered locations within nearby Russian Wilderness, and both populations are more than 50 miles distant from the next closest stand in southern Oregon, according to Ronald Lanner in *Conifers of California*. Despite existing at the extreme southern limit of their range, the trees seem to be thriving. Identify them by their narrow spire shape, strongly aromatic crushed needles, and close resemblance to red fir. Within the lakes amphibians thrive: Frogs, tadpoles, and the ubiquitous, orange-bellied roughskin newt all entertain along the shorelines. In early October, cattle graze here as well.

Continuing west toward the Marble Mountains, the trail climbs steeply up the slopes and offers superlative views of the entire basin before attaining the divide and reaching a junction with the PCT (7.1/6400´). From the ridge, the entire drainage of Wooley Creek reveals itself within a horseshoe of peaks dominated west-southwest by granite Medicine Mountain (6837´). From its headwaters here, Wooley Creek plummets more than 5000 feet through dense, undisturbed forest to join the Salmon River 20 miles away. Its entire pristine watershed is protected within the wilderness.

Once on the ridge, turn right and follow the PCT descending gently northwest to a four-way junction (8.6/6230´), where you continue straight toward Marble Rim. Right leads down into Marble Valley, the possible shortcut or return route mentioned above. Left drops down in just over

a mile to Big Elk Lake, visible southwest in an open grassy area. Now climbing again toward the marble slopes, the trail remains below the divide until it reaches the low, treeless notch along Marble Rim (8.7/6480´).

Part of the complex geologic mix of the Klamath Mountains, the Marble Mountains most likely originated more than 200 million years ago from coral reefs surrounding an ancient, offshore island or landmass. Over the millennia, the reefs' skeletal remains collected in thick layers that eventually solidified into the sedimentary rock, limestone. Smashed into North America, the limestone was transformed to marble and exposed by erosion to form the spectacular cliffs before you. North, Rainy Valley trails away more than a thousand feet below. Southeast are the jagged peaks of the highest mountains in the wilderness, and the Trinity Alps (Hike 54) can often be seen on the distant southern skyline. Return as you came via Sky High Lakes Basin or take the Marble Valley shortcut.

Nearest Visitors Center: Scott River Ranger Station, (530) 468-5351, located in Fort Jones by the intersection with Scott River Rd., is open 8 AM–4:30 PM Monday through Friday.

Backpacking Information: No wilderness permit is necessary, but a valid campfire permit is required, obtainable at any national forest visitors center. Sites are abundant in the Sky High Lakes Basin.

Nearest Campground: Free overnight camping is permitted in sites around the trailhead. Otherwise, try Indian Scotty Campground (28 sites, $10) at the Lovers Camp turnoff from Scott River Rd.

Additional Information: www. fs.fed.us/r5/shastatrinity

HIKE 56

Castle Dome

The Granite Castle

Highlights	Jagged thrusting pillars of granite
Distance	5.4 miles round-trip
Total Elevation Gain/Loss	2300´/2300´
Hiking Time	3–5 hours
Optional Map	USGS 7.5-min. *Dunsmuir*
Best Times	April through October
Agency	Castle Crags State Park
Difficulty	★★★★

Raking the sky, a jagged protrusion of granite bursts from the slopes above Interstate 5. Needle-sharp spires, bulbous domes, a mania of fantastical granite blades, Castle Crags is unlike anywhere else in California. Add to this views of Mt. Shasta and you have a hike that must be done.

The Hike follows the steep trail to Castle Dome (4966´), a tall rounded peak in the middle of Castle Crags. Unlike trails in nearby high-elevation areas, the hike here usually becomes free of snow by April and does not receive snowfall again until November. While summer months are crowded, spring and fall offer increased

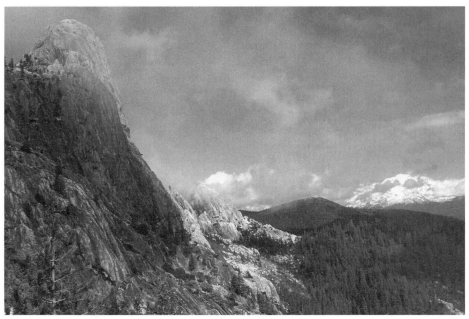

Castle Dome and distant Mt. Shasta

Castle Dome

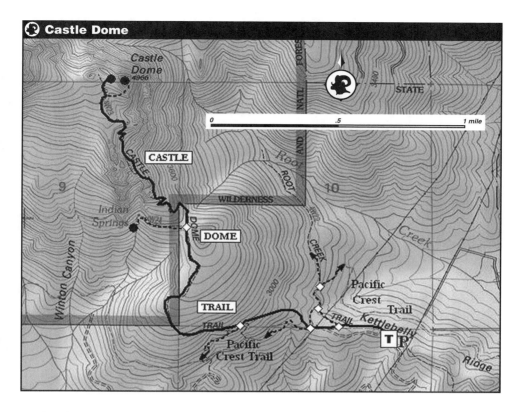

solitude and views of a snow-mantled Mt. Shasta. While no water is available at the trailhead, sources can be found by the visitors center, in the campground, and halfway at Indian Springs.

To Reach the Trailhead: Take the Castella off-ramp from Interstate 5 and head west, immediately turning right into Castle Crags State Park. Turn right past the entrance station toward Crags Trail and Vista Point and proceed 2 miles, passing the campground before reaching the parking lot at the road's end—RVs and trailers are not allowed on this steep and narrow road. There is a day-use fee of $6.

Description: From the trailhead at the west end of the lot (0.0/2580´), the level double-track trail begins climbing among second-growth Douglas firs, incense cedars, bigleaf maples, alders, ponderosa pines, black oaks, and poison oak to quickly reach a junction with Root Creek

Trail—bear left and continue on Castle Crags Trail. After a few switchbacks, the trail crosses the Pacific Crest Trail beneath some power lines (0.4/2680´) and continues climbing. Canyon live oak begins to appear and the small Indian Creek drainage is visible below you to the west, before a gradually rising traverse brings you to the junction with Bob's Hat Trail (0.6/2910´)—continue upward on Castle Crags Trail. Crossing into Castle Crags Wilderness, the rising trail briefly levels out on the eastern slope of Indian Creek, and offers the first tantalizing glimpses of granite crags and the deep east-west drainage of Castle Creek. Formed between 170 and 225 million years ago when the Klamath Mountains and Sierra Nevada were joined as one continuous mountain range, the granite of Castle Crags closely resembles the rock of the eastern Sierra Nevada in both age and composition.

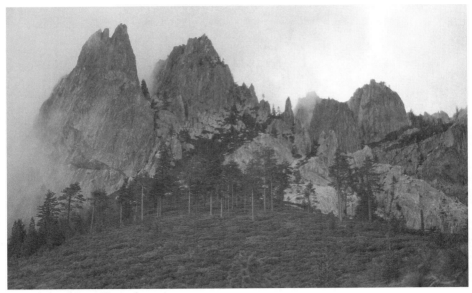

Jagged thrusting pillars of granite

At the posted junction for Indian Springs (1.5/3560´), a brief and highly recommended side trip leads to a series of lush springs emerging from the hillside and dribbling out of cracks in a mossy 25-foot-high block of granite. Back on the main trail, the route gets rocky and steep, switchbacking rapidly as sugar pine and increasing manzanita line the path. Mt. Shasta soon appears for the first time beyond the sheer east face of Castle Dome. The fire lookout on top of Mt. Bradley (5556´) is visible between the two.

Weaving through jagged pillars of granite surmountable only by climbing spiderpeople, the trail, occasionally hewn into solid rock, begins to diverge into a maze of use paths near the top. The wider main trail is generally easy to follow; it terminates at a fenced overlook with a view into the deep crevice between Castle Dome and the neighboring crags. The thick ground cover of the upper crags is primarily manzanita and huckleberry oak; the trees are sugar and ponderosa pine. The summit of Castle Dome (2.7/4966´) can be bagged from the south with some precarious scrambling—follow the easiest route up the south face and wrap around to the east. Return the way you came.

Nearest Visitors Center: Castle Crags State Park Visitors Center, (530) 235-2684, located at the park entrance, is open 8 AM–6 PM daily May through September and sporadically in October through April.

Backpacking Information: While not allowed within the state park, backcountry camping is allowed within Castle Crags Wilderness—no wilderness permit is needed. A few possible sites exist around Castle Dome, but there is no water above Indian Springs.

Nearest Campground: Castle Crags State Park Campground has 76 sites ($15–$20, depending on season). Reservations are recommended in the summer; call (800) 444-7275 or visit www.reserveamerica.com.

Additional Information: www.parks.ca.gov

HIKE 57

Heart Lake

Lighthearted

Highlights	The quick and easy Shasta-Trinity experience
Distance	1.8 miles round-trip
Total Elevation Gain/Loss	700´/700´
Hiking Time	1–2 hours
Optional Map	USGS 7.5-min. *Seven Lakes Basin*
Best Times	June through October
Agency	Shasta-Trinity National Forest
Difficulty	★★

Just north of Castle Crags Wilderness, tiny Heart Lake perches among boulders and trees high above Castle Lake. The massif of Mt. Shasta looms beyond, a great geographic transition easily observed without the physical punishment of other nearby hikes.

The Hike climbs past Castle Lake to reach Heart Lake, an easy hike with easy access that provides a quick sample of the region's geography. Fishing for brook and rainbow trout is popular in deep Castle Lake. Water is available at the trailhead.

To Reach the Trailhead: Take the Mt. Shasta exit from Interstate 5 and head west, immediately turning left (south) at the stop sign by the fish hatchery. Continue straight on W. A. Barr Rd. for 2.6

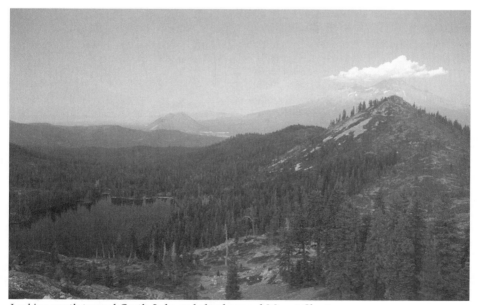

Looking north toward Castle Lake and cloud-capped Mount Shasta

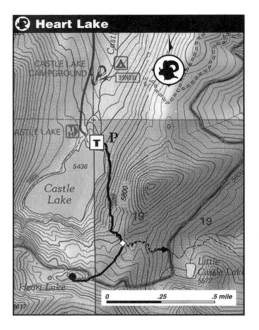

Heart Lake

miles, bearing left on Castle Lake Rd. at the Y-junction immediately after crossing the outflow from Siskiyou Lake. Castle Lake Rd. twists uphill for 7.5 miles to a large circular paved lot at the road's end.

Description: From the trailhead, drop down to Castle Lake (5436'). Known to the local Shasta-Wintun Indians as "Castle of the Devil," home of the evil spirit Ku-Ku-Pa-Rick, Castle Lake is one of the most extensively studied mountain lakes in all of California. Numerous informative placards highlight the work done here over the past 60 years. The wide trail strikes south along the lake's east shore among white fir and lodgepole pine, passing several heavily used primitive campsites before reaching a posted sign for Little Castle and Heart lakes.

The narrower trail begins to climb, traversing above Castle Lake and becoming increasingly rocky and root-strewn. Red fir begins to appear trailside, tantalizing views begin to appear between the peaks, and you soon crest the low divide above Castle Lake. The junction for Heart Lake is precisely at this divide. Continuing

straight on the obvious trail leads to Little Castle Lake in a quick half mile, but the unposted spur to Heart Lake strikes a hard right from the main trail and soon reaches its destination. Western white pine appear here, Mt. Eddy (Hike 58) is visible northwest through a notch in the ridge, and Mt. Shasta is apparent in its entirety.

Castle Lake is located at the eastern edge of the Klamath Mountains, a geologically complex range whose ancient rocks vary in age from approximately 80 to over 300 million years old. You are so close to the edge of this geologic province that you can see beyond it to the young rocks mantling Mt. Shasta, rocks formed less than 10,000 years ago. Here in the eastern Klamath Mountains, however, the peaks are composed primarily of the Trinity Complex—the largest exposure of ancient seafloor in all of North America. Yet the rocks around you are granite, the exposed surface of a small bubble of magma that rose through the older rock between 170 and 225 million years ago and solidified before reaching the surface. Castle Crags (Hike 56), a mere 6 miles south of here, represents the southern edge of this granite outcropping. The darker rocks of the Trinity Complex can be found mixed in with the lighter granite on your return trip. So back you go!

Nearest Visitors Center: Mt. Shasta Ranger District Office, (530) 926-4511, located in the town of Mt. Shasta at 204 West Alma St. (parallel to Lake St.), is open 8 AM–4:30 PM daily Memorial Day through Labor Day and Monday through Friday only the rest of the year.

Nearest Campground: Castle Lake Campground, located a half mile north of the lake on Castle Lake Dr. (6 sites, free, no water), is always full on weekends.

Additional Information: www.fs.fed.us/r5/shastatrinity

Mount Eddy

Seafloor Summit

Highlights	Killer views of Mt. Shasta and the Klamath Mountains
Distance	10.0 miles round-trip
Total Elevation Gain/Loss	2100´/2100´
Hiking Time	5–7 hours
Optional Maps	USGS 7.5-min. *South China Mountain* and *Mount Eddy*
Best Times	Mid-June through September
Agency	Shasta-Trinity National Forest
Difficulty	★★★★

Dwarfed by its towering neighbor, the rocky rise of Mt. Eddy may not immediately catch your attention but, if you want a secluded valley and a summit with sweeping 360-degree views, it should.

The Hike ascends Mt. Eddy (9025´) from the west, passing through a broad valley with easy access to Upper Deadfall Lake before steeply climbing to attain the summit. The high elevation of Mt. Eddy means that snow can linger well into June and return anytime in October. Crowds are unfortunately thick during the summer months, when as many as 60 cars can be found parked at the trailhead. Fishing is good in Upper Deadfall Lake and wildflowers are abundant in June and July. No water is available at the trailhead, but it can always be obtained from Deadfall Creek 2.5 miles from the trailhead.

To Reach the Trailhead: Take the Edgewood exit from Interstate 5—located 2 miles north of Weed—and go west. Just past the freeway, turn right and then quickly left in 0.2 mile to stay on Stewart Springs Rd. for 4.2 miles. At the wooden gate marking the entrance to Stewart Springs, turn right onto Forest Service Rd. 17. Proceed 9.5 miles on the paved road to the posted Parks Creek Trailhead on the left, just past the divide. An alternate trailhead can be found 1.4 miles farther down the road,

from a gravel lot at a sharp U-turn in the road. The trail leading from here follows Deadfall Creek along the valley bottom and avoids some areas of recent logging activity, joining the trail described below in 1.5 miles and adding an extra 750 feet of elevation gain to the hike.

Description: From the trailhead (0.0/6850´), the hike begins on the PCT and briefly parallels the road as it passes among Jeffrey pine, white fir, and western white pine. It then curves east to begin a long, gradually rising traverse above the valley that soon passes through an area of recent logging activity. As views open up, the glacial origin of the valley is readily apparent in its broad U-shape.

In season, wildflowers abound along the trail—please do not pick them. The reddish-brown rocks here are part of the Trinity Complex, the largest exposure of ancient seafloor found in North America. Accreted to the continent roughly 250 million years ago, these rocks weather to form a nutrient-deficient soil that provides habitat for many rare and unusual plants found only where such rocks are exposed. Let them live.

Reaching the valley floor, you come to a four-way junction (2.6/7230´). The PCT continues straight and the trail from the alternate trailhead joins from the right,

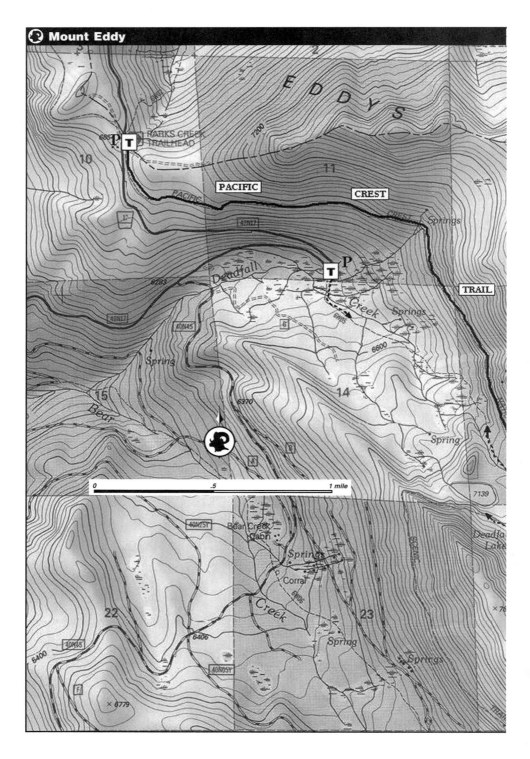

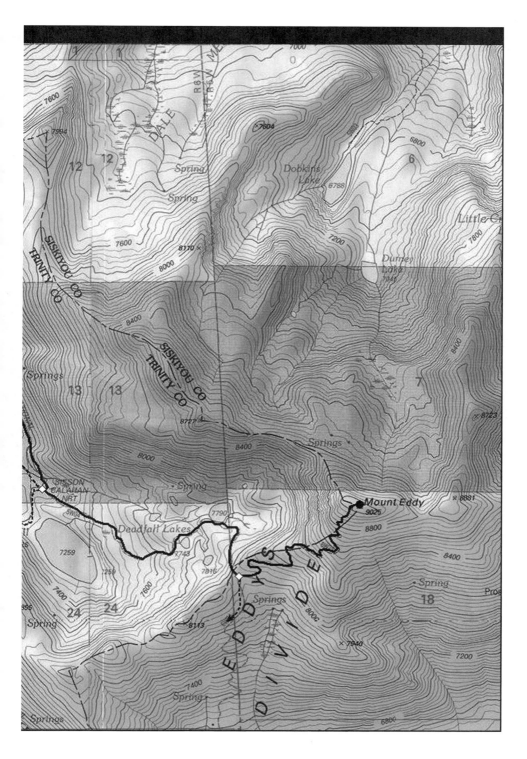

but you turn left toward Mt. Eddy, visible due east from here. Lodgepole pines now predominate. In 0.1 mile you reach an unmarked spur trail that splits right to Upper Deadfall Lake—fishing and swimming opportunities abound around the lakeshore.

Back on the main trail, your route quickly steepens where the trail switchbacks to reach several ponds in a small basin, the last source of water for this hike. As the trail continues to climb, an unusual stand of foxtail pine appears among mountain hemlock and western white pine.

Foxtail pine exists in two distinct populations separated by a gap of nearly 300 miles: one in the Klamath Mountains, of which the trees around you are the easternmost representatives; and one in the southern Sierra Nevada, found primarily in Sequoia and Kings Canyon national parks. How such a wide gap developed remains unresolved, but it seems likely that the two populations are remnants of a once extensive forest across California. Closely related to the ancient bristlecone pine (Hike 94), foxtail pines are able to survive in soils inhospitable to most other conifers. They are easily identified by the namesake needle clusters that extend densely along the branches.

Reaching a divide (4.0/8000′), you come to another junction—turn left and begin the grueling push to the top. The rocky path switchbacks more than a dozen times as it climbs the south ridge and provides increasingly airy views. Approximately halfway to the top, scrubby whitebark pines, the only conifer capable of surviving at such high elevations, have been twisted into krummholz form by the harsh elements. Ever-tightening switchbacks finally deposit you on the summit (5.0/9025′).

An old abandoned fire lookout blown over during the winter of 1998–99 crowns the summit, providing some shelter from windy conditions. The view is unbelievable. Mt. Shasta dominates the landscape east above the thin ribbon of I-5 and the perfect cone of Black Butte (6325′). To the west, a large stretch of the Trinity River drainage can be identified, and the distant peaks of the Trinity Alps (Hike 54) rake the skyline southwest. Due west are the mountains of Russian Wilderness, and Marble Mountain Wilderness (Hike 55) forms the skyline west-northwest. Return the way you came.

Nearest Visitors Center: Mt. Shasta Ranger District Office, (530) 926-4511, located in the town of Mt. Shasta at 204 West Alma St. (parallel to Lake St.), is open 8 AM–4:30 PM daily Memorial Day through Labor Day and Monday through Friday only the rest of the year.

Backpacking Information: A campfire permit is required. Besides a large campsite by Upper Deadfall Lake, the adventurous can sleep on the often-windy summit of Mt. Eddy.

Nearest Campground: There are several campgrounds along Hwy. 3, including Scott Mountain Campground, located 5 miles north of the junction of Hwy. 3 and U.S. Forest Service Rd. 17, and Eagle Creek Campground, 6 miles south of the junction (fee, water available). Hwy. 3 can be accessed from the trailhead by driving west on FSR 17 for 13 twisty miles.

Additional Information: www. fs.fed.us/r5/shastatrinity

HIKE 59

Hidden Valley

Mount Shasta

Highlights	The mountain. The views.
Distance	6.0 miles round-trip
Total Elevation Gain/Loss	2300´/2300´
Hiking Time	4–6 hours
Optional Maps	USGS 7.5-min. *McCloud* and *Mount Shasta*
Best Times	July through October
Agency	Mt. Shasta Wilderness
Difficulty	★★★★

An active volcano, Mt. Shasta towers over the landscape of Northern California and hides a secluded world of rock and snow on its southwest flank. Hidden Valley awaits. Mt. Shasta (14,142´) is part of the Cascade Range of volcanoes that extends from Northern California to northern Washington State, and includes such notable peaks as Mt. St. Helens and Mt. Rainier. With a volume of roughly 80 cubic miles, Mt. Shasta is substantial—the largest of the Cascade Range—and while its vents have been active for at least 100,000 years, the bulk of the current mountain has been constructed over only the past 10,000 years in a series of at least 13 separate eruptions. Hotlum Cone at the summit has erupted eight times during this period, covering the mountain and surrounding landscape with lava and debris flows. Its most recent eruption occurred in 1786 and there is no doubt that the mountain will flare again—current studies indicate that on average eruptions take place once every 250–300 years.

The Hike follows the popular trail to Horse Camp from Bunny Flat before continuing on an open cross-country traverse over loose and rocky slopes to Hidden Valley, a secluded depression offering outstanding views of the mountain. Because Mt. Shasta is primarily a mountaineer's

playground and Bunny Flat is the principal trailhead for the summit, crowds will be thick during mountain-climbing season (roughly April through July). The period following climbing season is best for hikers as crowds reduce drastically and the snow preferred by aspiring climbers melts off the trail. No water is available at the trailhead. Horse Camp has a freshwater spring and provides the hike's only water source.

To Reach the Trailhead: Take Interstate 5 to the town of Mt. Shasta and proceed east on Lake St. to join Everitt Memorial Hwy. and continue toward the mountain—Bunny Flat Trailhead is 12 miles from town on the north side of the road.

Description: At the trailhead (0.0/6900´), be sure to complete a self-issued day-use permit before striking out on the wide trail. Shasta red fir, manzanita, and lupine surround you as the trail climbs above a broad, dry meadow swept clean by the occasional heavy winter avalanche. Use trails crisscross the area—stay on the main trail and bear left at the next obvious junction.

Winding through open forest, the path curves west toward the edge of Avalanche Gulch, climbing more steeply now along the edge of a lateral moraine carved by recent glaciation. A trail from Sand Flat

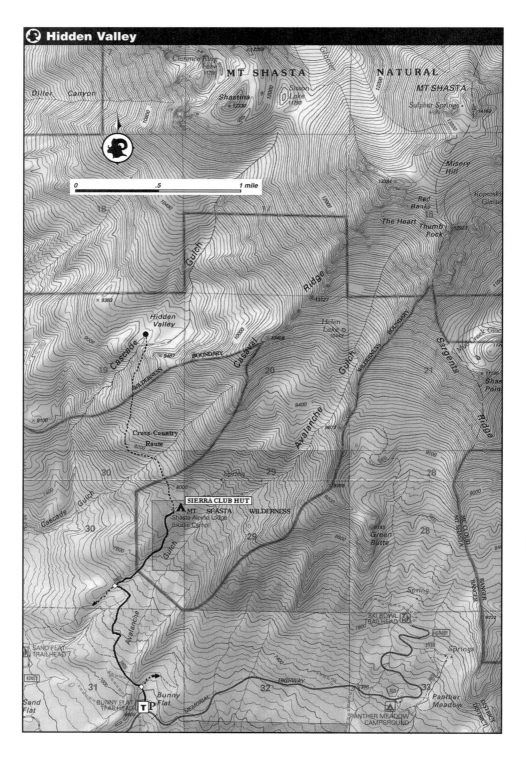

Hidden Valley

trailhead joins from the left (1.0/7330´) and you soon cross the wilderness boundary. The steady ascent leaves the shaded forest just before reaching the open vistas of Horse Camp (1.7/7880´). The Sierra Club hut located here is a historic shelter open to everyone for browsing, relaxing, and reflecting. The hut is manned by a seasonal caretaker until early October, and supplies are available here in the event of an emergency. The standard climbing route is visible northwest, winding east around the distinctive Red Banks near the top before reaching unseen Misery Hill and the final push to the summit. Campsites and well-marked trails crisscross the area around Horse Camp, and an excellent outhouse is nearby.

From Horse Camp, the route to Hidden Valley follows a generally distinct trail that has been marked in recent years by wands to minimize hiker impact. Please stay on the marked route—the loose slopes are easily scarred. The rocky route begins beyond the northern campsites and is clearly discernible as it immediately begins climbing north out of Avalanche Gulch. Lassen Peak (10,457´), the southernmost volcano of the Cascade Range, soon appears southeast beyond the eastern ridge of Avalanche Gulch. Cresting a rise, the trail levels out briefly in a flat bowl (2.0/8100´) where spectacular views west open up. The Eddys rise across the valley, with the high point of Mt. Eddy (9025´, Hike 58) visible just south of the perfect cone of Black Butte (6325´). Beyond Mt. Eddy, the distant skyline peaks of the Trinity Alps (Hike 54) can be picked out southwest on a clear day.

As the route begins climbing steeply out of the bowl, shrubby and twisted whitebark pines appear among the rocks, shrunken to krummholz form by the powerful elements so high on the mountain. The final trail section is less discernible, where the route scrambles above sheer Cascade Gulch to crest into barren Hidden Valley (3.0/9220´). Shastina (12,330´)

dominates to the north, a subsidiary cone formed between 9300 and 9700 years ago. The southern edge of Hidden Valley is part of Casaval Ridge, the sharp spine winding northwest toward the main summit, which offers some of the mountain's more technical routes when snow and ice are present. Return the way you came.

Nearest Visitors Center: Mt. Shasta Ranger District Office, (530) 926-4511, located in the town of Mt. Shasta at 204 West Alma St. (parallel to Lake St.), is open daily 8 AM–4:30 PM Memorial Day through Labor Day and Monday through Friday only the rest of the year.

Backpacking Information: A wilderness permit is required, and is available free anytime outside the Mt. Shasta Ranger District Office. A donation is requested for camping in the sites around Horse Camp ($5 per tent, $3 per person without tent). The only other options are the small sites in Hidden Valley, which don't have water. Be sure to follow the guidelines for the human waste pack-out program, if you are camping beyond an outhouse—supplies are available at the trailhead. While you will often find a community fire by the Sierra Club hut, no campfires are allowed elsewhere on the mountain.

Nearest Campground: Panther Meadows Walk-In Campground (10 sites, free, no water) is located 2 miles east of Bunny Flat Trailhead on Everitt Memorial Hwy. Also try McBride Springs Campground (10 sites, $10) on Everitt Memorial Hwy. Both are usually full during the summer, especially on weekends.

Additional Information: www. fs.fed.us/r5/shastatrinity and www. shastaavalanche.org

HIKE 60

North Gate

Northern Exposure

Highlights	The more removed north side of Shasta
Distance	4.0 miles round-trip
Total Elevation Gain/Loss	1600´/1600´
Hiking Time	3–5 hours
Optional Map	USGS 7.5-min. *Mount Shasta*
Best Times	July through October
Agency	Mt. Shasta Wilderness
Difficulty	★★★

California's largest glaciers spill north from the summit of Mt. Shasta, permanent icy expanses extending thousands of feet down the mountainside. The portal to the region is North Gate, removed from the bustle by a maze of dirt roads, access point for up-close views of glaciers and summit.

The Hike follows an obvious trail through an unusual whitebark pine forest to reach exceptional views of Shasta's upper north flank. The adventurous can continue for some distance up the mountain but the slopes require increasing technical skills and equipment above 10,000 feet. Because the area offers challenging mountaineering problems, climbers are plentiful here in late spring and early summer. As the snow melts away in July, climbing routes become hazardous; the region remains little visited until the following spring. No water is available at the trailhead or anywhere along this hike, once the snow has melted.

To Reach the Trailhead: Take Hwy. 97 north from Weed for 15 miles to Military Pass Rd. (Forest Service Rd. 43N19) and turn right. The route from here is rough, unpaved, and passes along a maze of logging roads. Follow FSR 43N19 for 4.5 miles to the junction with Andesite Logging Road and stay right. From this point to the trailhead, follow the roadside

direction signs to the trailhead, located 4 miles farther.

Description: Mt. Shasta (14,142´) is part of the Cascade Range of volcanoes that extends from Northern California to northern Washington State, and includes such notable peaks as Mt. St. Helens and Mt. Rainier. With a volume of roughly 80 cubic miles, Mt. Shasta is substantial—the largest of the Cascade Range—and while its vents have been active for at least 100,000 years, the bulk of the current mountain has been constructed over only the past 10,000 years in a series of at least 13 separate eruptions. Hotlum Cone at the summit has erupted eight times during this period, covering the mountain

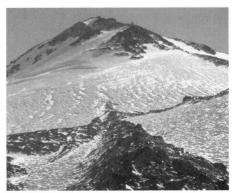

The alpine flanks of Mount Shasta

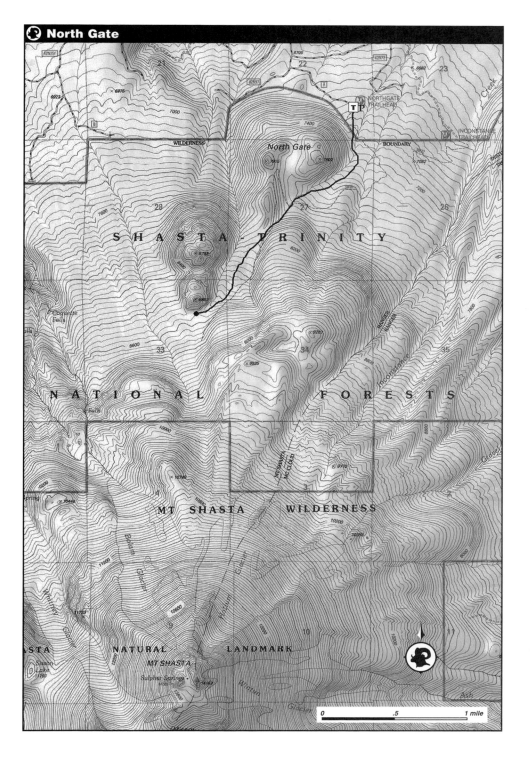

North Gate

and surrounding landscape with lava and debris flows. Its most recent eruption occurred in 1786 and there is no doubt that the mountain will flare again—current studies indicate that on average eruptions take place once every 250–300 years.

At the trailhead (0.0/7000´), be sure to complete a self-issued day-use permit before beginning on the dusty single-track trail. Mt. Shasta's summit looms over the trees from the parking lot but soon disappears as you pass beneath the branches of Shasta red fir and whitebark pine.

The trail ascends gently at first, but soon steepens noticeably as it climbs through a thick forest increasingly dominated by whitebark pine. Rarely attaining the size of the trees found here and seldom forming its own forest, whitebark pine is usually limited to shrubby growth just below tree line. It owes its existence to a unique symbiotic relationship with the Clark's nutcracker, a bird that harvests the pine seeds and caches them by the thousands in the ground for later consumption. Those left uneaten sprout, often forming thick clumps of trees from the bird's forgotten meal. The stubby, purple cones of whitebark pine usually glisten with sap, and their visibility at the end of sweeping upturned branches helps attract the nutcracker. Interestingly, the seeds will not drop of their own accord and must be harvested by these birds to plant future generations. Built like a small crow, a Clark's nutcracker can be identified by its light gray body and the white patches on its black wings and tail. Its call is a flat "khaa" or "khraa."

Where views first begin to open up (1.3/8000´) the trail levels out somewhat, and the broad rounded summit of the Whaleback (8528´) becomes visible nearby to the northeast. The path becomes faint as you proceed through a sandy valley littered with avalanche-swept trees—wands are usually placed to mark the route. Please follow the designated route as the fragile ecosystem here is easily scarred.

This hike ends where the broad valley curves west, providing an awesome view of Mt. Shasta (2.0/8550´). Looking south toward the summit, the broad expanses of Bolam Glacier (west) and Hotlum Glacier (east) merge into a large snow and ice field covering all angles of the upper mountain. Both are technical climbs with dangerous crevasses, requiring roped glacier travel for an ascent. Those feeling adventurous can continue south up the rocky slopes to 10,000 feet, but be aware that distances are deceiving—the top of the nearby slope here is 1500 feet farther up the mountain—and a summit pass is required to continue above 10,000 feet. Return the way you came.

Nearest Visitors Center: Mt. Shasta Ranger District Office, (530) 926-4511, located in the town of Mt. Shasta at 204 West Alma St. (parallel to Lake St.), is open daily 8 AM–4:30 PM Memorial Day through Labor Day and Monday through Friday only the rest of the year.

Backpacking Information: A wilderness permit is required, and is available free anytime outside the Mt. Shasta Ranger District Office. Campsites are plentiful in the upper valley. No water is available once the snow has melted. Campfires are prohibited.

Nearest Campground: There's nothing very close. Try the campgrounds on Everitt Memorial Hwy.: Panther Meadows Walk-In Campground (10 sites, free, no water), 2 miles east of Bunny Flat Trailhead, and McBride Springs Campground (10 sites, $10). Both are usually full during the summer, especially on weekends. Castle Lake Campground (6 sites, free, no water) is located a half mile north of the lake on Castle Lake Dr. and is always full on weekends.

Additional Information: www.fs.fed.us/r5/shastatrinity and www.shastaavalanche.org

HIKE 61

Sheepy Ridge

Tule or not Tule

Highlights	The land of a million birds
Distance	0.6 mile round-trip
Total Elevation Gain/Loss	180'/180'
Hiking Time	1 hour
Optional Map	USGS 7.5-min. *Hatfield*
Best Times	Year-round
Agency	Tule Lake National Wildlife Refuge
Difficulty	★

Tule (TOO-lee) Lake sits in the Klamath Basin, a region of vast wetlands providing habitat for 353 species of birds. Many are migratory, stopping over to rest and refuel before continuing on their journeys. Geese, swans, and ducks of all types pass through, peaking in numbers during March and early November and swelling the number of birds in the Klamath Basin to more than 1 million. Winter is a magical time—Tule Lake freezes over and raptors of all kinds congregate here. From December through February, the Klamath Basin hosts the largest concentration of bald eagles in the contiguous U.S.—more than 500 can be present in the Basin—and Tule

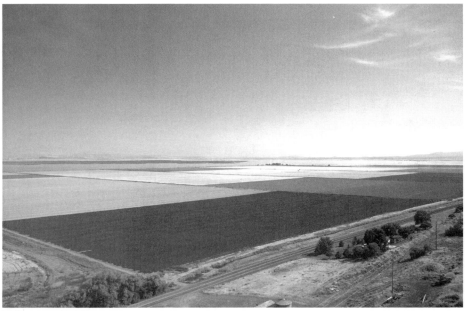

Tule or not Tule?

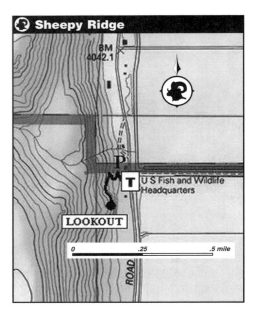

Lake is one of the best spots to observe them. During the summer resident ducks and other waterbirds raise their young, livening the area with their darling broods. Options for bird watching include an auto tour, self-guided canoe trails, and reservable photo blinds. The visitors center (see below) has all the details.

The Hike climbs Sheepy Ridge behind the Klamath Basin Wildlife Refuges Visitors Center, an easy hike that is primarily an introduction to adventuring around Tule Lake. It offers broad views of the landscape from an unusual stone hut perched above the sheer cliffs. The exposed trail is scorching during summer months, so sun protection is essential. While snow can cover the trail in the winter, the Tule Lake region is worth visiting year-round for its ever-changing seasonal birdlife. Water is available at the trailhead.

To Reach the Trailhead: Take East-West Rd. west from the town of Tulelake on Hwy. 139. In 4.8 miles, turn left on Hill Rd. to reach the visitors center in 0.5 mile.

The trail starts in the upper parking lot. Approaching from Lava Beds National Monument, take Hill Rd. 9.3 miles north from the park road—the junction is located immediately west of the Lava Beds north entrance station.

Description: Pick up an interpretive brochure at the trailhead before you begin. Climb through rabbit brush and sage, making three switchbacks before traversing over to the stone lookout at the trail's end. Constructed by the Civilian Conservation Corps in 1938, the enclosed hut offers respite from the sun's blistering rays.

Sheepy Ridge was formed as the adjacent land to the east slipped downward along a long, linear fault, forming a north-south ridge that extends more than 10 miles south into Lava Beds National Monument. Looking south down the ridge, notice the several cinder cones east of its terminus. The farthest east is Schonchin Butte (Hike 62). The collapsed form of Medicine Lake Volcano (Hike 64) occupies the distant southern skyline. As you face east, the perfect squares of reclaimed wetland surround Sump 1-A and the northern section of Tule Lake. The hills of Oregon recede into the northern distance.

Nearest Visitors Center: Klamath Basin National Wildlife Refuges Headquarters and Visitors Center, (530) 667-2231, is open 8 AM–4:30 PM Monday through Friday and 10 AM–4 PM on weekends and holidays.

Nearest Campground: Indian Well Campground (water, 43 sites, $10) is located 0.5 mile from the Lava Beds National Monument Visitors Center.

Additional Information: www.fws.gov/klamathbasinrefuges

HIKE 62

Schonchin Butte

Scorchin' Schonchin

Highlights	A sweeping vista of volcanic wasteland
Distance	1.4 miles round-trip
Total Elevation Gain/Loss	500´/500´
Hiking Time	1–2 hours
Optional Map	USGS 7.5-min. *Schonchin Butte*
Best Times	Year-round
Agency	Lava Beds National Monument
Difficulty	★

Lava Beds National Monument is a land smothered by recent lava flows, pocked with cinder cones, devoid of all surface water. A world both hostile and fascinating, it's almost entirely visible from the fire lookout atop Schonchin Butte (5253´).

This is an active volcanic area. The entire landscape was formed less than 1 million years ago when lava spilled across the surface and smothered it beneath thick flows of black basalt. Much of the lava originated in Medicine Lake Volcano to the west, but several vents within the monument have been active during the past 10,000 years. The Modoc Plateau is a part of the Earth's crust that is undergoing extension, thinning and cracking in places as it is pulled apart. These cracks allow liquid basalt from the Earth's interior to well up onto the surface, creating the lava flows and cinder cones seen in the monument today.

Schonchin Butte is a cinder cone that was produced by an active vent sometime during the past 10,000 years. As a new fissure allows magma to rise toward the surface, ground water is overheated, blowing large chunks of rock into a distinct cone shape around the surface opening. Once the actual magma reaches the surface it typically pours out at the base of the cone,

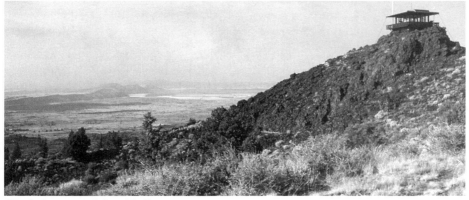

Fire lookout atop Schonchin Butte

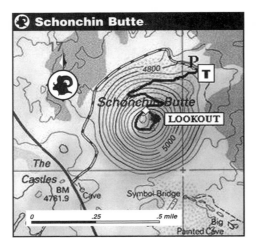

Schonchin Butte

4800

P T

Schonchin Butte

LOOKOUT

5000

The Castles o
BM
4761.9   Cave   Symbol Bridge

0   .25   .5 mile

Big
Painted Cave

flowing with gravity over the land. Schonchin Butte and the Schonchin Lava Flow, which flowed north over the heart of the monument, are textbook examples. This type of eruption is generally small and short-lived, producing a volcano in miniature that rarely erupts again.

The Hike climbs Schonchin Butte via a well-maintained trail to the summit fire lookout, an easy hike with several, strategically located rest benches. While the hike is partly shaded, the sun is intense during summer months on the exposed portions of trail. The monument is open year-round and receives light snowfall from November through April. Despite the intense sun, Lava Beds receives most visitors during summer months, making the rest of the year preferable for a hike. No water is available at the trailhead or anywhere along the way.

To Reach the Trailhead: Take Hwy. 139 northwest from Hwy. 299—the turnoff is just west of Canby. In 29 miles, turn west onto Hwy. 97. When you reach a fork in 2.7 miles, bear right onto Hwy. 10 and drive 10 miles to the monument border. From here, the visitors center is 4 miles and the turnoff for Schonchin Butte 6.2 miles. (Approaching from the north, the turnoff is 7.3 miles south of the north entrance station.) The unpaved road reaches the trailhead

parking area in 1 mile and is easily passable for all vehicles, though RVs and trailers are not recommended due to the tight turnaround. There is a $10 entrance fee, which is valid for seven days.

Description: From the trailhead (0.0/4800′), the wide path traverses up the north flank of the cone. Juniper, sage, rabbit brush, and mountain mahogany cover the slopes, and the fire lookout is visible above you. After two switchbacks, the trail forks. While both paths lead to the summit, the left is more direct, but the right traverses around the old cinder crater providing good views of the lookout's precarious roost. Go for the loop!

A wooden railing rings the lookout and you may have the opportunity to converse with the seasonal worker that staffs this active facility. Placards identify the surrounding landmarks, including Glass Mountain (Hike 64) and Mt. Shasta (Hikes 59–60). The fresh-looking, razor-sharp rocks of the Schonchin Lava Flow cover the ground below you to the north, barely colonized by plant life after thousands of years of erosion. Hidden among the cracks at the flow's northern end is Captain Jack's Stronghold, where a small band of Modoc Indians successfully resisted army attack for over six months by using the maze of caves and passageways in the lava flow. Lasting from November 1872 until June 1873, the Modoc War was the last Indian war fought in the U.S.

Nearest Visitors Center: Lava Beds National Monument Visitors Center, (530) 667-8113, is open daily 8 AM–6 PM in summer and 8:30 AM–5 PM rest of the year.

Nearest Campground: Indian Well Campground (water, 43 sites, $10) is located 0.5 mile from the visitors center.

Additional Information: www.nps.gov/labe

HIKE 63

Valentine Cave

The Underground

Highlights	Spelunking in a lava tube
Distance	0.5 mile round-trip
Total Elevation Gain/Loss	Negligible
Hiking Time	1 hour
Optional Map	USGS 7.5-min. *Schonchin Butte*
Best Times	Year-round
Agency	Lava Beds National Monument
Difficulty	★

Feel the cool inky darkness of a cave below a scorching volcanic desert. Lava tubes are formed as the sides and surface of a lava flow solidify, covering with hardened basalt the liquid rock that still courses inside. Once the flow stops, the lava drains away and leaves a hollow tube with several distinctive features inside. Lavicles are formed when liquid rock drips from the ceiling and solidifies. Benches found on the tube walls represent decreasing surface levels brought on by reductions in flow volume. Roof collapse typically exposes the lava tubes, which can wind underground for miles through passages of varying widths.

The Hike is the only one in the book that goes underground, following spacious Valentine Cave to its terminus well beyond the reach of the sun's rays. It's a good introduction to the 700-plus caves of Lava Beds, most of which are challenging to explore. It is short and easy but requires taking important precautions. Sturdy nonslip shoes are essential, and long pants and a warm pullover are recommended. Carry two sources of light with you at all times, but do not use gas or carbide lanterns. The visitors center provides flashlights free of charge during the day and sells simple, plastic hard hats, although Valentine Cave has ceilings sufficiently

high for you to walk upright. With its cool, constant, year-round temperature, Valentine Cave provides welcome respite from summer heat and winter chill, and is open all year long. No water is available at the trailhead.

To Reach the Trailhead: Take Hwy. 139 northwest from Hwy. 299—the turnoff is just west of Canby. In 29 miles, turn west onto Hwy. 97. When you reach a fork in 2.7 miles, bear right onto Hwy. 10 and

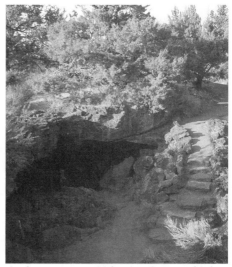

At the entrance to Valentine Cave, cool inky darkness awaits.

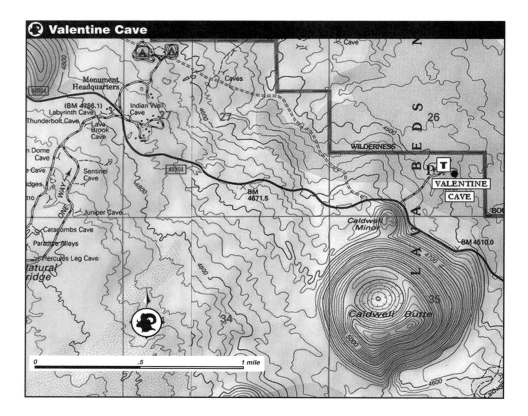

drive 10 miles to the monument border. From here, the visitors center is 4 miles. There is a $10 entrance fee, which is valid for seven days. Continue on the park road (Hwy. 10) 1.7 miles southeast of the visitors center and turn left toward Valentine Cave, reaching a substantial parking lot in 0.2 mile. Approaching from the south, the turnoff is 2 miles northwest of the park boundary.

Description: A paved trail leads 50 feet to the cave entrance, ringed by junipers and sagebrush. The collapsed blocks preserve solidified pahoehoe (puh-HOY-hoy), a ropy type of lava flow formed by basaltic magma. The magma associated with Mt. Shasta and the Cascade Range forms blocky, slow-moving flows known as aa (ah-ah). After immediately splitting around a large pillar, the cave resumes its tubelike shape in increasing darkness.

Lavicles cover the ceiling and benches. The cave narrows abruptly in the back, terminating in a small crawl space that continues a few feet farther. If the cave is empty of other visitors, turn out your lights to experience utter darkness.

Nearest Visitors Center and Campground: Lava Beds National Monument Visitors Center, (530) 667-8113, is open daily 8 AM–6 PM in summer and 8:30 AM–5 PM the rest of the year.

Nearest Campground: Indian Well Campground (water, 43 sites, $10) is located 0.5 mile from the visitors center.

Additional Information: www. nps.gov/labe

HIKE 64

Glass Mountain

Obsidian

Highlights	A recent lava flow laced with volcanic glass
Distance	1.0 mile or less round-trip
Total Elevation Gain/Loss	50´/50´
Hiking Time	1 hour
Optional Maps	USGS 7.5-min. *Medicine Lake* and *West of Kephart*
Best Times	Mid-June through September
Agency	Modoc National Forest
Difficulty	★

Lava cooled so fast it turned to glass. Medicine Lake Volcano is larger in mass than nearby Mt. Shasta, yet its slopes are so gradual as to be almost unremarkable. It is a shield volcano formed from basaltic lava, an extremely broad mountain very similar to those of the Hawaiian Islands. Measuring 15 miles east-west by 25 miles north-south with a surface area greater than 900 square miles, it is a prominent landmark of the Modoc Plateau.

Unlike the towering stratovolcano of Mt. Shasta, Medicine Lake Volcano hardly appears intimidating. This is because the entire top of the mountain collapsed approximately 100,000 years ago in a block 4 miles wide by 6 miles long, forming a large depression, or caldera. Smaller volcanoes welled up along the circular fracture, spilling lava both into the caldera and down the slopes of the mountain.

Glass Mountain, the most recent flow in the Medicine Lake complex, spilled down the volcano's east flanks less than 1000 years ago. Liquid magma is a soup of chemicals unformed and without

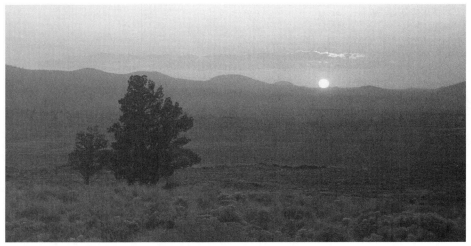

The sun sets behind the remnants of Medicine Lake Volcano.

Glass Mountain

To Reach the Trailhead: Take Hwy. 97 west from Hwy. 139 for 20 miles to unpaved Forest Service Road 43N99 on the right, the first of three possible turnoffs for Glass Mtn. (Approaching from the west, the turnoff is 4.8 miles east of the junction of Hwys. 49 and 97. Don't be tempted by the GLASS MOUNTAIN signs you see at the first two turnoffs at 1.1 miles and 3.9 miles from the junction.) As you head north on FSR 43N99 astonishing views of the flow appear before you reach a small, posted pullout at its base, 3.9 miles from Hwy. 97.

Description: From the trailhead (7050´) head up the obvious path. The lava flow has been worked by heavy machinery and numerous paths wind this way and that. While none of them really go anywhere, they make for considerably easier walking than over the jagged piles of rock. Obsidian is visible everywhere, glinting in the sunlight, interlaid with enormous amounts of gray pumice. A few, scattered lodgepole and western white pine pioneer this moonscape. Mt. Hoffman (7913´) is almost due west and Red Shale Butte (7834´) is south, easily identified by the bare red nubbin at its summit. These mountains are two of the smaller volcanoes that welled up along the fracture zone after the mountaintop collapsed. Glass Mtn. (7622´) is the bluff visible north, the highest point on the lava flow. Wander as much as you like, but don't lose your bearings in the maze of trails.

structure. Most lava flows are extruded slowly enough for the assorted chemicals to gradually cool and form discrete crystals, but occasionally the molten rock cools so quickly that it hardens unchanged, forming black glass, or obsidian. This transformation occurred at Glass Mountain. Native Americans prized obsidian's sharp edges for knives and arrowheads; at least four different tribes collected here, trading to neighboring tribes more than a hundred miles away.

The Hike is an opportunity to wander around on a recent lava flow and see obsidian in its natural state, though collecting it is prohibited. This is a remote part of California and odds are that you won't encounter anybody else, regardless of when you come. This hike is at a relatively high elevation for the region—above 7000 feet—and snow can fly as early as October. No water is available at the trailhead or on the lava flow.

Nearest Visitors Center: Doublehead Ranger District Office, (530) 667-2246, just southeast of the town of Tulelake on Hwy. 139, is open 8 AM–4:30 PM Monday through Friday.

Nearest Campground: There are four campgrounds around Medicine Lake (72 sites total, $7 per vehicle).

Additional Information: www. fs.fed.us/r5/modoc

Mount Vida

The Farthest Reaches

Highlights	A quiet mountaintop in the farthest corner of Northern California
Distance	3.2 miles round-trip
Total Elevation Gain/Loss	800´/800´
Hiking Time	2 hours
Optional Map	USGS 7.5-min. *Mount Bidwell*
Best Times	Mid-June through October
Agency	Modoc National Forest
Difficulty	★★

Four miles from Oregon, twelve miles from Nevada. In this remote northeast corner of California, in the northern reaches of the Warner Mountains, on top of Mt. Vida, get away from it all.

The Hike climbs Mt. Vida (8224´) via High Grade National Recreation Trail, an easy ascent along a disused jeep road that ends with a short off-trail jaunt to the summit. In this far corner of the state it is highly unlikely that you will encounter anybody regardless of when you come, although hunters travel the region in fall. Snow can linger here until late June. This is an extremely hot, dry area and summer months can be sweltering. Sun protection is always important. No water is available at the trailhead or anywhere along the hike.

To Reach the Trailhead: It is necessary to travel some rough roads. The final 2.9 miles climb 1200 feet on a very rocky road, and should not be attempted if you are overly concerned about your low-clearance vehicle. To get there take Hwy. 395 to the Forest Service Rd. 2 turnoff, 0.9 mile south of the Oregon border. Head 5.6 miles east on mostly unpaved FSR 2 to an unposted junction—0.4 mile after the posted turnoff on the right for Poison Lake and 0.7 mile before the Lily Lake Picnic Area. Those unwilling to drive the final

section can park here and make the arduous walk to the trailhead. Otherwise, turn right (south) and begin climbing. After 1.2 miles, bear left at the fork and continue 0.7 mile before bearing right toward Little Lily Lake at the next fork. Continue straight 0.4 mile later, where a road branches right toward the Sunset Mine. You reach a sign for the High Grade Trail 0.5 mile farther where the forest opens up—park by the roadside. While the road continues, motor vehicles are prohibited beyond this point. It is also possible to reach the trailhead from the east by taking FSR 2 west from Ft. Bidwell for 12.5 miles to the unposted junction described above, but it is a rough and rocky option.

Description: From the trailhead (0.0/7600´) continue on the road. Passing through dense fields of corn lilies, it offers good views of nearby Mt. Vida. The route briefly descends before climbing steeply back on the ridgetop—now with views west of giant Goose Lake. Continuing south, the road soon makes its closest approach to Mt. Vida (1.3/8000´) before arcing away west. Leave the road here and proceed by the easiest off-trail route to the summit ridge of the mountain.

From the summit, look southeast and stare down the trinity of Upper, Middle,

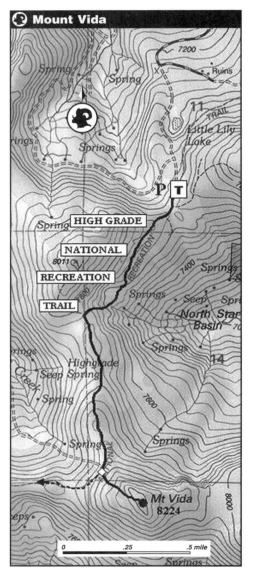

block dropped along parallel faults relative to the adjacent landscape, creating a basin hemmed in by sheer escarpments and covered with sediments washed down from the surrounding mountains. This is the defining geography of the Basin and Range Province, a distinct geologic region that essentially begins here and continues east to Utah. The valley floor is more than 3500 feet beneath you on Mt. Vida and, presumably, still dropping.

On the skyline due south are the mountains of South Warner Wilderness (Hikes 66–67). Looking northeast below you, serene North Star Basin is a small piece of wonderful wilderness, with the long plateau of Mt. Bidwell (8290´) rising beyond the basin. West beyond Goose Lake is the broad volcanic expanse of the Modoc Plateau, with the collapsed ring of Medicine Lake Volcano (Hike 64) clearly identifiable west-southwest. When you're ready, go back the way you came!

Nearest Visitors Center: Warner Mountain Ranger District Office, (530) 279-6116, is located in Cedarville on the east side of the Warner Mountains and open 8 AM–4:30 PM Monday through Friday. Also try the Modoc National Forest Supervisor's Office, (530) 233-5811, located immediately west of Alturas on Hwy. 299 and open 8 AM–5 PM Monday through Friday.

Backpacking Information: A valid campfire permit is required. Because campsites are hard to find, this trip is better done as a dayhike.

Nearest Campground: Cave Lake Campground (6 sites, free), 0.3 mile past the Lily Lake Picnic Area (see above). Fishing is good at both lakes.

Additional Information: www.fs.fed.us/r5/modoc

and Lower Alkali lakes, each encrusted with salt left by evaporating water. Enclosed on the east by the peaks of Nevada, they sit trapped in a graben, a valley formed through extension of the Earth's crust. Also known as a "pull-apart basin," Surprise Valley was formed when a large

HIKE 66

Mill Creek Valley

Welcome to the Warners

Highlights	Mill Creek Valley and the enigmatic Washoe pine
Distance	3.8 miles round-trip
Total Elevation Gain/Loss	750′/750′
Hiking Time	3–4 hours
Optional Map	*South Warner Wilderness* by the U.S. Forest Service
Best Times	Mid-June through October
Agency	South Warner Wilderness
Difficulty	★★

Not many people have even heard of South Warner Wilderness, and even fewer have been there. A mountain range in miniature, it is remote, rugged, beautiful, and still largely untraveled.

The Hike provides an easy introduction to South Warner Wilderness, following Slide Creek Trail as it climbs a small rise to descend into wonderfully open Mill Creek Valley. With its large aspen groves, the valley could make an ideal fall hike—rustling golden leaves, perfect weather, and solitude. Colors peak in early to mid-October. The hike's only drawback is the grazing cattle in the valley from July through September. This region was used for cattle and sheep grazing long before it was designated an official wilderness, and this use was permitted to continue under the 1964 Wilderness Act—yet another reason to come in October. Snow usually flies by November. Water is available near the trailhead in Soup Spring Campground.

To Reach the Trailhead: Take Hwy. 64 east from the town of Likely on Hwy. 395. In 10 miles, bear left on Hwy. 5 by a sign for Mill Creek Lodge. Proceed 3 miles to the turnoff for Mill Creek Campground. The paved road goes right, but you continue straight on the unpaved but easily traveled gravel road. Continue 1.7 miles to an unposted Y-junction—bear right. Take the turnoff for Soup Spring Campground 5.6 miles past this junction and proceed 0.4 mile to the trailhead parking lot on your left.

Description: After signing the register at the trailhead (0.0/6800′), begin hiking along an old road lined with large gray boulders. Mule's ears, white firs, and Jeffrey pines are all around. This is also a good place to begin looking for the rare Washoe pine. Closely related to ponderosa and Jeffrey pine, Washoe pine *(Pinus washoensis)* was only recognized as a separate species in 1938. Its habitat is limited to a few locations in northeastern California and western Nevada, with this region of the Warner Mountains nurturing the densest collection of specimens. It closely resembles its two relatives, possessing needles in bundles of three and developing yellowish plates on its trunk similar to those

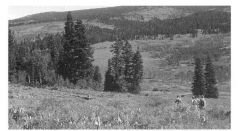

Hikers descend into Mill Creek Valley.

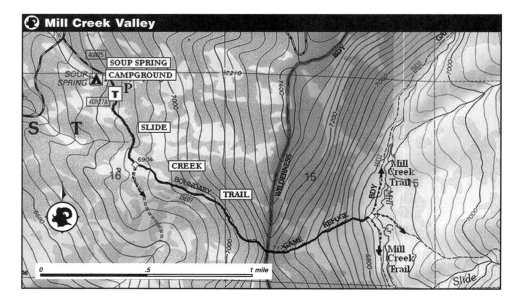

of ponderosa pines. Their cones identify them, however. Smooth to the touch, they look like Jeffrey pine cones but are noticeably smaller—only 2–4" long instead of 5–10". The wood resin produced by Washoe pine is also chemically distinct from that of Jeffrey pine and the two rarely hybridize. Genetically, it is more closely related to Rocky Mountain ponderosa pine; some experts speculate that it is a recent genetic offshoot from that population. According to Ronald Lanner in *Conifers of California*, its exact origin remains unknown.

The wide road quickly reaches a fork by four wooden posts—go left through the posts. Now single-track, the trail alternately passes through thick forest and open areas populated with sagebrush, rabbit brush, juniper trees, and more Washoe pines. Cresting the ridge (1.3/7150´), you enter South Warner Wilderness and begin descending into Mill Creek Valley. Views of the rolling topography quickly open up as you leave the forest. Eagle Peak (9892´), the highest peak in the wilderness, rises from the opposite side of the valley. Reaching mellifluous Mill Creek (1.9/6750´) the path intersects Mill Creek Trail, which heads both upstream and down. Neither

direction leads to any immediate destination but both are pleasant rambles. Go as far as you desire before returning the way you came.

Nearest Visitors Center: Warner Mountain Ranger District Office, (530) 279-6116, is inconveniently located in Cedarville on the east side of the Warner Mountains and open 8 AM–4:30 PM Monday through Friday. Also try the Modoc National Forest Supervisor's Office, (530) 233-5811, located immediately west of Alturas on Hwy. 299 and open 8 AM–5 PM Monday through Friday.

Backpacking Information: No wilderness permits are needed, but a valid campfire permit is required. There are campsites along Mill Creek.

Nearest Campground: Very close to the trailhead is Soup Spring Campground (8 sites, fee in summer but free after Labor Day).

Additional Information: www. fs.fed.us/r5/modoc

HIKE 67

Patterson Lake

Heart of the Warners

Highlights	The heart of South Warner Wilderness
Distance	10.2 miles round-trip
Total Elevation Gain/Loss	2900´/2900´
Hiking Time	8–12 hours
Optional Map	*South Warner Wilderness* by the U.S. Forest Service
Best Times	Mid-June through October
Agency	South Warner Wilderness
Difficulty	★★★★

Here's a hike to the heart of a small piece of mountain paradise.

The Hike climbs to Patterson Lake (9040´) through Pine Creek Basin, a strenuous trip that packs in all the wilderness has to offer, from soaring raptors to crystalline creeks, from sweeping panoramic vistas to the largest lake in the wilderness. The hike's second half, climbing out of Pine Creek Basin, is steep, sustained, and shadeless—skin-frying conditions during the summer months. Those looking for a shorter excursion should make the 4.6-mile round-trip to the Pine Creek crossing, a less demanding hike to a wonderful picnic spot. October is the nicest time to visit as aspens turn gold and weather is ideal. Snow can linger well into June along upper sections of the trail. While no water is available at the trailhead, Pine Creek is soon accessible.

To Reach the Trailhead: Take Hwy. 64 east from the town of Likely on Hwy. 395. In 9 miles, bear left on Hwy. 5 by a sign for Mill Creek Lodge. Proceed 3 miles to the turnoff for Mill Creek Campground. The paved road turns right but you continue straight on the unpaved but easily traveled gravel road for 1.7 miles to an unposted Y-junction—bear left and continue on Hwy. 5 for 5.3 miles to the posted turnoff for Pine Creek Trail. Turn right, reaching the parking lot at the road's end in 1.4 miles.

Approaching from the north, take Parker Creek Rd. (Hwy. 56) east from Alturas for 14 miles to where Hwys. 31 and 5 split. Head south on Hwy. 5 for 10.5 miles to the Pine Creek Trail turnoff.

Description: An information sign and register mark the start of the trail. From the trailhead (0.0/6800´) the single-track trail passes through thick white fir where babbling Pine Creek can be heard unseen below you. The firs increase in size and are joined by large ponderosa pines as you cross into the wilderness by an idyllic stream confluence. Fill your water bottles here because the trail next travels away from the creek, seldom approaching it.

Becoming progressively steeper, the trail passes near several, shallow, swampy lakes before reaching the open meadows of Pine Creek Basin (2.3/7400´). While the trail crosses the creek and reenters the trees, you should continue a short distance ahead to an ideal picnic spot by a small bend in the creek. Of volcanic origin, Warner Mountains' rocks were formed from ash and lava flows extruded on the landscape roughly 30 million years ago. Within the past 2 million years, glaciers carved the upper mountain reaches and formed the broad bowl of Pine Creek Basin.

Back on the main trail, you begin the long brutal climb to the ridgecrest above.

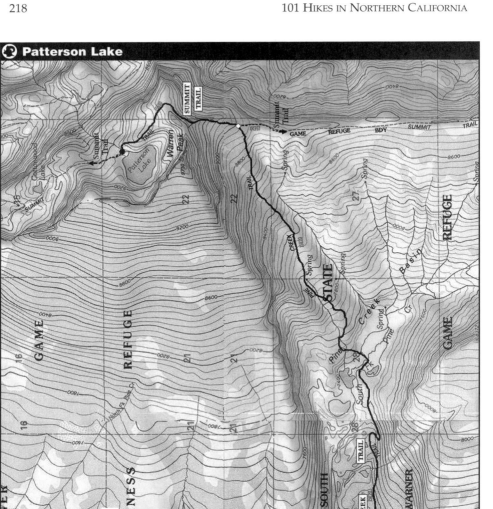

Patterson Lake

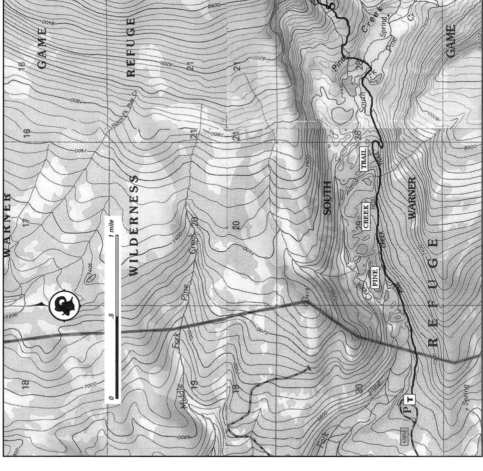

Views become increasingly expansive as the exposed path climbs through sagebrush, mule's ears, and spring-fed patches of corn lilies. A few isolated whitebark pines dot the slopes. Mt. Shasta's distinct cone more than 100 miles west becomes visible near the top before you reach the ridge and the junction with the Summit Trail (4.2/9000′).

Views east suddenly open up and the deep basin of Surprise Valley lies below you, brimming with the salt-encrusted trinity of Upper, Middle, and Lower Alkali lakes. Enclosed by Nevada peaks to the east, the lakes fill depressions in a graben, a valley formed through extension of the Earth's crust. Also known as a "pull-apart basin," it occurs when a large block of crust drops along parallel fault lines relative to the adjacent landscape. This is the defining geography of the Basin and Range Province, a distinct geologic region that essentially begins here and continues east to Utah. Surprise Valley is more than 4000 feet below you on the Summit Trail and, presumably, still dropping. Eagle Peak (9892′), the highest peak in the Warner Mountains, is visible almost due south.

Turning north, the trail continues to climb before finally cresting a rise and dropping 300 feet to Patterson Lake (5.1/9715′). Exceedingly deep and green, Patterson Lake was formed 1.8 million years ago through glacial erosion. Backed by the sheer layered cliffs of Warren Peak (9710′), it boils with rainbow trout and is excellent for fly fishing. Rest and rejuvenate here before returning the way you came.

Nearest Visitors Center: Warner Mountain Ranger District Office, (530) 279-6116, is inconveniently located in Cedarville on the east side of the Warner Mountains and open 8 AM–4:30 PM Monday through Friday. Also try the Modoc National Forest Supervisor's Office, (530) 233-5811, located immediately west of Alturas on Hwy. 299 and open Monday through Friday 8 AM–5 PM.

Backpacking Information: No wilderness permit is needed, but a valid campfire permit is required. Campsites are located around Patterson Lake and in the Pine Creek Basin.

Nearest Campground: Soup Spring Campground is located a few miles to the south (8 sites, fee in summer but free after Labor Day). When approaching from the south bear right instead of left at the unposted Y-junction and proceed 5.6 miles to the campground turnoff.

Additional Information: www. fs.fed.us/r5/modoc

HIKE 68

Burney Falls

Burney Man

Highlights	A perennial waterfall unlike any other
Distance	1.2 miles
Total Elevation Gain/Loss	200´/200´
Hiking Time	1 hour
Optional Map	USGS 7.5-min. *Burney Falls*
Best Times	April through November
Agency	McArthur-Burney Falls Memorial State Park
Difficulty	★

Imagine a volcanic cliff 129 feet high. Over its lip twin waterfalls cascade into an iridescent pool. Springs gush from its face, showering lush vegetation with spray while birds dart through rainbow refractions of light. This is Burney Falls.

The unusual multitiered falls result from two distinct geologic layers stacked on top of each other. The upper layer is the porous Burney Basalt, which allows water to easily percolate to the nonporous formation underneath. Both layers are exposed in the cliff face, where water pours forth in a constant year-round flow. The volume of Burney Creek, spring fed less than a mile above the falls, varies little with season; the entire system gushes a steady 100 million gallons of water a day. The moist corridor below the falls is an ecologic oasis, harboring species not normally seen in the Modoc Plateau. Oregon oak, Douglas fir, vine maple, flowering currant, and bear clover are at the far limit of their respective ranges, accompanied by the more typical assortment of Jeffrey pine, black oak, and manzanita. The fish of nearby Lake Britton attract osprey and bald eagles, sometimes seen soaring overhead.

The Hike is an easy loop that descends to viewpoints of Burney Falls and explores the ecology of Burney Creek with the help of interpretive placards. The park is open year-round, but snow may cover the trail from Thanksgiving until April. Crowds are extremely heavy from Memorial Day through Labor Day. Fishing is popular (but challenging) in Burney Creek, although strict regulations govern the stretch of water below the falls. Above the falls, standard regulations apply and the fishing is just as good. Water is available at the trailhead.

To Reach the Trailhead: Take Hwy. 89 north for 5 miles from the junction of Hwys. 89 and 299 to the park entrance.

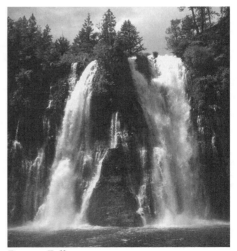

Burney Falls

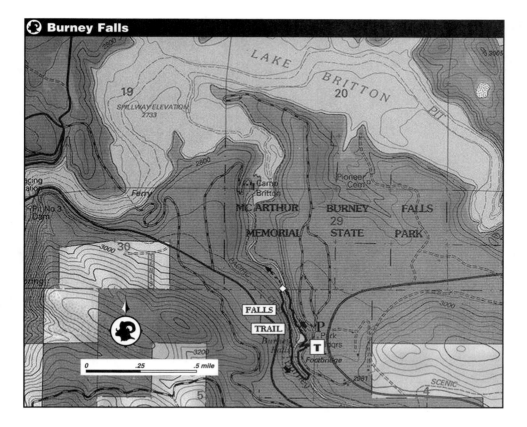

Burney Falls

There is a day-use fee of $6 per vehicle. Park in the lot across from the visitors center.

Description: From the parking lot, descend to the falls along the wide paved path, enjoying the cool 65°F temperature near the bottom. Continue downstream on the paved trail below large piles of broken Burney Basalt. Notice the springs that continually gush from the opposite streambank, indicating surface exposures of the geologic formation below the basalt. Cross the first bridge and continue on the dirt trail that heads an additional 50 yards downstream and splits—go left on the Falls Trail. Heading uphill away from the creek, the trail quickly reaches the level of the falls. Although unseen, the falls sound louder and more powerful here. Cross the river above the falls on a bridge (memorialized by visitors' chisel marks) to where the trail once again divides. Head left (downstream) to another parking lot where a rock-lined pedestrian path paralleling the road gets you back to the starting point. A half mile upstream from the bridge, the riverbed springs make an interesting side trip.

Nearest Visitors Center: Park visitors center, (530) 335-2777, is open daily in summer 10 AM–4 PM.

Nearest Campground: The state park campground has 128 sites ($15–20 depending on season). Reservations are recommended in the summer; call (800) 444-7275 or visit www.reserveamerica.com.

Additional Information: www.parks.ca.gov

HIKE 69

Magee Peak

Thousand Lakes Volcano

Highlights	The remote rim of an extinct volcano plus backcountry lakes
Distance	12.0 miles round-trip
Total Elevation Gain/Loss	3200´/3200´
Hiking Time	5–7 hours
Optional Map	*Ishi, Thousand Lakes, and Caribou Wildernesses* by the U.S. Forest Service
Best Times	July through September
Agency	Thousands Lakes Wilderness
Difficulty	★★★★

Thousand Lakes offers a less-traveled wilderness in the Modoc Plateau, complete with alpine lakes and sweeping mountain summits. Here you can contemplate the construction and destruction of a volcano from atop an eroding crater rim.

Spawned from the same volcanic activity that created Lassen Peak, Thousand Lakes Volcano has not been active in historical times. Although it was likely created within the past million years, it has been dormant long enough for a glacier to eat away its northeastern slopes and leave a horseshoe of peaks around the former crater. One of them, Crater Peak (8683´), is the highest point in Lassen National Forest. Thousand Lakes Wilderness is small, only 16,335 acres, and does not have one thousand lakes—more like a dozen.

The Hike ascends Magee Peak (8549´), one of the peaks along the volcano's summit rim, passing several lakes along the way. Two of them, Everett and Magee, are located roughly midway and make a worthwhile destination for those unprepared for the full ascent. The approach described here from Cypress Trailhead in the northwestern corner of the wilderness receives lighter use than Tamarack Trailhead farther east. While this approach adds about 500 feet of elevation gain, it

avoids the popular but less exciting Lake Eiler area. You are more likely to encounter equestrians than hikers on this trail. Fishing is worthwhile throughout the wilderness. No water is available at the trailhead and none can be easily obtained for the first 3.5 miles and 1600 feet of ascent.

To Reach the Trailhead: Prepare yourself to cover some dirt roads. Take Hwy. 89 north from the junction of Hwys. 89 and 44 in Old Station for 11.8 miles to the turnoff for Forest Service Rd. 26, located 0.3 mile past the Hat Creek Work Center. Approaching from the north, the turnoff is located 1.6 miles south of the Hat Creek Fire Station and post office. Reset your odometer at the turnoff and head west on the unpaved road to the first junction (mile 3.6)—bear right to continue on FSR 26. Turn left at the next junction (mile 5.3), still continuing on FSR 26. At mile 8.3, turn left onto FSR 34N60 and follow it to the road's end at mile 11.0. The information sign at the head of the parking area marks the trailhead.

Description: From the trailhead (0.0/5520´), you pass through stands of sugar pine, red and white fir, juniper, and Jeffrey pine before quickly crossing rocky and seasonally dry Eiler Gulch. From here, a steady climb brings you into the

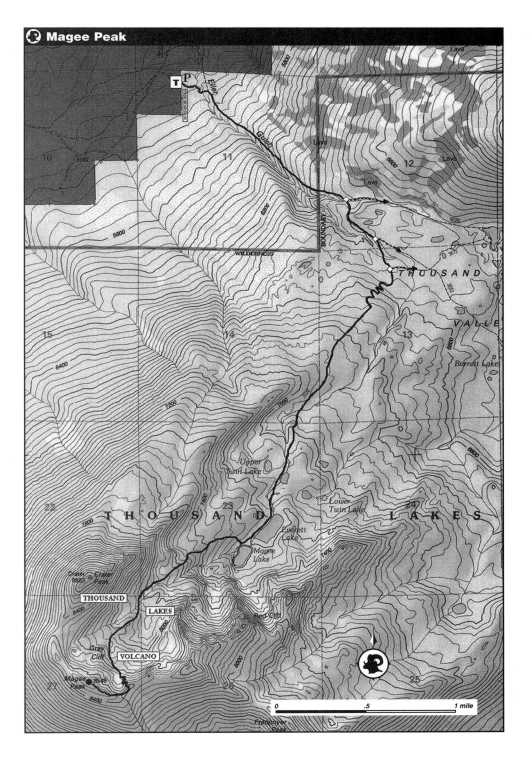

wilderness. Shortly after the weathered boundary sign (1.0/6240´) the trail levels out and reaches a junction (1.2/6330´)—go right toward Barrett and Magee lakes. A left turn would bring you to large but shallow Lake Eiler, a side trip not recommended unless you are desperate for water. Crossing Eiler Gulch, bear right again at two, subsequent, nearby junctions and stay on the trail (3E04) toward Magee Peak.

The trail switchbacks steeply southwest before leveling out in a forest where western white and lodgepole pine enter the mix. Mountain hemlock can also be identified near the lakes. After a long, level stretch and a brief climb, you pass dried-up Upper Twin Lake and soon reach Everett Lake (3.6/7180´). Magee Lake is next, accessed by going left on the unposted spur trail after Everett Lake. Both lakes are pretty and deep, good for relaxing and swimming.

Now climbing again, you enter the heart of the ancient volcano with Crater Peak towering above to the west. The trees are now almost exclusively mountain hemlock, although a smattering of whitebark pine can also be seen. The views become more expansive as you ascend up-canyon past the prominent red outcrops to the east, climbing nine steep switchbacks on the loose upper slopes to finally reach the summit ridge (5.3/8400´). Traverse west along the ridge to stand on top of Magee Peak (5.5/8549´).

As you look northeast, the scouring force of the glacier that carved this volcano is obvious. The broad valley formed by the glacier turns east below Freaner Peak (7485´), a satellite vent of the same volcanic complex. Fredonyer Peak (8054´) is the summit on the ridge extending due east from the crater rim. Lassen Peak (10,457´) is an easy landmark to the south, and Chaos Crags (Hike 70) are visible below its northern flanks. The ridge extending west from Lassen Peak ends in Brokeoff Mtn. (9235´, Hike 71), the highest remnant of Mt. Tehama. This ancient volcano once rose above present-day Lassen Volcanic National Park and was probably contemporary with Thousand Lakes Volcano. Return the way you came.

Nearest Visitors Center: Hat Creek Visitors Center, located in Old Station at the junction of Hwys. 89 and 44, is open late April through Memorial Day weekend 9:30 AM–4 PM, Memorial Day through mid-September daily 9:30 AM–4 PM, and mid-September through mid-December Friday through Sunday 10 AM–4 PM. The Hat Creek Ranger District Office, (530) 336-5521, is located in Fall River Mills on Hwy. 299 and is open Monday through Friday 8 AM–4:30 PM.

Backpacking Information: No wilderness permit is required but a valid campfire permit is necessary. Both Everett and Magee lakes have good campsites.

Nearest Campground: Honn Campground (6 sites, $8, no water) is 2.1 miles south of the turnoff for FSR 26 on Hwy. 89.

HIKE 70

Chaos Crags

Jumble-laya

Highlights	An ephemeral frog pond below a 2000-foot-high jumble of volcanic rock
Distance	4.0 miles round-trip
Total Elevation Gain/Loss	1050'/1050'
Hiking Time	2–3 hours
Optional Map	USGS 7.5-min. *Manzanita Lake*
Best Times	Mid-June through September
Agency	Lassen Volcanic National Park
Difficulty	★★

Roughly 1000 years ago, lava was extruded from Lassen Peak's northern flank. Too viscous to flow downhill, it piled up as giant domes of solid rock covered in loose rubble—Chaos Crags. A minor explosion about 300 years ago along Chaos Crags' northwestern slope triggered a huge landslide that traveled more than 2 miles to dam Manzanita Creek and form Manzanita Lake. Dubbed the Chaos Jumbles, the chaotic remains of the slide are plainly evident today.

The Hike climbs from the northwest corner of the park to tiny Crags Lake at the base of Chaos Crags. The "lake" is really a small pond fed only by snowmelt, which slowly evaporates over the course of the summer. Although largest in late June, it's never really big enough to be nice for swimming. Depending on conditions, it can be completely dry by August or remain as a tiny puddle throughout the season. Visitation here is relatively light, especially compared to other national parks. No water is available at the trailhead.

To Reach the Trailhead: Take Hwy. 89 to the Loomis Museum in the northwest corner of the park, located 0.4 mile east of the Manzanita Lake Entrance Station. There is a $10 entrance fee for Lassen Vol-

canic National Park, valid for seven days. At the east end of the museum parking lot, turn south on the road to Manzanita Lake. The trailhead is almost immediately on the left in 0.1 mile. If there is no space for your vehicle here, park in the museum lot and walk to the trailhead.

Description: The path, running within earshot of rushing Manzanita Creek, is initially outlined with large volcanic boulders. Jeffrey pine and white fir compose this open forest. The trail soon arcs away from the creek into dense trees and shortly passes a lush spring, which feeds a brook lined with alder trees. Sugar pine and red fir begin to appear. A few scattered Douglas firs can be identified, too, by their distinctive cones around you on the ground. The trail next ascends adjacent to the hummocky moonscape of Chaos Jumbles, occasionally visible through the trees. Chaos Crags increasingly loom east above the treetops, where the trail enters more open terrain carpeted with manzanita scrub. You pass through lodgepole pine a few hundred feet before breaking out into a rough boulder field with epic views of Chaos Crags.

The final stretch to Crags Lake (6630') is the most challenging, a 100-foot descent through sand and loose rock. Hundreds

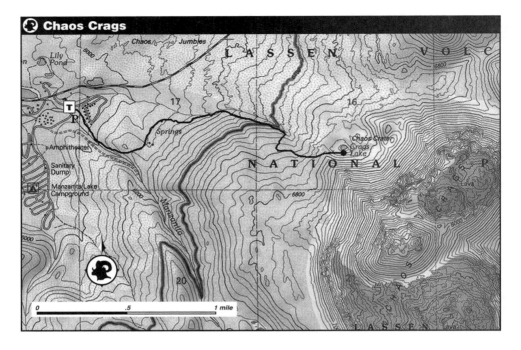

of tadpoles inhabit the lake and many mature frogs lurk along the moist shore, hurtling themselves behind nearby rocks at the approach of the curious hiker. Most trees here are sugar pines, although a few white firs and Jeffrey pines can be seen. A small chokecherry sits above the east end of the pond. Also known as Chaos Crater, this basin was created from the blast that triggered the massive landslide of Chaos Jumbles. Above, the pink scree slopes of Chaos Crags are deceptively high (not recommended for exploration); it's 1900 feet from the lake to the top of the highest promontory at 8530 feet.

Nearest Visitors Center: Loomis Museum and Visitors Center, (530) 595-4444 ext. 5180, is open 9 AM–5 PM daily mid-June through September and weekends only Memorial Day until mid-June.

Nearest Campground: Manzanita Lake Campground (179 sites, $18) is located on the south side of Manzanita Lake.

Additional Information: www.nps.gov/lavo

HIKE 71

Brokeoff Mountain

Tehama's Edge

Highlights	The eroded lip of an ancient volcano and far-reaching views of contemporary volcanoes
Distance	7.4 miles round-trip
Total Elevation Gain/Loss	2600´/2600´
Hiking Time	4–6 hours
Optional Map	USGS 7.5-min. *Lassen Peak*
Best Times	July through September
Agency	Lassen Volcanic National Park
Difficulty	★★★★

While everybody likes to climb Lassen Peak, try Brokeoff Mountain instead—a less-traveled peak with views every bit as exceptional.

Brokeoff Mountain (9235´) is the highest remnant of the former Mt. Tehama, a huge stratovolcano, which began erupting 600,000 years ago and grew to be over 11 miles wide at its base. Erosion and structural collapse wasted the volcano core once major activity stopped 200,000 years ago, leaving only the volcanic slopes. Lassen Peak (10,457´) was formed from more recent eruptions along the eroded eastern flanks of Mt. Tehama some 11,000 years ago.

The Hike climbs Brokeoff Mountain from the park road near the south entrance station, a strenuous trip flush with wildflowers in July and early August. Snow can linger a long time in Lassen Volcanic National Park, and usually does not disappear on this trail until very late June or early July. While less popular than the Lassen Peak Trail, this hike still receives ample use during the summer. No water is available at the trailhead but sources are plentiful along the first half of the hike.

To Reach the Trailhead: Take Hwy. 89 to the park's southwest edge. The trailhead is 0.4 mile south of the entrance station on the west side of the road. Parking is opposite the trailhead. There is a $10 entrance fee for Lassen Volcanic National Park, valid for seven days. Those approaching from the south are still required to pay at the entrance station.

Description: From the trailhead (0.0/6600´), you immediately start climbing through dense alder thickets. After crossing a small stream, the trail breaks out into a more open forest of red fir, incense cedar, and western white pine. The rocky pyramid of Brokeoff's summit is a beacon already visible northwest above the trees as you continue upward to rejoin the earlier stream. Paralleling the water, the trail crosses a small creek outlet (1.2/7460´) from tiny, unseen Forest Lake, and then starts to climb more rapidly. As you gain elevation, mountain hemlock appear and soon views open up—Lake Almanor is visible southeast and Forest Lake just below you. Leaving the creek (and your last water source), you traverse below the imposing southeast face of Brokeoff Mtn., making a few switchbacks among dense mats of lupine before cresting the mountain's south ridge (2.4/8400´). On a steady ascending traverse northwest, you have good views west across the Great Central Valley. All the trees here are mountain

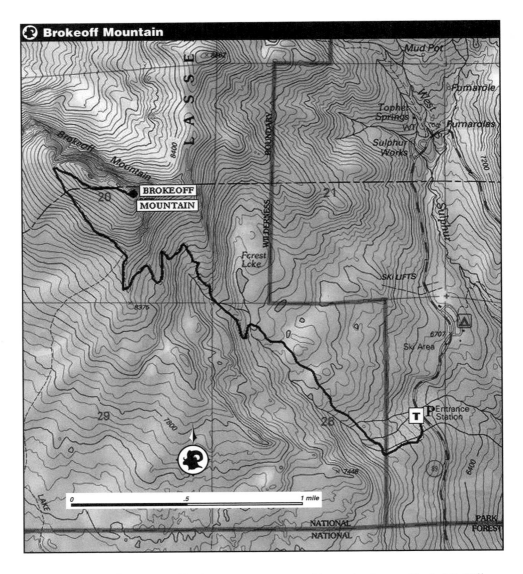

Brokeoff Mountain

hemlock, most bursting with tiny cones. Near the ridgetop, the trail cuts back east, passing below a satellite summit before finally reaching the top (3.7/9235´). A few scraggly whitebark pines and an anomalous, krummholz Jeffrey pine are growing from the rocky hillside just below the summit.

Grab a seat on the flat summit and admire the view. Looking northeast, Mt. Diller (9087´) is the highest peak between you and imposing Lassen Peak. Mt. Diller is another remnant of Mt. Tehama; the bands exposed below its western ridge are hardened flows that once coursed down the western flanks of the long-gone volcano. North beyond these bands are Chaos Crags (Hike 70) and more distant Thousand Lakes Volcano (Hike 69). Turning east-southeast, Mt. Conard (8204´) is the bare sandy-looking ridgetop across the deep valley of Mill Creek. Some 200,000 years ago, the towering summit of Mt. Tehama rose between you and Mt. Conard directly above today's Sulphur Works, the parking lot of which is visible more than 2000 feet below. When you're ready, back down you go!

Nearest Visitors Center: The Kohm Yah-mah-nee Visitor Center, (530) 595-4480, is located in the southwest entrance of the park off of Highway 36 on Highway 89. Open daily year-round. Park headquarters is in Mineral, (530) 595-4444, located on Hwy. 36 about 5 miles west of the junction of Hwys. 89 and 36 south of the park and open 8 AM–4:30 PM Monday through Friday.

Backpacking Information: While backpacking is allowed on this hike, the lack of good campsites makes it less appealing than dayhiking. A wilderness permit is required and can be obtained at the visitors centers, as well as at the southwest entrance station and the Loomis Museum and Visitors Center, (530) 595-4444, ext. 5180. Loomis Visitors Center is open mid-June through September daily 9 AM–5 PM, open weekends only Memorial Day until mid-June.

Nearest Campground: Southwest Campground (21 sites, $14) is a walk-in campground by the southwest entrance station. The Summit Lake campgrounds in the center of the park are the closest drive-in options.

Additional Information: www.nps.gov/lavo

HIKE 72

Devils Kitchen

Baking with the Devil

Highlights	Geothermal action away from the crowds
Distance	5.0 miles round-trip
Total Elevation Gain/Loss	700'/700'
Hiking Time	2–3 hours
Optional Map	USGS 7.5-min. *Reading Peak*
Best Times	Mid-June through September
Agency	Lassen Volcanic National Park
Difficulty	★★

California lives, breathing outward in hissing fumaroles and fetid mudpots! While most experience bubbling volcanic activity along the mobbed trail to Bumpass Hell, you should come—away from the crowds—to Devils Kitchen.

Underneath Lassen Volcanic National Park, at least 6 miles deep, is a large body of molten rock. Groundwater encountering it is heated to extraordinary temperatures, sometimes in excess of 500°F. Kept in liquid form by intense pressures found at such depths, the superheated water rises and flashes to steam near the surface. Boiling pools and billowing fumaroles are the result. Most of the hot water rises vertically to Bumpass Hell, but several substantial lateral flows exist, including the one spewing out at Devils Kitchen.

The Hike is an easy one, following Hot Springs Creek to a substantial area of geothermal activity. It is a quieter section, accessed far from the main park road and receiving light use. A great early summer hike for wildflowers, it generally receives light use in the fall. While no water is available at the trailhead, Hot Springs Creek is accessible early on.

To Reach the Trailhead: Take Hwy. 36 to Chester and turn north on Feather River Drive—the turnoff is across from Plumas Bank in the east end of town. In 0.7 mile,

bear left at the fork to stay on Feather River Rd. Drive 5.7 miles to another fork. Bear right and follow Warner Valley Road 10.6 miles to the trailhead parking lot, located on the left immediately past Warner Valley Campground. The last 3.1 miles are unpaved. A $10 entrance fee is due at the self-pay entrance station just inside the park boundary.

Description: At the trailhead (0.0/5670'), brochures are available for Boiling Springs Lake Nature Trail, a 3-mile interpretive trail to Cold Boiling Lake that parallels this hike for a short distance to Stop 9. Our trail begins on the Pacific Crest Trail and immediately heads to Hot Springs Creek, briefly following it before crossing a rusting metal bridge and heading slightly upslope. A hot spring can be seen flowing directly out of the ground at Stop 8, the water almost too hot to touch. This water, along with that from other nearby hot springs, flows into the baths at Drakesbad Guest Ranch visible across the broad meadow. Unfortunately, the baths are for guests only.

At Stop 9 the trail reaches a four-way junction (0.3/5730') by a large incense cedar. The Cold Boiling Lake Nature Trail and PCT head left, straight leads to Drake Lake, but you turn right and head back downslope. You reach another junction

Devils Kitchen

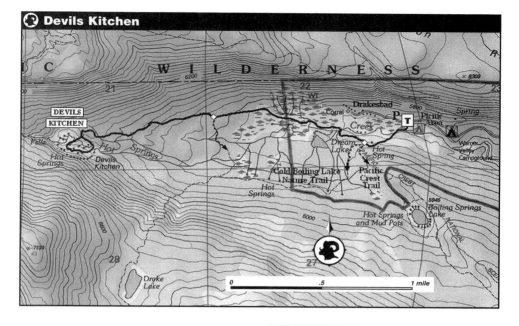

immediately prior to recrossing the creek. Turning left here leads to Dream Lake, a nearby shallow pond where beavers can sometimes be spotted, but you continue straight across the alder-choked stream and enter the wide, open meadow. A few paths from the ranch join your trail, now winding along the north side of the meadow. You reenter a dense forest of predominantly white fir (1.1/5760´) and soon reach another junction. An optional return trail splits left to join the trail leading to Drake Lake. A slow and gentle climb ahead toward Devils Kitchen ends by a hitching post atop a small rise, where the sulfuric stench of geothermal activity first assaults your nose.

A 0.5-mile loop trail runs through Devils Kitchen, with informative placards and a stern warning not to go off the trail. Enjoy the fantastic hues of technicolor rock, accompanied by the dull roar of venting fumaroles and the musical bass of bubbling mudpots.

Nearest Visitors Center: Warner Valley Ranger Station, located just east of Warner Valley Campground, is open sporadically—try knocking on the door. Farther away is Loomis Museum and Visitors Center, (530) 595-4444, ext. 5180, which is open 9 AM–5 PM daily mid-June through September and weekends only Memorial Day until mid-June.

The Kohm Yah-mah-nee Visitor Center, (530) 595-4480, is located in the southwest entrance of the park off of Highway 36 on Highway 89. Open daily year-round. Park headquarters is in Mineral, (530) 595-4444, located on Hwy. 36 about 5 miles west of the junction of Hwys. 89 and 36 south of the park and open 8 AM–4:30 PM Monday through Friday.

Nearest Campground: Warner Valley Campground (18 sites, $14) is located 0.5 mile east of the trailhead.

Additional Information: www.nps.gov/lavo

HIKE 73

Deer Creek

Ishi's World

Highlights	A remote world of rugged cliffs and canyons
Distance	2.0 miles
Total Elevation Gain/Loss	750'/750'
Hiking Time	1–2 hours
Optional Map	*Ishi, Thousand Lakes, and Caribou Wildernesses* by the U.S. Forest Service
Best Times	Spring and fall
Agency	Ishi Wilderness
Difficulty	★★★

Here, dark basalt cliffs compose inaccessible canyons—a place that once sheltered Ishi, the last of the Yahi Indians. Before the Gold Rush, the Yahi occupied a vast region in the foothills southwest of Lassen Peak. By 1865 nearly the entire Yahi nation had been wiped out, the victim of disease and ruthless extermination by encroaching settlers. Only a tiny band survived, disappearing into the rugged terrain around Mill and Deer creeks in 1872. They lived in traditional fashion—hunting with bow and arrow and gathering what the land provided—but their numbers slowly dwindled. By the early 1890s Ishi and only four others remained, living in a tiny settlement perched on a narrow ledge 500 feet above the creek. When surveyors stumbled across Ishi fishing with a harpoon in the river in 1908, the Yahi survivors fled into the surrounding hills. But by the year's end only Ishi still lived.

The Hike is a short exploratory loop of Deer Creek, once the center of the Yahi people and later Ishi's final refuge. In order to complete the loop, it is necessary to ford Deer Creek—be prepared for waist-deep water on the crossing year-round. The creek swells with snowmelt and can be impassable during spring and early summer—try the easier out-and-back ad-

venture along the more scenic north side during these times. Spring is the best time to visit, when wildflowers and pleasant

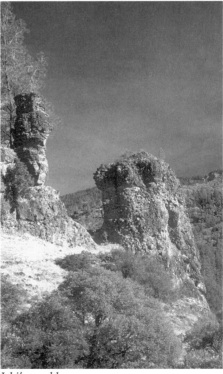

Ishi's world

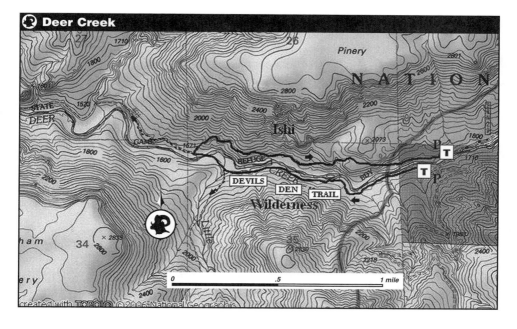

temperatures are common. Summers are brutally hot and should be avoided, but mild weather returns in the fall. Fishing is possible in Deer Creek but special restrictions apply—check current regulations. Beware poison oak and ticks in the brush. Due to the difficulty of access, crowds are light here. Water is available from Deer Creek.

To Reach the Trailhead: You'll need a high-clearance four-wheel-drive vehicle and a good map; the area is laced with logging roads and it is easy to get lost. (The U.S. Forest Service map for Lassen National Forest is recommended.) Take Hwy. 36 to the small community of Paynes Creek and head south on Plum Creek Rd. In almost 9 miles, turn right on unpaved Ponderosa Way (Forest Service Rd. 707B), located 0.5 mile past the turnoff for FSR 774A. Remain on Ponderosa Way (also posted as FSR 28N29) for the next 21 miles to reach Black Rock Campground. Continue for another 5 miles past the campground and bear right and then immediately right again to remain on increasingly rough 28N29, which you'll fol-

low for the next 15 miles to Deer Creek. The southern trailhead is located by the Ishi Wilderness information signs just before the bridge. The northern trailhead is immediately across the creek.

Description: From the southern trailhead (0.0/1700´), the hike begins on Devils Den Trail and immediately crosses a small creek. In 0.1 mile, you pass a small wilderness boundary placard hammered to a ponderosa pine; the trail stays left, away from the creek. Douglas firs, canyon live oaks, black oaks, incense cedars, California bays, ponderosa pines, and alders compose this low-elevation forest, with a thick undergrowth of blackberries, wild grapevines, toyon, and poison oak. On this north-facing slope, plants are protected from the heat of the sun's rays, and even delicate ferns survive in the dribbling stream gullies.

The river remains largely inaccessible where the trail climbs two switchbacks, traversing briefly 100 feet above the river before descending steeply to cross Little Pine Creek. After this crossing, Devils Den Trail turns abruptly upslope away from the water, but you follow the faint path that heads toward Deer Creek. Reaching the river by a pleasant swimming hole, continue downstream to the long riffle located above the next pool. This is the crossing (1.3/1550′).

Once on the other side of Deer Creek, follow the grassy clearing uphill to find the trail. On these drier south-facing slopes, the vegetation changes dramatically. Juniper, blue oak, and gray pine are common away from the river. California buckeye, redbud, and live oak grow closer to the water. While the trail continues 12 miles downstream, your route turns up-canyon and immediately begins climbing above the river through a bizarre world of volcanic cliffs and pillars.

Over the past million years, ancient volcanoes near today's Lassen Volcanic National Park sent periodic mudflows coursing across the land. A jumble of rocks, mud, and ash, the mudflows solidified in layers, which were later exposed as Deer Creek eroded through them. Threading two impressive pillars, the trail descends briefly and then climbs, making a long traverse through a dense forest of ponderosa pine, black oak, and manzanita before descending abruptly to the trailhead.

As you soon will, Ishi left this wilderness and entered the modern world.

Found in a corral outside of Chico, he became an overnight sensation and attracted the attention of anthropologists at the University of California. Brought to San Francisco on August 9, 1911, Ishi lived a mostly private life in the Museum of Anthropology until his death in March 1916 from tuberculosis.

Nearest Visitors Center: Chester-Almanor Ranger Station, (530) 258-2141, is located on Hwy. 36 just west of Chester and open 8 AM–4:30 PM Monday through Saturday.

Backpacking Information: A wilderness permit is not needed, but a valid campfire permit is required. There are numerous campsites downriver along Deer Creek.

Nearest Campground: Black Rock Campground (6 sites, stream water only) is about 20 miles from the trailhead on Ponderosa Way, or FSR 28N29.

Additional Information: www.fs.fed.us/r5/lassen/recreation/wilderness/ishi

HIKE 74

Big Chico Creek

Bidwell Did Well

Highlights	Bountiful valley woodlands and a basalt gorge
Distance	3.5 miles round-trip
Total Elevation Gain/Loss	600′/600′
Hiking Time	3–5 hours
Optional Maps	USGS 7.5-min. *Richardson Springs* and *Paradise West*
Best Times	Spring and fall
Agency	Bidwell Park
Difficulty	★★

Bidwell Park provides a living diorama—a glimpse of the bounty and rich diversity of life that once flourished in the Great Central Valley. It's also good for swimming.

In 1905 John and Annie Bidwell donated this land to the city of Chico for the public's use and enjoyment. The third largest municipal park in the country after New York's Central Park and Portland's Forest Park, it is a beautiful tract along Big Chico Creek, a lush riparian alley winding through dry oak woodlands. Fremont cottonwoods, California bays, willows, Oregon ash, white alders, California box elders, bigleaf maples, and California

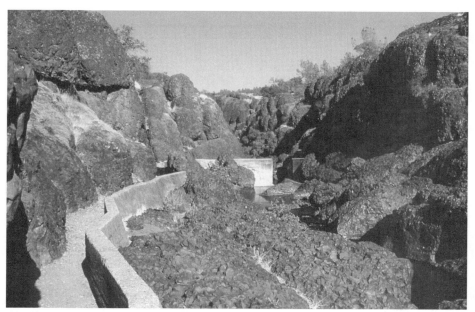

Big Chico Creek pools and pours through volcanic basalt.

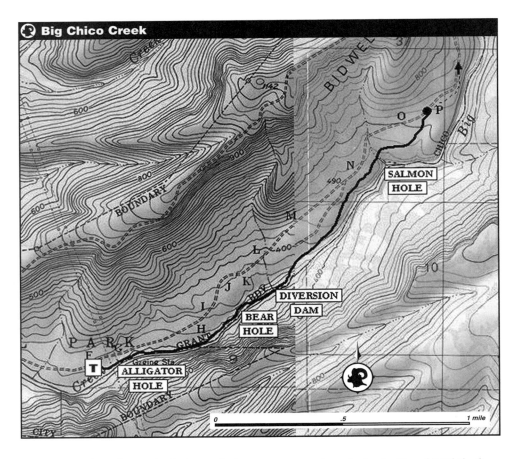

sycamores line the creek; their trunks are interwoven by the twisting tendrils of wild grapevines. Valley oaks, blue oaks, interior live oaks, canyon live oaks, gray pines, California buckeyes, black walnuts, and Chinese stink trees thrive on the dry slopes away from the creek. Flowers and some trees offer seasonal displays of color, and birdlife abounds year-round. In Upper Bidwell Park, sheer canyons carved through erosion-resistant basalt result in wild formations of rock, stripped clean of soil and plant life for long sections.

The Hike winds along Big Chico Creek in Upper Bidwell Park, passing through lush creekside vegetation before threading up through basalt outcroppings to the canyon rim and park road. (A bicycle or vehicle left at Parking Lot P would facilitate

an easy return to the trailhead.) While the hike can be done year-round, it is sizzling in the summer months with daily highs hovering around 100°F. Fall and spring provide the most ideal temperatures. Sun protection is always worth having. Fishing is prohibited in Big Chico Creek. No water is available at the trailhead.

To Reach the Trailhead: Take Hwy. 99 in Chico to the East 8th St./Hwy. 32 off-ramp and head east on E. 8th St. for 2 miles to Chico Canyon Rd. Turn left and go 0.6 mile to Centennial Ave. Turn right, and 0.5 mile farther turn right again onto Wildwood Ave., immediately beyond the sign for Upper Bidwell Park. After 1.9 miles of road, with speed bumps by the golf course, you reach a gate closed on Mondays and after rainy days. If you're here on those days, park in nearby Parking Lot E and walk the short distance to the trailhead. The trailhead is in Parking Lot F, 0.7 mile past the gate on the right. The last 0.4 mile is unpaved.

Description: From the parking lot (0.0/300´), take the widest, most obvious trail down to the creek and begin heading upstream. Throughout this hike numerous use paths branch this way and that, but the main trail close to the stream is generally obvious. A posted spur trail soon leads down to the Day Camp swimming area, overshadowed by layered basalt—a pancake stack—exposed near the top of the opposite cut bank.

Known as the Lovejoy Basalt, it's a result of volcanic flows 18 million years old that originated somewhere east of present-day Susanville. With no intervening mountains present at the time, the flows coursed southwest, nearly reaching the present site of Winters in the middle of the Great Central Valley. Existing rocks in what is now Bidwell Park were coated with a thick layer of erosion-resistant basalt. The underlying rocks compose the Chico Formation, formed approximately 75–100 million years ago just offshore from the continental edge. Sediments washed into the sea were deposited in beds thousands of feet thick, becoming shale and sandstone over time. Where exposed by the down-cutting of Big Chico Creek, this formation provides good soil for the rich plant life around you.

Continuing upstream, you soon reach Bear Hole (0.7/300´), where there's a remarkable change in scenery. Here the creek has not eroded through the Lovejoy Formation and instead flows through surprising basalt formations bare of most vegetation. Numerous signs warn of the swimming hazards in this treacherous section. From here, it is possible to walk along the creek a short distance on the remains of an old cement flume. Passing through a narrow basalt gorge with sheer, 40-foot walls, the flume ends at an old diversion dam. A mildly precarious stairway requires a bit of scrambling to get to here. An alternative stretch of trail skirts this section along the canyon rim.

Now at the top of the stairs, follow the shadeless trail along the canyon rim to an overlook of Salmon Hole (1.6/530´), a deep, accessible swimming spot in the gorge below. Beyond this point, the canyon below becomes wider and difficult to access. It's possible to continue to the northern reaches of Upper Bidwell Park, but this hike—having sampled what the park offers—ends where the trail rejoins the park road at Parking Lot P. Return the way you came or via the park road.

Nearest Visitors Center: Chico Creek Nature Center, (530) 891-4671, is located on E. 8th St. 1 mile east of the Hwy 99 off-ramp and open 11 AM–4 PM Tuesday through Sunday.

Nearest Campground: Woodson Bridge State Recreation Area (37 sites, $11–14 depending on the season) is located 20 miles northwest of Chico along the banks of the Sacramento River. Take South Ave. 3 miles west of Vina on Hwy. 99.

Additional Information: www.bidwellpark.org

HIKE 75

Middle Fork Feather River

Wild Feather

Highlights	Deep wilderness, untouched forest, and a crystalline river
Distance	7.0 miles round-trip
Total Elevation Gain/Loss	2900´/2900´
Hiking Time	4–6 hours
Optional Map	USGS 7.5-min. *Haskins Valley*
Best Times	Mid-July through September
Agency	Plumas National Forest
Difficulty	★★★★★

Not an easy hike, this is an introduction to Middle Fork Feather River country, perhaps the deepest, least hospitable wilderness in California. Below the bridge on Quincy-La Porte Rd., the Middle Fork Feather flows inaccessible to vehicles for over 30 miles, as it rushes below steep canyon slopes 2000–3000-feet high. Numerous mines dotted the region in the past, and many of today's trails (including this one) are their former access roads. The geology of the Feather River region is in-

credibly complex. Exposed rocks range in age from approximately 150 million years to over 400 million years, making the mix far older than the typical Sierra Nevada granite. This hike descends into one of the most poorly understood geologic provinces in California, a jumble of metamorphosed blocks accreted to North America approximately 250 million years ago.

The Hike follows Little California Trail, which drops 2450 feet along a seldom-used jeep road to a point just above the river.

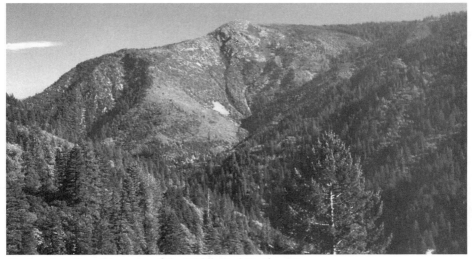

Go deep into the wild canyon of the Middle Fork Feather River.

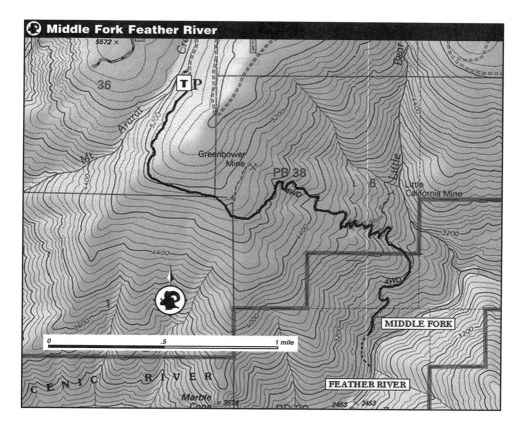

The remaining 300 feet of descent is a harrowing bushwhack. It is highly unlikely that you will see anybody else, regardless of when you go. Fishing is excellent with native rainbow trout particularly abundant. There is no water at the trailhead or anywhere before the bottom.

To Reach the Trailhead: Take Bucks Lake Rd. west from Quincy (the turnoff is downtown by the courthouse) toward Meadow Valley. In 9.5 miles turn left onto Big Creek Rd. and proceed 6.8 miles to Forest Service Rd. 60. This is the end of the pavement. Reset your odometer and turn left. Reaching a fork at mile 1.9, bear left on FSR 23N19. Beyond the Lookout Rock Trailhead, the road reaches a T-junction at mile 4.3—go right on FSR 23N55. You reach an unposted four-way junction at mile 6.6; those with low-clearance vehicles should park here and walk to the

trailhead. The rest can turn left and go 0.8 mile to the trailhead, in a small lot where the road narrows. A sign warns would-be motorists that the road beyond this point is steep, narrow, and four-wheel-drive only.

Description: From the trailhead (0.0/5330´), follow the jeep road, briefly passing through a thick forest of dogwoods, red firs, and sugar pines, and then along a level, more-open stretch lined with manzanita. You get the best views of the hike along this early section. Curving east into tree cover, the trail passes several large ponderosa pines and Douglas firs, and soon begins its steep, unrelenting descent. As the elevation drops switchback by switchback, the vegetation slowly changes. Sugar pines and red firs quickly disappear, replaced by increasing numbers of incense cedars, ponderosa pines and, especially, black oaks. Canyon live oaks can be seen near the bottom.

The jeep road abruptly terminates in a forest of black oak, where there's a table hammered to a tree (3.2/2750′). The barely discernible trail continues beyond the washout gully that blocks the road. With a keen eye pick out the path traversing slowly downward through thick brush. Watch your footing on the steep slopes in this section. Before long, a discernible path bears off, dropping more directly down toward the river (3.5/2450′). Although challenging, it's rewarding to explore the Middle Fork Feather River both up- and downstream . . . at least for a little bit.

Nearest Visitors Center: Mt. Hough District Ranger Station, (530) 283-0555, is located 3 miles north of Quincy on Hwy. 70 and open 8 AM–4:30 PM Monday through Friday.

Backpacking Information: A valid campfire permit is required. There are a few campsites where the jeep road ends.

Nearest Campground: There are numerous campgrounds around Bucks Lake. Consult the Plumas National Forest map.

HIKE 76

Sierra Buttes

Look Out

Highlights	A fire lookout with hundred-mile views
Distance	11.0 miles round-trip
Total Elevation Gain/Loss	3200´/3200´
Hiking Time	8–10 hours
Optional Map	USGS 7.5-min. *Sierra City*
Best Times	July through September
Agency	Tahoe National Forest
Difficulty	★★★★

Sierra Buttes soar; powerful monoliths of naked rock burst from the sylvan terrain of the North Fork Yuba River. Atop their highest peak a tower perches—a lookout for wildfire with commanding views.

Part of a complicated geologic puzzle, the rocks of Sierra Buttes were probably formed during the eruptions of ancient undersea volcanoes some 350 million years ago. Accreted to North America more than 200 million years ago, their resistance to erosion has left them exposed as naked mountains today.

The Hike is a long, challenging ascent of Sierra Buttes from Lower Sardine Lake and provides the full Sierra Buttes experience of scenery, lakes, and summit vista. Two alternative access trails—one via the Pacific Crest Trail, one via Tamarack Lakes—offer shorter routes to the summit. Both these trails miss out on the exceptional views of Sierra Buttes above Sardine Lakes, however. Via the Pacific Crest Trail, the round-trip to the summit is 4.6 miles with an elevation gain/loss of 1600 feet. Via the Tamarack Lakes, the round-trip is 6.2 miles with an elevation gain/loss of 2300 feet. With two vehicles or one vehicle and a bicycle, you can begin at Lower Sardine Lake and exit via the PCT, sparing your knees considerable downhill compression. Snow can linger deep into

June and the trail is usually not snow-free until July. While the Sardine lakes are an extremely popular fishing destination with heavy crowds all summer long, only a small percentage of people are on the trail. Fishing is possible at the Tamarack lakes and both are planted with fingerling trout. Water is available near the Lower Sardine Lake Trailhead but not at the two alternative trailheads. Sources are scarce along the trail—the Tamarack lakes near that trailhead are your only sure bet.

To Reach the Trailhead: Take Hwy. 49 to Bassetts Station, located 5 miles east of Sierra City and 15 miles west of Sattley. Turn north onto Gold Lake Rd., proceed 1.3 miles, and turn left toward Sardine and Packer lakes. In 0.3 mile the road forks: Left leads to the lower trailhead, right to the two upper trailheads. Going left, the trailhead is 0.1 mile farther on the right just before Lower Sardine Lake Campground, and is signed TAMARACK CONNECTION TRAIL 12E08. Going right at the fork, you reach a Y-junction in 2.7 miles by the Packer Lake day-use area—go left and stay on Forest Service Rd. 93. The Tamarack Lakes Trailhead is a short 0.2 mile ahead and the PCT Trailhead a steep and winding 2.1 miles farther.

Description: From the Lower Sardine Lake Trailhead (0.0/5770´), the wide and

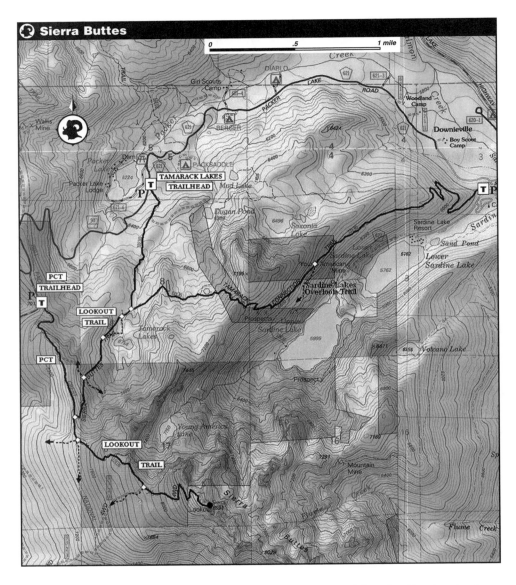

rocky trail begins climbing through manzanita, Douglas firs, Jeffrey pines, white
firs, and incense cedars. The lookout tower
is barely discernible to the naked eye,
perched on top of the mountain's highest
point. The trail soon climbs a ridge, crossing briefly to the eastern side before returning to begin the fabulous traverse above
Sardine lakes. Dazzling Sierra Buttes overshadow the emerald waters of Upper and

Lower Sardine lakes, lending inspiration
to your feet as you approach the grueling
ridgetop ascent. Along the way, you pass
the junction for the Sardine Lakes Overlook Trail (1.7/6500´). After powering up
the steep switchbacks to attain the ridge
(2.3/7050´), you descend briefly and pass
two small ponds before reaching the junction with the Lookout Trail (3.2/6720´).
Those approaching from Tamarack Lakes

Trailhead join here; you turn left (southwest) on the wide four-wheel-drive road to immediately reach Lower Tamarack Lake. The trail forks just past the lake: Left leads down to nicer Upper Tamarack Lake, right is the continuation of the hike. The upper lake is good for some very brisk swimming.

Now on posted Tamarack Connection Trail 12E30, you climb steadily southwest and cross a wide logging road halfway to the ridgetop. The lookout becomes visible southeast between the peaklets before three switchbacks bring you to the ridgetop. The junction with the PCT (4.0/7350´) is located by a large, twisted western white pine. Those approaching from the PCT Trailhead join here, where your trail continues southeast up toward the summit. Winding steeply through large boulders, you stay near or along the ridgecrest and begin the final push to the top. Note your route as it can be difficult to spot on your return, especially when lingering snow obscures the track. The icy, turquoise water of Little America Lake lies below, the lookout sits above, and mountain hemlock grows all around you, climbing the four-wheel-drive access road to the top. Following it up eight switchbacks, you then reach the stairs—as if you weren't tired enough—and 141 steps later you reach the top (5.5/8591´).

The interior of the seasonally staffed lookout is off-limits, but the walkway that surrounds it is open for 360-degree views. The northeast corner of this precarious roost actually juts out into the void beyond the summit cliffs! On a reasonably clear day, Lassen Peak (10,457´) is visible more than 70 miles away on the northwest horizon, the peaks of Desolation Wilderness appear far to the south-southeast, and the Coast Ranges rise beyond Sutter Buttes and the Great Central Valley (a distance of more than 100 miles). Return as you came, or by one of the two alternate routes.

Nearest Visitors Center: Yuba River Ranger Station, (530) 288-3232, is located 7 miles north of North San Juan and 23 miles south of Downieville on Hwy. 49 and is open 8 AM–4:30 PM Monday through Friday.

Backpacking Information: A campfire permit is required. The only campsites along this hike are around Tamarack Lakes and receive heavy use.

Nearest Campground: Sardine Campground (25 sites, $20) at Lower Sardine Lake and Packsaddle Campground (14 sites, $20) near Packer Lake both provide water. More primitive Berger and Diablo campgrounds (7 and 18 sites respectively, $16) are on the road to Packer Lake and lack water.

Additional Information: www.fs.fed.us/r5/tahoe

HIKE 77

Middle Fork Yuba River

The Middle Yuba

Highlights	The peaceful Yuba watershed
Distance	2.0 miles round-trip
Total Elevation Gain/Loss	1200′/1200′
Hiking Time	3–4 hours
Optional Maps	USGS 7.5-min. *Alleghany* and *Graniteville*
Best Times	May through mid-November
Agency	Tahoe National Forest
Difficulty	★★★

Difficult to access, this diminutive fork of the larger Yuba system was once swarming with miners during the height of the California Gold Rush. Ditches were dug, the river dammed, flumes constructed, lumber milled, towns built, and not a stone left unturned in the fervent quest for gold. Today only the gurgling river remains.

The Hike descends steeply to the river via a spotty, overgrown, and unmaintained trail. The river can be shallow, but numerous deep pools provide opportunities for swimming and fishing. It is very unlikely that you will encounter anybody regardless of the time of year you are visiting. No water is available at the trailhead or anywhere before the river itself. *This is an area rife with abandoned mine shafts and tunnels. Be cautious when traversing cross-country on the slopes as collapsed mines can create pitfalls beneath the litter of the forest floor. Never, ever go into an abandoned tunnel!*

To Reach the Trailhead: Take Hwy. 49 north from Nevada City. After driving 4 miles beyond the South Fork Yuba's crossing, turn right onto Tyler Foote Rd. going toward North Columbia and Malakoff Diggins State Park. In 8.7 miles the road reaches a Y-junction; continue straight on Cruzon Grade Rd. for another 5.5 miles. Leave the paved road where it swings south at the

posted turnoff for Malakoff Diggins, and proceed straight ahead on the washboard surface of Backbone Rd. Bear right on Snow Tent Rd., where Backbone Rd. quickly forks left, and go 11 miles to the (easily missed) fenced Graniteville cemetery on the road's south side. Directly across the road from the cemetery is an unmarked four-wheel-drive road. If you have a low-clearance vehicle, park here and walk the short distance to the trailhead. Otherwise, turn left on the road and proceed 0.3 mile to a fork—bear right to immediately reach a four-way intersection. Turn left down the very steep, rocky, and overgrown path, which terminates in a small lot after 0.3 mile. Be aware

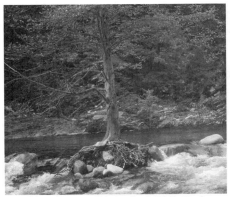

An alder clings to life in the Middle Fork Yuba River.

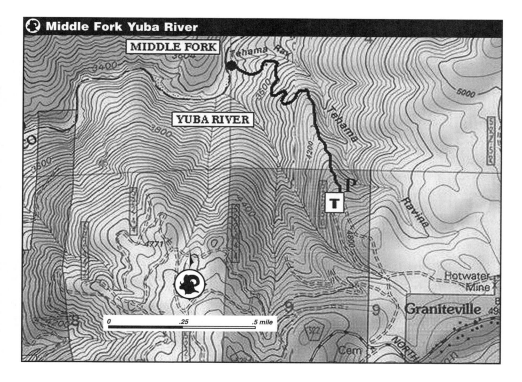

Middle Fork Yuba River

that the final section of road crosses private property.

Description: From the lot (0.0/4530′), the trail is almost indiscernible. It descends north—straight down—along the ridge below you for 600 feet. Although sketchy in spots, the trail becomes somewhat more distinct as you go—just stay on top of the ridge. Without a turn the trail plummets downward, soon reaching a small stand of Douglas firs on a ridge bump (0.3/4200′). Clear views southwest reveal the undeveloped Middle Yuba drainage. The trail veers obviously west 300 feet farther down—keep your eye out. Passing through dense forest, this overgrown section of trail is, nonetheless, generally easy to spot. If you find yourself off-trail, retrace your steps to find the path; the slopes are dangerously steep. Look for a few, particularly large sugar pines before you finally reach the river (1.0/3340′). Douglas firs, ponderosa pines, black oaks, bigleaf maples, and canyon live oaks line the riverbanks. Ex-ploratory adventures await upstream and down. Return the way you came.

Nearest Visitors Center: North Bloomfield Ranger Station, (530) 265-2740, is located in Malakoff Diggins State Historic Park and open 9 AM–5 PM daily in summer and 10 AM–4 PM weekends only the rest of year. Yuba River Ranger Station, (530) 288-3232, is located 7 miles north of North San Juan and 23 miles south of Downieville on Hwy. 49 and open 8 AM–4:30 PM Monday through Friday.

Backpacking Information: A valid campfire permit is required. Campsites exist along the river.

Nearest Campground: Shooter Hill Campground (30 sites, $15) is in Malakoff Diggins State Historic Park.

HIKE 78

North Fork American River

The Mother Lode

Highlights	Gold Rush echoes and the North Fork chasm
Distance	8.5 miles one-way
Total Elevation Gain/Loss	2300′/2600′
Hiking Time	5–7 hours
Optional Map	USGS 7.5-min. *Duncan Peak*
Best Times	May through October
Agency	Tahoe National Forest
Difficulty	★★★★

The North Fork American River tumbles west through the Sierra foothills, slicing through the heart of California's Gold Country. Despite running parallel to the busiest highway in the Sierra Nevada (Interstate 80), this stretch of river receives surprisingly light use. The fact that it rushes through a precipitous canyon a half mile deep may have something to do with it.

In 1848, gold was discovered at Sutters Mill on the South Fork American River above Sacramento. Within two years, thousands of gold-seekers were poking and prodding every unturned rock in the American River drainage. The surrounding slopes were denuded, mines dug; fortunes were made and lost. After the gold petered out, the remote canyons were left to nature. Mine shafts and memories are all that remain along this hike.

The Hike approaches the North Fork from the south on Beacroft Trail, descends steeply to reach the river, follows it 2.2 miles downstream to Mumford Bar, and then climbs just as steeply to Mumford Bar Trailhead. Since the two trailheads are separated by 5 miles of paved road, leave either a car or a bicycle at the end trailhead. While the hike can be completed in either direction, beginning on Beacroft Trail, described below, spares you an extra

100 feet of climbing. Due to the easy trailhead access and close proximity to major population centers, you will likely see a few people (though not many). Fishing is good. No water is available at either trailhead and none is available before canyon bottom. *This is an area rife with abandoned mine shafts and tunnels. Be cautious when traversing the slopes cross-country, as collapsed mines can create pitfalls beneath the litter of the forest floor. Never, ever go into an abandoned tunnel!*

To Reach the Trailhead: Take the Forest Hill Road exit from Interstate 80, just east of downtown Auburn. Proceed east on Forest Hill Rd. for 34 miles to the substantial Mumford Bar Trailhead lot—your terminus. Drive a bike or car to the smaller (and more easily missed) Beacroft Trailhead lot 5 miles farther along the road to begin your hike.

Description: The posted trailhead (0.0/5450′) is at the end of the very rough road that strikes north from the main Beacroft parking area. Climbing very briefly, the trail then begins its descent into the canyon. If thick vegetation obscures views for most of the drop, it allows passage through two distinct plant communities. Above 4000 feet is the coniferous woodland community, where red firs, sugar pines, and Douglas firs are the dominant

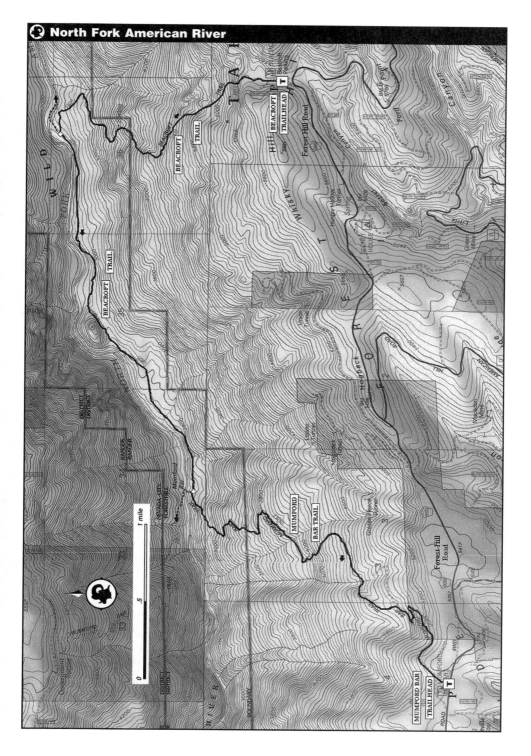

trees. Below 4000 feet, the vegetation changes to that of the foothill woodlands community. Incense cedars and ponderosa pines replace the higher-elevation conifers, and black oaks, manzanita, California bays, bigleaf maples, and canyon live oaks appear everywhere. This ecological transition zone extends the length of the western Sierra Nevada between roughly 3000 and 5000 feet.

Almost exactly 1000 feet down (1.0/4400´), the trail passes through an open area with dizzying views up-canyon. The geology of the area is extremely complex, resulting from the accretion of an offshore landmass to North America approximately 250 million years ago. Part of this landmass likely contained the gold of California's mother lode, redistributed throughout the region in the scattered pockets so fervently hunted by prospectors.

Continuing to the bottom, the trail reaches a junction (2.4/2860´), where the river is readily accessible as it races through a chute 10 feet deep—a great swimming hole. From here, head downstream 2.5 miles to the junction for Mumford Bar Trail. The trail runs among trees parallel to the broad riverbed. The river can be accessed at various points; it is possible to walk along the river itself for stretches to rejoin the trail later on.

Immediately prior to reaching the junction (4.9/2650´), you pass the Mumford Bar Cabin, built around 1900 and currently being repaired by the U.S. Forest Service. From here, the Mumford Bar Trailhead is only a few thousand feet above and a couple dozen switchbacks away. Once trailside views into the canyon disappear, it's only 500 more feet of gain to the parking lot (8.5/5250´).

Nearest Visitors Center: Forest Hill Ranger Station, (530) 367-2224, is located 15 miles east of I-80 on Forest Hill Rd. and open 8 AM–5 PM Monday through Saturday in summer and 8 AM–4:30 PM Monday through Friday the rest of the year.

Backpacking Information: This is an excellent overnight trip with numerous campsites along the river. A valid campfire permit is required.

Nearest Campground: Mumford Bar Trailhead Campground (5 sites, no water, free) is near the hike's western trailhead. Robinson Flat Campground (7 sites, water, free) is 5 miles east of the Beacroft Trailhead on Forest Hill Rd.

Additional Information: www. fs.fed.us/r5/tahoe

HIKE 79

Rubicon River

Gone on the Rubicon

Highlights	The crystalline Rubicon River
Distance	6.0-plus miles round-trip
Total Elevation Gain/Loss	500´/500´
Hiking Time	1–5 hours
Optional Maps	USGS 7.5-min. *Bunker Hill* and *Robbs Peak*
Best Times	May through October
Agency	Eldorado National Forest
Difficulty	★★

Originating in Desolation Wilderness, Rubicon River flows through beautiful, unspoiled Sierra foothills on its way to join the Middle Fork American River. Hiking beside this river—clear as glass and emerald green—is a peaceful experience.

The Hike is an exploration of a small stretch of Rubicon River that flows for 10 miles without road access. Running along slopes parallel to the river, the trail provides views into some deep gorges, as well as opportunities to scramble down and explore along the river. There is no end destination for this hike—this description goes 3 miles upstream but you can continue past this point, or turn around earlier without missing any significant sights. The first 1.5 miles of trail are the most dramatic. This hike can be done virtually year-round as snow usually does not fall here until January. Fishing is fair to good, with the water clarity often making for challenging conditions. No potable water is available at the trailhead but the river is easily accessible.

To Reach the Trailhead: Take Hwy. 49 south from Auburn to the junction with Hwy. 193 in Cool and turn east. Proceed 12.7 miles to the Georgetown stop sign and turn left on Main St., which becomes Forest Service Rd. 1 (also known as Wentworth Springs Road) on the other side

of town. Follow FSR 1 for 20 miles to the junction with FSR 2 and turn left. The road descends and crosses the Rubicon River in 5 miles. Immediately past the bridge, there is a small unmarked dirt road on the right. Those with low-clearance vehicles should park here by the paved road. The others can take the rough road 0.4 mile to a parking area by the river. The unposted trailhead is halfway down this road, marked by five 1-foot-high wooden posts.

Description: From the trailhead (0.0/3390´), climb past an angler's survey box and begin your hillside traverse among black oaks, canyon live oaks, ponderosa pines, incense cedars, and Douglas firs. Fragrant bear clover fills in the understory. The early section also crosses a geologic divide, passing briefly over metamorphic rocks before reaching the more typical granite of the Sierra Nevada. Early on look for schist and other metamorphic rocks in the creekbeds that the path crosses.

Climbing high above the river, the trail peaks at a clearing (1.0/3710´), which offers views up-canyon and of the opposite slopes rising more than 2000 feet above the river. It then drops back down; where the trail bottoms out you pass a spur trail to the river (1.7/3600´), one of only two, good access points. A few, small white

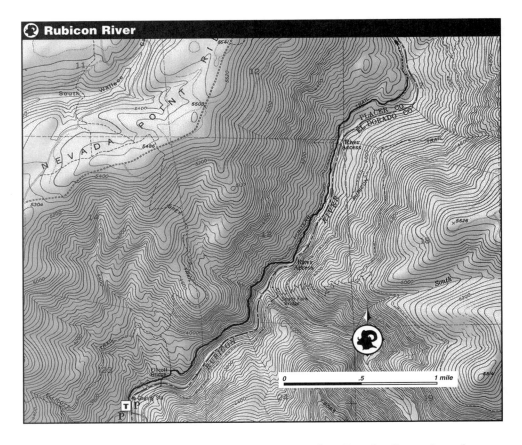

Rubicon River

firs can be spotted as you continue along the more level trail and the canyon slopes become more gradual. Near a significant creek gully where the riverbed is clearly visible, you pass the next river access point. Large, healthy representatives of in-

cense cedars, Douglas firs, and ponderosa pines grow along the trail's upper section; it is possible to continue all the way to Hell Hole Reservoir, a 10-mile one-way journey from the trailhead. Turn around whenever you'd like.

Nearest Visitors Center: Georgetown Ranger Station, (530) 333-4312, located 3.6 miles east of the Georgetown stop sign on FSR 1, is open 8 AM–4:30 PM daily May through November and Monday through Friday only December through April.

Backpacking Information: While it is legal to backpack on this hike (valid campfire permit required), finding good campsites can be a challenge.

Nearest Campground: Stumpy Meadows Campground (39 sites, $15) is located 12 miles east of Georgetown on FSR 1. There are a few primitive use sites near the trailhead parking area.

Additional Information: www.fs.fed.us/r5/eldorado

HIKE 80

Mount Tallac

Tallac Attack

Highlights	Views encompassing all of Lake Tahoe and much of Desolation Wilderness
Distance	9.2 miles round-trip
Total Elevation Gain/Loss	3400´/3400´
Hiking Time	6–8 hours
Optional Maps	*Desolation Wilderness* by the U.S. Forest Service, *Desolation Wilderness & Vicinity* by Wilderness Press
Best Times	July through September
Agency	Desolation Wilderness
Difficulty	★★★★

Mt. Tallac soars above Lake Tahoe's southwest shore, a landmark peak beckoning fit hikers to its lofty summit. From the top, Lake Tahoe and the heart of Desolation Wilderness spread out below you.

In this land of exposed granite, Mt. Tallac (9735´) is a dark, metamorphic anomaly. A roof pendant, the mountain is a remnant of the landscape that existed prior to the intrusion of the Sierra Nevada granite. Formed near the ancient continental margin of North America 200–120 million years ago, the rocks of Mt. Tallac are a complex mix of volcanic flows above metamorphosed sea-floor sediments. While these rocks once covered the surrounding landscape, erosion has exposed the underlying granite, leaving only a few small remnants on the highest peaks.

The Hike quickly and steeply ascends Mt. Tallac via the most direct route from Lake Tahoe's southwest shore, passing Floating Island and Cathedral lakes along the way. Mt. Tallac is in Desolation Wilderness, an incredibly popular area that is heavily traveled all summer long until Labor Day. In September, the weather remains delightful and crowds all but disappear—the optimal time for your "Tallac Attack." Snow lingers well into June on

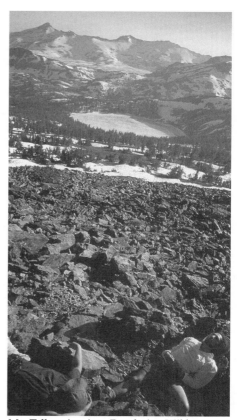

Mt. Tallac view into Desolation Wilderness

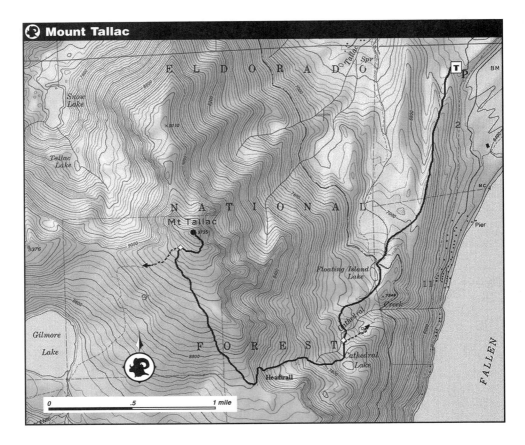

the trail's upper reaches and can return as early as October. No water is available at the trailhead. Cathedral Creek, about halfway up the mountain, provides a reliable trailside source.

To Reach the Trailhead: Take Hwy. 89 north of the junction of Hwys. 50 and 89 in South Lake Tahoe for 3.5 miles to the posted turnoff for the Tallac Trailhead on the left. Approaching from the north on Hwy. 89, the turnoff is 2 miles south of Eagle Point Campground. From Hwy. 89, it is a short 1.2 miles on the access road to the large trailhead parking lot—bear left at the first fork and right at the second.

Description: All dayhikers are required to obtain a wilderness permit, available free at the big information sign by the start of the trail (0.0/6500′). Immediately climbing, the trail ascends through Jeffrey pines,

white firs, and manzanita to quickly obtain the top of the ridge that hems in Fallen Leaf Lake, visible below you to the east. As glaciers advanced from the mountains toward Lake Tahoe in the recent geologic past, they pushed rocky debris in front of them like giant bulldozers, depositing it alongside to form lateral moraines (parallel ridges along the glacier edges) and terminal moraines at the points of farthest advance. Remaining after a glacier melted, moraines formed natural basins that filled with large lakes. Fallen Leaf Lake is an outstanding example, as is Emerald Bay, joined to Lake Tahoe because its terminal moraine is slightly lower than Tahoe's current water level.

Views of Mt. Tallac's eastern flanks are constant until the trail drops west below the ridgetop, briefly parallels Tallac Creek, and enters Desolation Wilderness a few hundred yards before reaching Floating Island Lake (1.4/7230´). Named for the large grassy mats that occasionally break off from its shores and float about, the shallow lake once contained a floating island buoyant enough to float six men, according to Barbara Lekisch in *Tahoe Place Names*.

The trail crosses Cathedral Creek before reaching a junction (2.3/7580´) where a steep trail climbing from Stanford Sierra Camp on Fallen Leaf Lake joins from the left. Cathedral Lake (2.5/7620´) makes a wonderful rest stop, and good views can be had from its eastern rim. Continuing, the rocky trail steepens and makes a few switchbacks on the way to a glacial cirque dotted with drooping mountain hemlocks (2.9/8200´). A tall, wizened western white pine stands between you and the rocky slopes of Mt. Tallac. The small creek here is your last opportunity to obtain water.

Snow can remain on the east-facing headwall late in the season and obscure the already difficult-to-distinguish track—the correct route runs along the headwall's northwest side. Once you're on top of the slope (3.2/8550´), the broadly sloping southwestern flank of the mountain is revealed. Pink phlox hug the ground as the trail veers northwest parallel to the ridge, reaching the summit via a short, posted trail (4.6/9715´).

The jagged summit makes for difficult seating but get comfortable, you'll want to savor the view. The stretch of land from Emerald Bay (Hike 81) to the Stateline casinos was once filled with rivers of ice, a spectacular scene to imagine. As you look southwest down into Desolation Wilderness, the irregular shape of island-studded Lake Aloha (8116´) sits below the peaks of the Crystal Range, and perfectly round Gilmore Lake lies immediately below you. Return the way you came.

Nearest Visitors Center: Lake Tahoe Visitors Center at Taylor Creek, (530) 543-2674, is located 2.7 miles north of the junction of Hwys. 50 and 89 in South Lake Tahoe on Hwy. 89 and is open 8 AM–5:30 PM daily in summer and weekends only in the fall. In the off-season, contact the Forest Supervisor's office in South Lake Tahoe, (530) 543-2600, which is open 8 AM–4:30 PM Monday through Friday.

Backpacking Information: Campsites are extremely limited on this hike. Only a few small sites exist near Cathedral Lake; your best options are the broad southwest shoulder of Mt. Tallac above the headwall or the somewhat more distant Gilmore Lake. Wilderness permits are required for all overnight stays, and there is a $5 per person recreational fee (with an additional $5 for two or more nights). Permits can be obtained at the above visitors centers or the Pacific Ranger District Office, located 22 miles east of Placerville on Hwy. 50 and open 8 AM–4:30 PM Monday through Friday and on most weekends.

Desolation Wilderness has a quota system for specific backcountry zones; 4 permits are available for the area around Cathedral Lake, 6 for the upper slopes, and 18 for the Gilmore Lake area. Half the spots are first-come, first-served; the other half can be reserved by calling (530) 647-5415 anytime after the third Thursday in April ($5 reservation fee).

Nearest Campground: Campgrounds line Lake Tahoe's shore. The closest are Eagle Point Campground (100 sites, $25) and Fallen Leaf Campground (205 sites, $20).

Additional Information: www.fs.fed.us/r5/ltbmu

HIKE 81

Lake Tahoe

Tahoe Bliss

Highlights	Tahoe shores, Emerald Bay, and Vikingsholm
Distance	6.6 miles one-way
Total Elevation Gain/Loss	1150'/850'
Hiking Time	3–5 hours
Optional Map	USGS 7.5-min. *Emerald Bay*
Best Times	Mid-June through September
Agency	D. L. Bliss and Emerald Bay state parks
Difficulty	★★

Lake Tahoe needs no introduction. Despite the thick development elsewhere, this pristine shoreline allows us to experience the majesty of what Tahoe must have once been.

The Hike is a one-way journey along Lake Tahoe's shoreline from D. L. Bliss State Park to Emerald Bay State Park along the Rubicon Trail. Swimming, sunning, and fishing are all possible diversions, and fairy-tale Vikingsholm awaits in enchanting Emerald Bay. While it can be completed in either direction, the hike description proceeds south from D. L. Bliss, saving Emerald Bay for the latter half of the day. Either a car shuttle is required for this hike, or you can take public transportation (see below) back to the entrance of D. L. Bliss. Be aware that the trailhead is a 2.3-mile road walk from the D. L. Bliss park entrance. This trail is very crowded

in summer, so arrive before 10 AM to get a spot in the small trailhead parking lot. After the lot has filled, check the small, unposted parking spaces 1.1 miles from the entrance—you can easily connect with the trail from there. If they too are full, the only available parking is along Hwy. 89. Water is available at the trailhead.

To Reach the Trailhead: Take Hwy. 89 to the entrance for D. L. Bliss State Park. Approaching from the south, it is 4 miles past Eagle Point Campground. From the north, it is 5.5 miles past Meeks Bay Campground. From the entrance station, follow signs toward Camps 141–168 and, at the final intersection, bear right toward the Rubicon Trail parking lot. There is a $6 day-use fee.

Public transportation is available from late May through early October on the Emerald Bay Shuttle; call (530) 541-7548 or

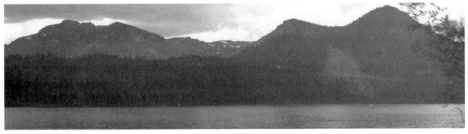

Emerald Bay

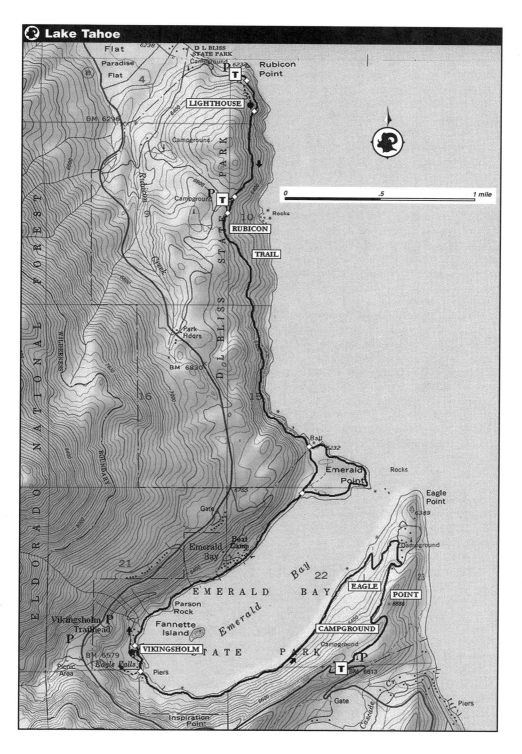

visit www.bluego.org. From around 10 AM until 6 PM, buses run a regular hour-long loop from Camp Richardson Resort to D. L. Bliss State Park and back, stopping at the Eagle Point Campground entrance and Vikingsholm parking area. Connections to and from South Lake Tahoe can be made at Camp Richardson.

Description: From the parking lot (0.0/6260´), the single-track trail strikes south among white firs, huckleberry oaks, and manzanita. At the immediate junction for the lighthouse trail, continue straight to quickly obtain your first views of Tahoe's distinctive, clear, aquamarine-tinted water below you. While reduced from its historic clarity of 120 feet deep, objects can still be seen to 75 feet in places! Along this early section of trail, numerous use paths branch down toward the lake. Lake access ends after the trail reaches a mildly precariously section protected by a chain-link fence (0.3/6330´) and slowly begins climbing. Osprey nest along this stretch and can occasionally be spotted until their departure in mid-August. By the time you reach the second junction for the lighthouse trail (0.4/6430´), the lake is 200 feet below. Resembling a modified outhouse, the lighthouse makes for an easy 0.1-mile side trip.

Turning inland, the trail continues to climb and suddenly offers magnificent views southwest of snow-frosted Mt. Tallac (Hike 80). Two large spur trails from the alternate parking lot in D. L. Bliss soon join the route in a dense forest of white firs (0.9/6520´), just before the trail crests at 350 feet above the lake. From here the trail slowly descends, passing among the bleached debris of a 1982 avalanche before reaching the lakeshore near Emerald Point (2.5/6230´). The trail forks: Left goes around the small peninsula's perimeter to worthwhile Emerald Point and the mouth of Emerald Bay, while right shortcuts to the bay proper. The flat peninsula is the terminal moraine of the glacier that carved Emerald Bay and pinedrops, horsetails,

ferns, and large Jeffrey pines sprout in the lush, sandy soil.

Veering southwest along the shores of Emerald Bay, the trail widens, passing Boat Camp before winding through the jumbled remains of a 1980 landslide (stay along the lake) to reach the Vikingsholm complex at the head of the bay (4.4/6230´). Considered the most authentic reproduction of Scandinavian architecture in the U.S., Vikingsholm was completed in 1929 without damaging any of the site's beautiful trees. Lora J. Knight spent summers here until her death in 1945, entertaining guests both onshore and in the teahouse on Fannette Island, in the middle of Emerald Bay. Donated to the state in 1958, the site now houses a visitors center, ferry dock, and other tourist-friendly facilities. The sod roof still sprouts flowers and regular tours inside Vikingsholm are offered daily in summer for a $5 fee. A steep trail climbs 1.0 mile and 800 feet to the Vikingsholm parking lot on Hwy. 50. From here, continue on the newly constructed trail running along the bay's southeast shore.

This quiet section is almost entirely level, climbing 300 feet only at the end to terminate at the campfire circle in upper Eagle Point Campground (6.3/6500´). It is an easy uphill through the campground to the parking spaces on Hwy. 50.

Nearest Visitors Center: D. L. Bliss Visitors Center, (530) 525-9529, is open 9 AM–4 PM daily Memorial Day through mid-October. Vikingsholm Visitors Center, (530) 525-8529, is open 9 AM–4 PM daily Memorial Day through September.

Nearest Campground: Eagle Point and D. L. Bliss campgrounds ($20–35, depending on season and site) are large, but they both regularly fill during the summer.

Additional Information: www.parks.ca.gov

HIKE 82

Grouse Lake

Muh-KULL-uh-mee

Highlights	Splitting granite gorges and remote Grouse Lake
Distance	11.0 miles round-trip
Total Elevation Gain/Loss	2500′/2500′
Hiking Time	6–8 hours
Optional Map	*Mokelumne Wilderness* by the U.S. Forest Service
Best Times	Mid-June through September
Agency	Mokelumne Wilderness
Difficulty	★★★★

Unlike most of the High Sierra, little-traveled Mokelumne Wilderness is a land more renowned for its deep river gorges than its soaring mountains. Experience here the sweep and variety of a rolling granite landscape topped with volcanic peaks and sliced by canyons thousands of feet deep.

The Hike follows a ridge west from the popular Blue lakes to isolated Grouse Lake, perched in a magnificent granite bowl near the chasm formed by Summit City Creek. The trail passes Granite Lake in 1.8 miles, a somewhat traveled fishing destination for the numerous anglers that ply the waters of the Blue lakes area. Fishing is

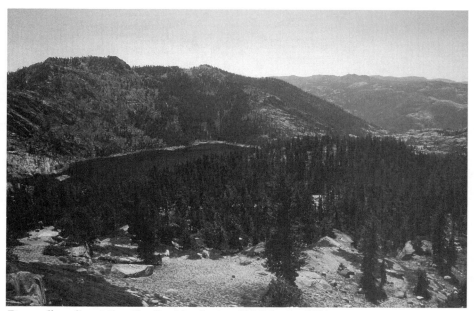

Deep valleys dissect the ridge-lined landscape of Mokelumne Wilderness.

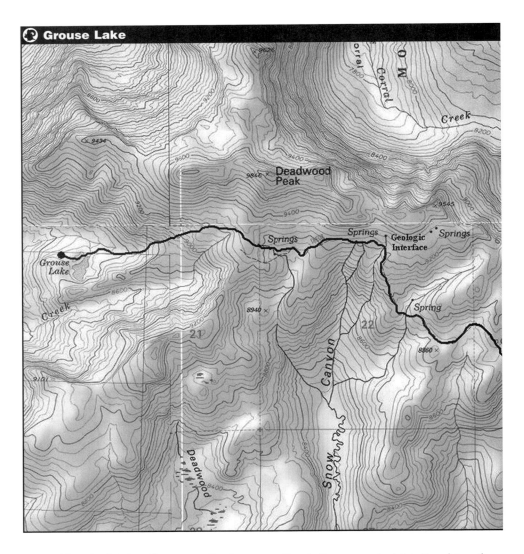

Grouse Lake

possible at both lakes. Snow usually clears by late June, with July and August the best months for wildflowers. While no water is available at the trailhead, faucets can be found in the nearby campgrounds around the Blue lakes.

To Reach the Trailhead: Take Blue Lakes Rd. (Forest Service Rd. 015) south from Hwy. 88—the posted turnoff is 6.6 miles east of Carson Pass. The paved road ends in 7.3 miles and you reach the junction for the Tamarack Lake Trailhead 3.7

miles farther—go straight. Reaching the Mokelumne Hydroelectric Project 1 mile later, the road becomes paved again; bear right and drive 1.9 miles toward Upper Blue Lake dam. The trailhead lot is on your left past Lower Blue Lake Campground (within eyeshot of Upper Blue Lake dam).

Description: From the parking lot (0.0/8140´), the trail immediately passes along a seasonal creek beneath a thick cover of lodgepole pine and mountain

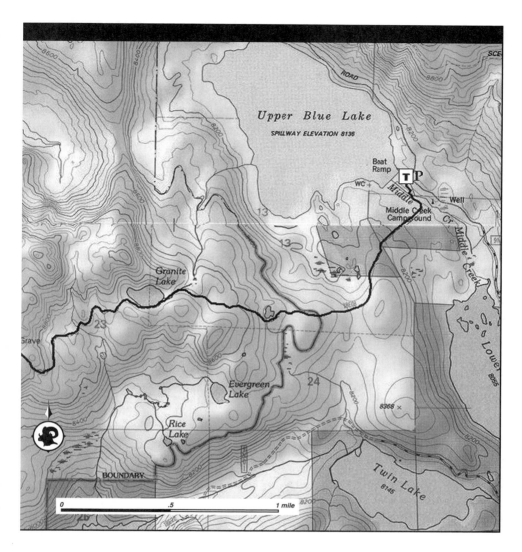

hemlock. Corn lilies, alpine asters, and a variety of other seasonal wildflowers decorate the moist understory along this early section of trail. Veering west, the trail crosses a stream and diverges in three directions: Go left (downstream), paralleling the stream briefly before angling away from it. As you gradually climb to Granite Lake, western white pines replace the lodgepole pines and you soon cross into Mokelumne Wilderness. Behind you, the Nipple (9342´) is visible immediately

northeast, the rocky turret of Jeff Davis Peak (8960´) east-northeast, and the dark brown ridge of pyramidal Raymond Peak (10,014´) and more distant Reynolds Peak (9679´) southeast. All these darker peaks are remnants of ancient volcanic flows that intermittently coursed over the rolling granite landscape of Mokelumne Wilderness during the past 30 million years. Today's rivers have eroded through most of these overlying volcanic rocks to reach the granite bedrock, but the higher peaks remain capped by these reddish-brown flows.

Ringed by broken hills of granite, pretty Granite Lake (1.8/8700') is a pleasant spot for a breather and offers good fly-fishing. Passing its western edge, the trail forks—head away from the lake. Cresting a small rise, you get the first views of the deep canyon of North Fork Mokelumne River. A few Sierra junipers can be identified as the now undulating trail slowly climbs to a distinct granite/volcanic interface near the ridgetop, passing several easy side trips to spectacular views south. Immediately prior to reaching the darker volcanic rocks (4.0/9220'), the trail passes below a striking illustration of the local geology. Along the interface above, granite boulders can be seen protruding from an eroding shell of loose volcanic rock, graphic evidence that the first lava flows pooled around and covered earlier existing features.

Traversing above meadow-filled Snow Canyon, the trail crosses several lush gullies, fed by springs emerging from the interface. Approaching the edge of the Snow Canyon watershed, the trail becomes indistinct; you encounter a triangular meadow bordered by several springs. Follow the farthest spring approximately 50 feet before crossing it near the edge of the exposed granite. The route is marked with small rock piles where it crests a slight ridge into the Grouse Creek drainage. Grouse Lake soon becomes visible over 600 feet below you. The trail descends quickly to meet it (5.5/8540'), passing through a healthy forest of western white pine and mountain hemlock on its way down. Note your route as you descend; it looks considerably different on the ascent.

Go beyond the west shore of Grouse Lake for views southwest of Mokelumne Peak (9334') and the tantalizing upper cliffs of the Summit City Creek gorge. Return the way you came.

Nearest Visitors Center: The local Chamber of Commerce runs an excellent visitors center in Markleeville, (530) 694-2475, that is open 8 AM–4 PM daily May through December, with reduced hours the rest of the year. A closer source of information is the U.S. Forest Service Carson Pass Information Center, located at the pass itself, which is open approximately 9 AM–5 PM daily during the summer.

Backpacking Information: There are campsites at Grouse Lake. Wilderness permits are required and can be obtained at the trailhead, at Carson Pass during open hours, or anytime at the register outside of the Markleeville visitors center.

Nearest Campground: PG&E runs 3 campgrounds around Upper and Lower Blue lakes (73 sites, $15–20); call (916) 386-5164.

Additional Information: www.fs.fed.us/r5/eldorado

HIKE 83

Hiram Peak

The Forgotten Sierra

Highlights	The summit of Hiram Peak and the heart of Carson-Iceberg Wilderness
Distance	2.4 miles round-trip
Total Elevation Gain/Loss	1250′/1250′
Hiking Time	2–3 hours
Optional Map	*Carson-Iceberg Wilderness* by the U.S. Forest Service
Best Times	Mid-June through September
Agency	Carson-Iceberg Wilderness
Difficulty	★★★

Forgotten Carson-Iceberg Wilderness is a little-visited landscape of volcanic peaks that straddles the central Sierra between Yosemite and Lake Tahoe. Set apart, Hiram Peak (9795′) provides summit views extraordinaire of the high wilderness heartland.

The Hike is a short, steep, easy-to-follow cross-country route from Highland Lakes Campground to the top of Hiram Peak. The region receives light use with the majority of visitors fishing at Highland Lakes. Snow usually clears by late June; July and August are the best for wildflowers. Water is available at the trailhead.

To Reach the Trailhead: Take Hwy. 4 toward Ebbetts Pass and bear south on Highland Lakes Rd.—the posted turnoff is 17 miles east of Bear Valley Road and 1.3 miles west of Ebbetts Pass. Approaching from the east, the turn is an easily missed hairpin on the left, so pay close attention. Unpaved Highland Lakes Rd. is passable for all vehicles and winds for 5.8 miles to its terminus at Highland Lakes Campground. Hiram Peak is plainly visible southeast of the campground on the opposite side of lower Highland Lake. Located behind Site 31 in the eastern half of the campground, the trailhead is indicated by a small wooden trail sign.

Description: From the trailhead (0.0/8670′), follow the obvious route upward through red firs and western white pines before breaking out onto an open hillside. Seasonal wildflowers here include mariposa lilies, explorer's gentian,

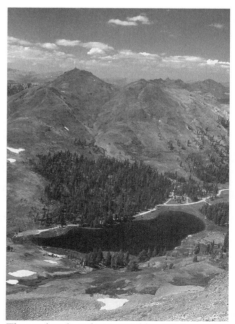

The road ends at lower Highland Lake on the edge of Carson-Iceberg Wilderness.

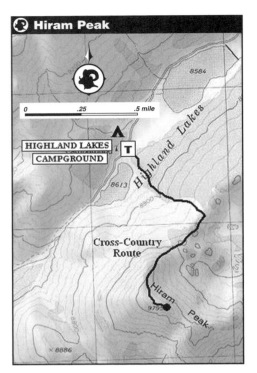

wild carrots, lupine, and mule's ears. Weaving along the forest edge, the trail begins to fan out and disappear as the summit of Hiram Peak comes into view to the south. Continue to the ridgetop above you (0.5/9130'), and then traverse south to the base of the talus slopes. As you begin your ascent, use paths make clambering up the slopes somewhat easier. You soon reach the ridge that bends southeast and leads you to the summit (1.2/9795'). You pass a few stumpy, twisted whitebark pines along the way to the top.

Beginning some 30 million years ago, intermittent volcanism covered the land of today's Carson-Iceberg Wilderness in layers of lava, mud flows, and volcanic debris; the region surrounding Hiram Peak is a complex composite of these flows. Feast on the view and admire the headwaters of three major California rivers. Looking east, the closest mountain is Arnot Peak (10,054'), part of the Sierra Divide. Its northeastern slopes are the headwaters of Wolf Creek, whose glacially carved valley can be seen trailing off northeast to join the Carson River. Flowing to the Stanislaus River, Disaster Creek drains the western flanks of Arnot Peak and is visible in the tarn-dotted open basin below you to the northeast. Looking south, the towering massif of Airola Peak (9942') and mostly hidden Iceberg Peak (9781') split the headwaters of Arnot Creek (east) and Highland Creek (west). Highland Creek flows into visible Spicer Meadows Reservoir before also joining the Stanislaus River. The two Highland lakes to the north actually mark a significant watershed between the Mokelumne River, fed by the upper lake, and the Stanislaus River, fed by the lower lake. On the horizon, the peaks of Mokelumne Wilderness (Hike 82) lie northwest and the mountains of Emigrant Wilderness (Hike 84) rise southeast. Return the way you came.

Nearest Visitors Center: Alpine Ranger Station, located 1.3 miles east of Bear Valley Rd. in a small hut by Hwy. 4, is open sporadically Thursday through Monday 8 AM–4:30 PM in season. A more reliable information source is the Calaveras Ranger District Office, (209) 795-1381, located in Hathaway Pines on Hwy. 4 and open 8 AM–5 PM Monday through Saturday.

Backpacking Information: A wilderness permit is required, obtainable at the above ranger stations during business hours. While there are no campsites along this hike, options do exist east of Hiram Peak along the cross-country route toward Arnot Creek.

Nearest Campground: Highland Lakes Campground at the trailhead has 35 sites ($8).

Additional Information: www.fs.fed.us/r5/stanislaus/calaveras

HIKE 84

Deadman Lake

Blue Canyon

Highlights	The volcanic High Sierra— solitude among falls, creeks, lakes, and peaks
Distance	4.5 miles round-trip
Total Elevation Gain/Loss	1700´/1700´
Hiking Time	3–5 hours
Optional Map	USGS 7.5-min. *Sonora Pass*
Best Times	July through September
Agency	Emigrant Wilderness
Difficulty	★★★

Emigrant Wilderness receives only the smallest fraction of the hordes that descend upon neighboring Yosemite National Park. Blue Canyon lies in a most remote corner of the wilderness. Solitude anyone?

Above 9000 feet near the Sierra Divide, Blue Canyon exists in a landscape of volcanic rubble unusual in this land of naked granite. Roughly 10 million years ago, a period of volcanism centered east of today's Sonora Pass smothered the landscape beneath numerous flows of mud and molten rock. Today these looser volcanic sediments have largely been eroded away, but sections still remain north of Yosemite near the Sierra crest. The layered, multihued bands exposed in the rocks and cliffs of Blue Canyon are part of these geologic remnants.

The Hike winds upward through Blue Canyon along the headwaters of Blue Canyon creek, passing starkly beautiful waterfalls en route to a couple of vibrantly blue lakes—Blue Canyon Lake and Deadman Lake. The single-track trail is steep and rocky, the lakes are surrounded by loose talus slopes, and the final mile to Deadman Lake is cross-country. Due to the high elevation, snow lingers deep into June and can return as early as October. While no

water is available at the trailhead, Blue Canyon creek is regularly accessible.

To Reach the Trailhead: Take Hwy. 108 toward Sonora Pass. The unposted trailhead is accessed from a small pullout on the south side of Hwy. 108. Approaching from the west, it is 2.1 miles past Chipmunk Flat dispersed camping area; your landmark is the distinctive waterfall where Blue Canyon Creek joins Deadman Creek and the pullout is immediately after the falls disappear from view. Approaching from the east, the trailhead is 2.8 miles past Sonora Pass (the pullout is 0.1 mile after the road begins its steepest descent from Sonora Pass). A dozen small lodgepole pines line the edge of the pullout, bare granite blocks sit across Hwy. 108 from it, and there is space for four cars.

Description: From the pullout (0.0/8920´), a discernible trail drops 40 feet to cross both Deadman Creek and the granite/volcanic geologic divide before quickly ascending the steep opposite slope to enter Blue Canyon. A few wilderness signs indicate you're on the right track as the trail winds through lodgepole pines and begins to offer views up-canyon. A use trail converges from the west side immediately before you cross a small feeder creek. Western white pines begin to

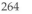

Deadman Lake

Carson-Iceberg Wilderness (Hike 83) are visible on the skyline.

Begin your cross-country adventure to Deadman Lake from here by ascending east toward the col of the long ridge, which lies between the small shark's-fin peak seen from the early sections of trail and the thumblike peak that juts from the ridge. Having obtained the ridgetop (1.8/10,300´), traverse north around the thumb on its east side and then scramble down over the tinkling piles of loose rock to reach the lake (2.2/10,484´). Barren, brilliantly blue, and ringed by naught but snow, rock, and lichen, Deadman Lake has a desolate beauty. Looking east, the nearby ridge marks the Sierra Divide and the routing of the Pacific Crest Trail. Return the way you came.

Nearest Visitors Center: Summit Ranger District Office, (209) 965-3434 and located in Pinecrest on Hwy. 108, is open daily 8 AM–5 PM and closed weekends and holidays October through May. Volunteer-staffed Brightman Flat Visitors Center is occasionally open also and is located 7 miles west of Kennedy Meadows' turnoff on Hwy. 108.

Backpacking Information: A wilderness permit is required, obtainable at the above visitors centers. The few campsites along this hike are bare and exposed, with Blue Canyon Lake offering the best sites. No quota is in effect for this trailhead.

Nearest Campground: Chipmunk Flat dispersed camping area (free, river water only) is 5 miles east of the turnoff for Kennedy Meadows on Hwy. 108. Numerous other campgrounds (44 and 17 sites respectively, $15) line Hwy. 108, including Baker and Deadman campgrounds at Kennedy Meadows.

Additional Information: www.fs.fed.us/r5/stanislaus

appear, easily identified by the deep red of their plated bark. The trail then swings away from the creek and begins steeply climbing, soon crossing the most significant feeder creek yet (0.8/9520´). Shortly thereafter, you come to a very sheer section of trail where the main path diverges in two directions—drop down to the creek and follow the obvious path alongside it. The trail next curves away from the creek and peters out immediately before reaching Blue Canyon Lake (1.5/10,037´). At the bottom of a rubble-filled glacial cirque, the sapphire lake offers a few, exposed campsites. Looking down-canyon, the peaks of

HIKE 85

Mono Lake

Mono Tufa

Highlights	Magical tufascapes
Distance	1.5 miles
Total Elevation Gain/Loss	Negligible
Hiking Time	1 hour
Optional Map	USGS 7.5-min. *Lee Vining*
Best Times	May through October
Agency	Mono Lake Tufa State Reserve
Difficulty	★

Explore the wild wonderland of Mono Lake—its water, tufas, and wildlife. Mono Lake sits in a natural basin where the sun evaporates 45 inches of fresh water annually, leaving large quantities of dissolved solids behind in the lake. Ongoing for over 700,000 years, this process has left Mono Lake exceptionally salty and alkaline—at present, with the lake being two times saltier than the ocean and 100 times more alkaline, 10 percent of it is dissolved solids. The water has a greasy, slippery feel and provides enough buoyancy to easily float a person.

Mono Lake currently has a surface area of approximately 70 square miles with an average depth of only 50 feet and a maximum depth of 150 feet. In 1941 the water-hungry city of Los Angeles began diverting four of the five streams that feed Mono Lake, which caused the lake level to drop more than 40 feet and upset the natural ecological balance. Concerned citizen groups took initiative in the 1980s to save the shrinking lake; in 1994 the State Water Resources Control Board ordered that Mono Lake be protected, and its level be raised 17 feet over the ensuing decades. With the lake recovering (the level still varies from year-to-year depending on the weather), current efforts now focus on how best to rehabilitate the lake environment.

Mono Lake's receded shoreline has exposed many of the spectacular tufa formations previously hidden beneath the lake's surface. Formed by a reaction between calcium-bearing freshwater springs that bubble up beneath the lake and the carbonate-rich lake water, the tufas are composed of solid calcium carbonate (limestone). A tufa tower grows upward from the lake bottom around the mouth of the spring until exposed above the surface of the lake. The towers of South Tufa Area were completely submerged prior to 1941 and will gradually return to the lake with rising water levels. Numerous active tufa towers continue to grow unseen beneath the lake today.

The lake's wildlife is as bizarre as the surrounding tufascapes. While the inhospitable water precludes survival of most aquatic life (there are no fish in Mono Lake), a few species thrive here in mindboggling numbers. The lake's winter algae bloom provides sustenance for the brine shrimp, which begin to hatch in the spring. By midsummer, an estimated 4 trillion tiny brine shrimp are swimming in the lake; Thousands of pounds are harvested annually for sale as tropical fish food. Brine fly pupae, the lake's other primary denizen, also depend on the algae for sustenance. During the summer, mature flies blanket

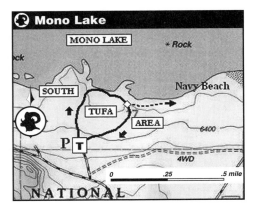

the lakeshore and produce harmless knee-high swarms when disturbed. The Kuzedika (Fly-Pupae Eaters), a band of the Paiute Tribe that once lived by the lake, harvested the fly pupae for food and trade. The size and color of brown rice grains, the prepared pupae taste like bacon bits. By late summer the algae is gone and the lake is once again clear and blue. Millions of birds pass through Mono Lake annually as they migrate, or winter here, consuming shrimp and flies as they go. Osprey nest on top of a few exposed tufa towers. Safe from predators, the osprey hunt in the nearby creeks and lakes.

The Hike is an easy stroll on the lake's south shore through surreal tufa formations. The trail is open and accessible during the snow-free months of the year, with heavy visitation throughout the summer months. Due to the area's popularity, this is not a hike for solitude seekers. No water is available at the trailhead or anywhere along the route. A swim in Mono Lake can be an unforgettable experience. Nearby Navy Beach offers the best opportunity and can be accessed either by hiking along the lakeshore or driving from the South Tufa Area. Avoid getting water in your mouth or eyes and be prepared for a salty, crusty coating on your body—no showers are available.

To Reach the Trailhead: Take Hwy. 395 south from Lee Vining for 6 miles to the Hwy. 120 junction. Follow Hwy. 120 east for 5 miles to the posted turnoff on your left for the South Tufa Area; a mile-long dirt road leads to the large trailhead parking lot. There is a $3 per person entrance fee.

Description: A 7-foot-wide asphalt path leads from the kiosk to the lakeshore, passing numerous tufa towers and soon providing your first opportunity to touch the lake water. The now single-track clay trail heads east from shore, winding through odd configurations of tufa and seasonal swarms of brine flies. While numerous paths wind through the brush, your route is clearly indicated. After turning away from the lake, the trail forks. Bearing left takes you on a longer return loop (an extra 0.5 mile) to the parking lot. Going straight brings you directly back.

Nearest Visitors Center: The outstanding Mono Basin Scenic Area Visitors Center, (760) 647-3044, is located on Hwy. 395 near Lee Vining, 1.3 miles north of the Hwy. 120 junction. It's open 9 AM–5:30 PM daily from May through October, with extended summer and weekend hours, and is closed in the off-season. Additionally, the Mono Lake Committee runs an information center in Lee Vining, (760) 647-6595, on the west side of Hwy. 395. Open daily year-round 9 AM–5 PM, with extended summer hours.

Nearest Campground: While there are no campgrounds around Mono Lake itself, numerous options exist south of Mono Lake along Hwy. 120 in Lee Vining Canyon and Hwy. 158 (the June Lake loop).

Additional Information: www. monolake.org

Nevada and Vernal Falls

Foaming Violent Thunder

Highlights	The raging river, incredible waterfalls, and spectacle of Yosemite
Distance	5.9 miles round-trip
Total Elevation Gain/Loss	1900´/1900´
Hiking Time	5–7 hours
Optional Map	USGS 7.5-min. *Half Dome*
Best Times	Mid-May through June
Agency	Yosemite National Park
Difficulty	★★★

Ah, Yosemite. Despite the crowds, despite the hassle, there is no other place on Earth like it. Go.

The Hike climbs from Yosemite Valley to the top of Nevada Fall, passing Vernal Fall along the way via the Mist Trail and returning on the John Muir Trail. The more water there is in the river, the more spectacular the hike—snowmelt increases its flow until the end of June, at which point it begins to decrease considerably. Exploding spray courses over the trail below Vernal Falls for much of the season, making good rain gear and waterproof boots useful but not essential to have. Crowds are somewhat lighter in May; otherwise they

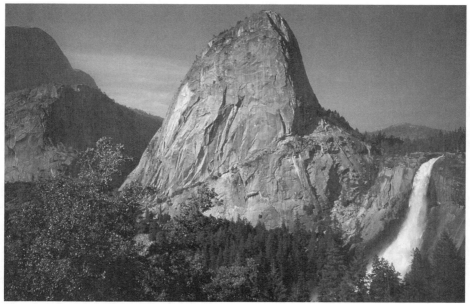

Nevada Fall explodes below Liberty Cap.

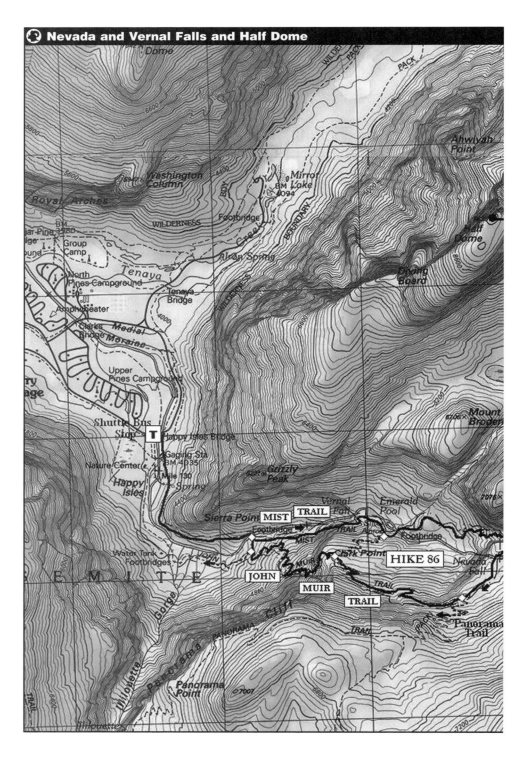

Nevada and Vernal Falls and Half Dome

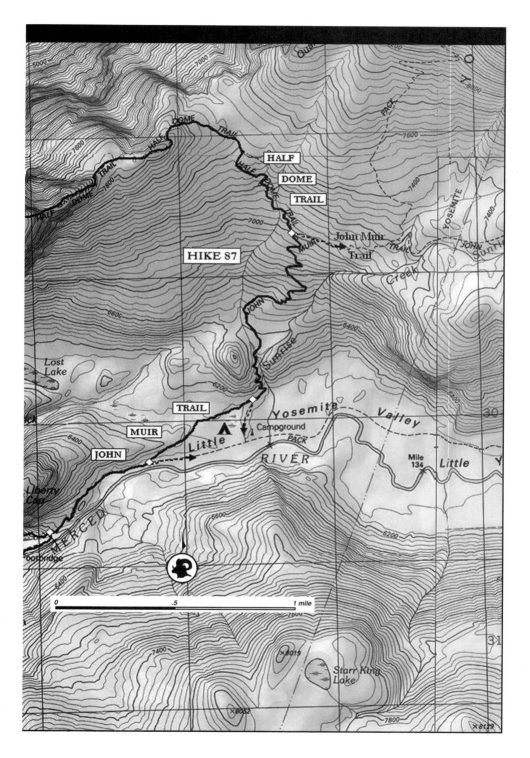

are unavoidable and, for some, perhaps overwhelming. With winter routes available, much of the hike can be done year-round—check conditions at the visitors center (see below). Water is available at the trailhead.

To Reach the Trailhead: Park in one of Yosemite Valley's day-use parking lots and take the free Yosemite Valley Shuttle Bus to Happy Isles Nature Center. There is a $20 entrance fee per vehicle for Yosemite National Park, valid for 7 days.

Description: From the bus stop (0.0/4030´), cross the Merced River bridge and head upriver on the 15-foot-wide superhighway of packed dirt to quickly reach the gigantic trailhead sign. Just beyond the sign, the trail winds up among huge granite boulders and closely parallels the now violent river. As you ascend, look for two of Yosemite's other landmark waterfalls—Upper Yosemite Fall is briefly visible behind you down-canyon before being cut off from view by Glacier Point,

and the wispy fall of Illilouette Creek to the Merced River can be momentarily seen cross-canyon.

Vernal Fall Bridge (0.8/4400´) provides your first views of the waterfall. Its smooth foaming curtain of water drops 317 feet and is dominated by two towering granite peaks—Mt. Broderick (6706´) left and Liberty Cap (7076´) just beyond it. Restrooms and a drinking fountain are available. Postings around the bridge indicate that, yes, the strong current can batter you to death against the rocks. Here, as everywhere along this hike, do not go in the water!

Climbing from the bridge, the trail quickly reaches a junction for the John Muir Trail (1.0/4440´)—continue straight up the Mist Trail. Billowing clouds of spray soon wash over the trail as it climbs through a lush garden of dripping greenery. You will get wet, so protect your camera! Just where the mist tapers out, you can peer into the heart of the fall over the top of a

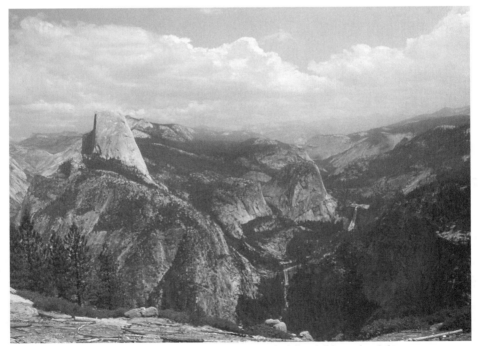

Half Dome from Glacier Point with Vernal and Nevada falls visible to the right

glistening rainbow, an unforgettable sight. Climbing to the top of the fall, the trail becomes steep and narrow; it traverses the face of a granite cliff, where hikers are protected by a metal guardrail. Surmounting this section, you reach a wide, open space above the fall where hikers dry out or sunbathe (1.5/5050′). Look over the lip of the fall at the Mist Trail below you. Do not be tempted to go in the river—almost every year some foolish person is swept over the fall and killed.

Continuing to Nevada Fall, parallel the river on any one of the many use paths to regain the main trail. Passing another short connector to the John Muir Trail, the trail crosses the river and climbs gradually to near the base of Nevada Fall. Here the mist is blown down-canyon rather than over the trail and forms a towering wall of spray visible through the trees. A short scramble would take you into the mist, but the fall itself is obscured if the river level is high.

With the sheer cliffs of Liberty Cap looming overhead, the trail then climbs 600 feet via nearly two dozen ever-tightening switchbacks to reach another junction with restroom facilities (2.3/6000′). To return to the trailhead go right on the John Muir Trail. In 0.2 mile you reach the top of Nevada Fall, where another restroom is available. You can access the cascade's protected lip via a short spur trail before the river crossing. Nevada Fall explodes, its water blown into swirling clouds that flow like an airborne river. Peering over the edge, buffeted by its winds, marvel at the torrent plummeting 571 feet to the rocks below.

The trail continues across the river and soon reaches a fork—go right. Traversing below the escarpment of Panoramic Cliffs, the John Muir Trail provides outstanding views of Liberty Cap and Nevada Fall, before descending along seemingly endless switchbacks to rejoin your earlier trail just above Vernal Fall Bridge (5.1/4440′). Halfway down, you have the option of retracing your steps on the Mist Trail by taking the posted connection to the top of Vernal Fall. Return to Happy Isles to end your day on the trail.

Nearest Visitors Center: Valley Visitors Center, located in Yosemite Village (Shuttle Bus Stops 5 and 9), is open 365 days a year. In summer it's open 9 AM–7 PM daily, with reduced hours the rest of the year. For general recorded information, call (209) 372-0200.

Backpacking Information: The closest backcountry camping is in Little Yosemite Valley, 0.5 mile past the top of Nevada Fall. See Hike 87 for more information on the hike to the area and the permit system and regulations.

Nearest Campground: Reservations are required from April through October for the three car-accessible campgrounds in Yosemite Valley. Reservations are available up to five months in advance, in blocks of one month at a time, with the next block becoming available on the 15th of each month. To make reservations, call (877) 444-6777 between 7 AM–9 PM (7 AM–7 PM November through February) or visit www.recreation. gov—you should make reservations as early as possible on the 15th. If you arrive without reservations in the Valley, try first-come, first-served Camp 4, a walk-in camping area (no individual sites, smaller groups will likely share the six-person sites with others). Otherwise head outside the Valley—try Tuolumne Meadows Campground in the morning and the U.S. Forest Service campgrounds just west of the park in the afternoon and evening.

Additional Information: www. nps.gov/yose

HIKE 87

Half Dome

The Burn

Highlights	Scaling Half Dome by cable with dizzying vertigo
Distance	16.4 miles round-trip
Total Elevation Gain/Loss	4800´/4800´
Hiking Time	10–12 hours
Optional Map	USGS 7.5-min. *Half Dome*
Best Times	Mid-June through September
Agency	Yosemite National Park
Difficulty	★★★★★

SEE MAP ON PAGES 268–269

There is no other hike in the world like this one.

The Hike is an extremely strenuous all-day affair that climbs to the summit of Half Dome from Yosemite Valley. The final stretch to the top is by a cable route so steep that you need to pull yourself up with both arms. Hikers should be in good shape and not suffer from acrophobia. Installed by the park once conditions allow, the cable route is usually up by Memorial Day and removed in early to mid-October. It is closed during the winter months. Sunscreen is essential for this hike as the bare rock of Half Dome provides no protection against the sun's burning rays. Crowds are constant all season long, although they're somewhat lighter after Labor Day. The trail gets congested by late morning, and the single-track cable route on top backs up by lunchtime. The earlier you start, the better.

To Reach the Trailhead: Park in one of Yosemite Valley's day-use parking lots and take the free Yosemite Valley Shuttle Bus to Happy Isles Nature Center. There is a $20 entrance fee per vehicle for Yosemite National Park, valid for 7 days.

Description: From the bus stop (0.0/4030´), cross the Merced River bridge and head upriver to quickly reach the gigantic trailhead sign. Just beyond the sign,

the trail winds up among huge granite boulders and closely parallels the now violent river. Vernal Fall Bridge (0.8/4400´) provides your first views of the waterfall. Its smooth foaming curtain of water drops 317 feet and is dominated by two towering granite peaks—Mt. Broderick (6706´) left and Liberty Cap (7076´) just beyond it. Restrooms and a drinking fountain are available. Postings around the bridge indicate that, yes, the strong current can batter you to death against the rocks. Here, as everywhere along this hike, do not go in the water!

Climbing from the bridge, the trail quickly reaches a junction for the John Muir Trail (1.0/4440´)—continue straight up the Mist Trail. Billowing clouds of spray soon wash over the trail as it climbs through a lush garden of dripping greenery. You will get wet, so protect your camera! Just where the mist tapers out, you can peer into the heart of the fall over the top of a glistening rainbow, an unforgettable sight. Climbing to the top of the fall, the trail becomes steep and narrow; it traverses the face of a granite cliff, where hikers are protected by a metal guardrail. Surmounting this section, you reach a wide, open space above the fall where hikers dry out or sunbathe (1.5/5050´). Look over the lip of the fall at the Mist Trail below you. Do not be tempted to go in the river—almost every year some foolish person is swept over the fall and killed.

Continuing to Nevada Fall, parallel the river on any one of the many use paths to regain the main trail. Passing another short connector to the John Muir Trail, the trail crosses the river and climbs gradually to near the base of Nevada Fall. Here the mist is blown down-canyon rather than over the trail and forms a towering wall of spray visible through the trees. A short scramble would take you into the mist, but the fall itself is obscured if the river level is high.

With the sheer cliffs of Liberty Cap looming overhead, the trail then climbs 600 feet via nearly two dozen ever-tightening switchbacks to reach another junction with restroom facilities (2.3/6000′). To continue toward Half Dome, head left, immediately passing the restroom on your way toward Little Yosemite Valley. Now gently climbing, the trail crests a small rise; it loses elevation for the first time where the top of Half Dome becomes visible northwest. Wide and sandy, the path rejoins the much calmer river before arcing away from it and passing the designated campground and seasonal ranger station on the right. Bear left at all junctions. Little Yosemite Valley is your last opportunity to get water for the next 1500 feet of elevation gain.

Turning north, your trail ascends upward through a dense red fir forest to reach the junction with the Half Dome Trail (4.8/7000′). While the John Muir Trail bears east here on its long journey to Mt. Whitney, you continue north to begin the ultimate ascent. You soon encounter a spring on the left where a small pipe conveniently diverts water for easy fill-up. Note that this nonpotable water must be purified; it is the last source on this hike. Views across Tenaya Canyon open up through the trees where the trail heads west to the base of the open slopes on the ridgetop (6.3/7900′).

Signs in many languages warn of the danger of lightning strikes. Take them seriously and do not proceed if thunderstorms are threatening. With your horizon clear, continue upward on the zigzagging stairway of granite blocks. As you pass twisted trees clinging to life in the nooks and crannies of bare rock, the trail gets progressively steeper. It soon crests a small rise and then drops to the bottom of the cable route (7.3/8410′).

Unless you arrive early, this final section will be a thin line of humanity creeping to the top. Blubbering acrophobes and exhausted hikers contribute to the line's slow pace; it can take upward of 30 minutes to reach the top. Be patient and savor this unforgettable experience while you wait. With both arms needed to pull yourself along, hand protection is important for preventing cable burn—a huge pile of mangled gloves found at the base of the cable route are free to use.

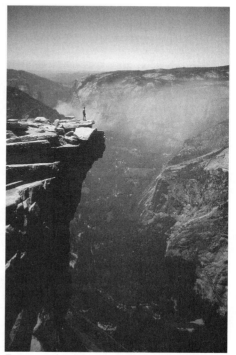

Dance with vertigo a vertical mile above Yosemite Valley.

The climb steepens on the upper section before finally reaching the end of the line (7.5/8810´). The actual summit (8838´) is at the north end.

Experience the dizzying vertigo of Half Dome as you creep toward the edge, staring almost 5000 feet down to the valley floor. Half Dome's northwest face is a vertical, 2000-foot sheer wall of granite, on which climbers can often be spotted. With unparalleled views from here, most of the southern half of the park is visible. Almost due north is Mt. Hoffman (10,850´), below which runs Tioga Road. Looking east beyond Little Yosemite Valley, the peaks of the Cathedral Range line the ho-rizon. Southeast are the spires of the Clark Range, all of which exceed 11,000 feet. Closer by, Clouds Rest (Hike 88) is immediately northeast along the ridge, with the bulges of Quarter Domes between it and Half Dome. If you look west down Yosemite Valley, many of the Valley's most prominent landmarks can be identified—Glacier Point is across the Merced River canyon and Cathedral Spires, El Capitan, and Yosemite Village are all visible.

Done reveling in this awe-inspiring place? Go back the way you came. For an alternate (and easier) descent, follow the John Muir Trail from Nevada Fall back to the Vernal Fall Bridge.

Nearest Visitors Center: Valley Visitors Center, located in Yosemite Village (Shuttle Bus Stops 5 and 9), is open 365 days a year, 9 AM–7 PM daily in summer, with reduced hours the rest of the year. For general recorded information, call (209) 372-0200.

Backpacking Information: Turning the marathon ascent of Half Dome into an overnight trip allows you to beat the morning rush on the cable route. Wilderness permits are required and there is a quota for this trailhead that always fills up. While 60 percent of the permits are subject to reservation, the other 40 percent are available on a first-come, first-served basis the day before or day of travel. To get a permit, be at a permit window the moment it opens (usually 7:30–8:30 AM), or make a reservation in advance by calling (209) 372-0740 Monday through Friday 8:30 AM–4:30 PM ($5 per person reservation fee). Permits can be obtained at the wilderness center adjacent to the Valley Visitors Center (opens 7:30 AM) and from permit stations at Tuolumne Meadows, Wawona, Big Oak Flat (just past the west entrance station on Hwy. 120), and Hetch Hetchy. Bear canisters are required and can be rented from the permit stations for $5 per trip. In Little Yosemite Valley, camping is allowed only at designated sites. Sleeping above 7600 feet on Half Dome is prohibited.

Nearest Campground: Reservations are required from April through October for the three car-accessible campgrounds in Yosemite Valley. Reservations are available up to five months in advance, in blocks of one month at a time, with the next block becoming available on the 15th of each month. To make reservations, call (877) 444-6777 between 7 AM–9 PM (7 AM–7 PM November through February) or visit www.recreation.gov—it is recommended that you make reservations as early as possible on the 15th. If you arrive without reservations in the Valley, try first-come, first-served Camp 4, a walk-in camping area (no individual sites, smaller groups will likely share the six-person sites with others). Otherwise head outside the Valley—try Tuolumne Meadows Campground in the morning and the U.S. Forest Service campgrounds just west of the park in the afternoon and evening.

Additional Information: www.nps.gov/yose

HIKE 88

Clouds Rest

Sky Walker

Highlights	Half Dome minus the madness
Distance	14.0 miles round-trip
Total Elevation Gain/Loss	2500′/2500′
Hiking Time	8–10 hours
Optional Map	USGS 7.5-min. *Tenaya Lake*
Best Times	Mid-June through September
Agency	Yosemite National Park
Difficulty	★★★★

Let's face it, Yosemite Valley is crazy. If the congestion there is too much for you, then you should be on the Tioga Road. And if you're on the Tioga Road, you should be climbing Clouds Rest.

The Hike ascends Clouds Rest (9926′) from Tenaya Lake, a steady climb with rewarding summit views of Half Dome and much of the national park. As throughout Yosemite, there will be people on the trail with you. However, there will be far fewer people than you would encounter on trails emanating from the Valley. Snow generally clears by mid-June, although it can linger into early July in years of deep snowpack. No water is available at the trailhead, and sources beyond Tenaya Creek can be non-existent late in the season.

To Reach the Trailhead: Go east on Tioga Rd. (Hwy. 120) to just west of Tenaya Lake in central Yosemite National Park, and park in the Sunrise Trailhead lot, located 33 miles east of Crane Flat and 9 miles west of Tuolumne Meadows Campground. There is a $20 entrance fee per vehicle for Yosemite National Park, valid for seven days.

Description: At the trailhead by the food storage lockers, the trail immediately splits—go left toward Sunrise High Sierra Camp. Passing among lodgepole pines, the wide concrete path soon becomes dirt. Skirting a pleasant meadow before crossing Tenaya Creek, the trail quickly reaches a junction for Tuolumne High Sierra Camp—bear right toward Sunrise.

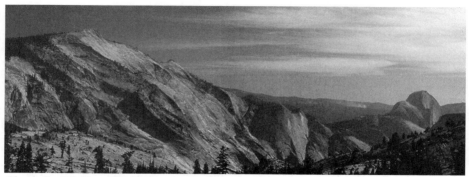

Clouds Rest (left) and Half Dome in the distance

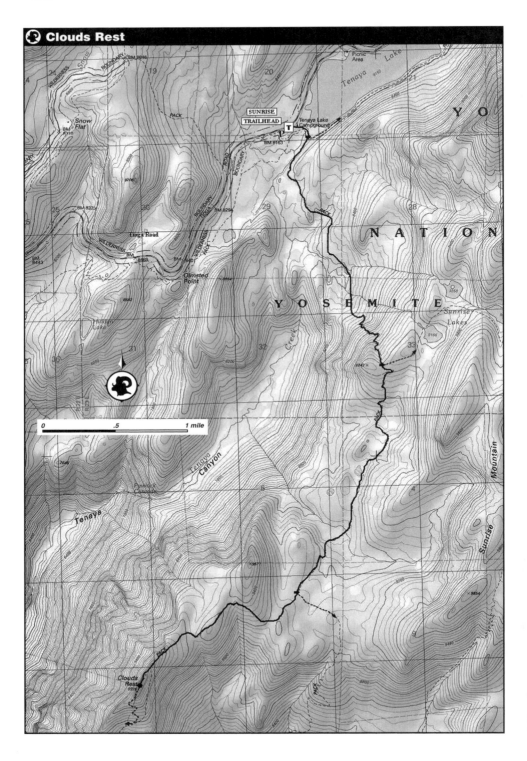

Clouds Rest

After briefly paralleling the creek, the trail curves south and passes on a long level stretch, weaving through boulders, lodgepole pines, and clearings seasonally flush with tiger lilies and other wildflowers. Red firs and western white pines appear as the trail climbs again; you soon find yourself switchbacking steeply to the top of a forested saddle. There is a four-way junction here—continue straight ahead. The unmarked trail that comes in from the right leads to surprise viewpoints of upper Tenaya Canyon. Left leads to the nearby Sunrise Lakes.

Descending south, the trail passes a shallow pond before crossing a small tributary of Tenaya Creek, which can run dry late in the season. This is your last source for water. Your route is a gentle rise from here to the next junction, where you continue straight ahead. The trail drops briefly before making a quick ascent to a broad saddle where views south are obscured by the trees . . . but not for long.

Continue along the ridgeline. Suddenly nothing impairs your view of the naked flanks of Clouds Rest shearing 4000 feet into Tenaya Canyon below. Sheets of exfoliating granite peel away from the slopes. The trail becomes indistinct the final 200 feet to the summit; take the broad granite runway directly along the ridgeline to the top (9926′).

Visible for the first time, Half Dome immediately draws your attention southwest. Those with binoculars can pick out the cable route's ant line on the northeast shoulder (Hike 87). Yosemite Valley winds away west below it all. Southeast beyond Little Yosemite Valley, the peaks of the Clark Range can be seen. Northeast on the skyline are the jagged pinnacles of Cathedral Range. North is Mt. Hoffman (10,850′), below which the Tioga Road winds around Tenaya Lake. Return the way you came.

Nearest Visitors Center: Tuolumne Meadows Visitors Center, (209) 372-0263, is open 8 AM–5 PM daily mid-June through mid-October, with occasional extended hours during peak times. For general Yosemite information, call the information center at (209) 372-0200.

Backpacking Information: Numerous campsites exist along or near this hike, although few have convenient access to water. Try Sunrise Lakes. There are no legal options on the summit. Wilderness permits are required and are most readily obtained from the permit station east of Tuolumne Meadows (open daily 8 AM–5 PM). There is a quota of 20 people for this trailhead and it always fills up. While 60 percent of the permits are subject to reservation, the other 40 percent are available on a first-come, first-served basis the day before or day of travel. To get a permit, be at the permit window the moment it opens, or make a reservation in advance by calling (209) 372-0740 between 8:30 AM and 4:30 PM Monday through Friday ($5 per person reservation fee).

Nearest Campground: Tuolumne Meadows Campground (304 sites, $20) opens once snow conditions allow and operates on a first-come, first-served basis until July 14. Beginning July 15, half the sites are subject to reservation; the other half remains first-come, first-served. Reservations can be made up to five months in advance, in blocks of one month at a time, with the next block becoming available on the 15th of each month. To make reservations, call (877) 444-6777 between 7 AM and 9 PM or visit www.recreation.gov. It is recommended that you make reservations as early as possible.

Additional Information: www.nps.gov/yose

HIKE 89

Mariposa Grove

Grizzly Giants

Highlights	The largest living things on Earth
Distance	5.8 miles
Total Elevation Gain/Loss	1100′/1100′
Hiking Time	3–4 hours
Optional Map	USGS 7.5-min. *Mariposa Grove*
Best Times	May through October
Agency	Yosemite National Park
Difficulty	★★

Incomparable, indescribable, unbelievable, the giant sequoias must be experienced firsthand. Visit the Valley only and you have seen but half the wonders of Yosemite.

The Mariposa Grove is one of the most northerly of 75 recognized giant sequoia groves that dot the western slopes of the Sierra Nevada. It is also the best known and most heavily visited. Not a spot for solitude, the grove receives hundreds to thousands of visitors daily. But most either select the narrated open-air tram tour, which putts along the paved roads of the grove, or walk but a short distance from the parking lot to the Grizzly Giant before returning to their vehicles, leaving the trails to far fewer people.

The Hike explores the entire grove by trail, and allows you to briefly escape the Yosemite bustle and peacefully commune with these giant trees. Mariposa Grove is open daily from approximately late April until late October when snow once again closes the 2-mile access road. Crowds are lightest in the evenings and early mornings. Water is available at the trailhead.

To Reach the Trailhead: Take the turnoff for the Mariposa Grove, located immediately inside the park just past the South Entrance Station on Hwy. 41, 35 miles (75 minutes) south of Yosemite Valley. Trailers

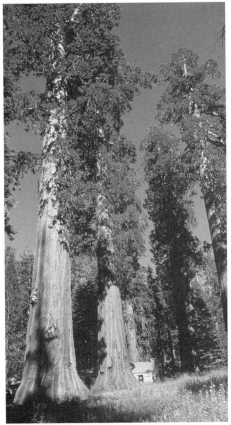

Upper Mariposa Grove and the Mariposa Grove Museum

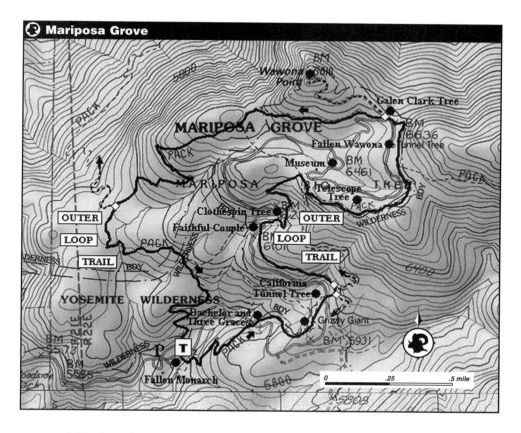

Mariposa Grove

are prohibited on the narrow 2-mile road to the parking lot, and RVs are not allowed between 9 AM and 4 PM. Despite its massive size, the parking lot is usually full by 10 AM during summer months. Additional parking is provided near the entrance station, and a free shuttle bus runs to the lot every 20 minutes during the busy season. There is a $20 entrance fee per vehicle for Yosemite National Park, good for seven days.

Description: To preserve the grove for future generations of trees (and visitors), do not take cones as souvenirs! From the parking lot, pass the gift shop and Tour Center on your way to the upper parking lot. The trail begins beside a kiosk where free brochures printed in five languages can be obtained (0.0/5600′). First head nearby to the Fallen Monarch, which is believed to have toppled more than 300 years ago. Crossing the road, you ascend numer-

ous oversized steps before recrossing the road by the Bachelor and Three Graces (0.5/5760′). Swelling in size near its base, the Bachelor provides a good example of what is known as a buttressed trunk.

The Grizzly Giant, fifth largest living thing on Earth, is next. Blackened and scarred, huge and grizzly indeed, its estimated age of 2700 years makes it one of the oldest living sequoias known. Just beyond it is the California Tunnel Tree, one of two trees in the grove tunneled by man, which poses a challenging physics problem of torque and balance. Walk through the tree, cross the road, and bear left at both trail junctions. The trail follows the road and soon reaches the Faithful Couple (1.5/6140′), a pair of enormous trees sutured together for more than 50 feet. The posted trail continues across the road to the Clothespin Tree, so named because

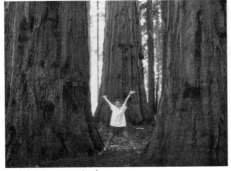

Celebrate sequoias!

of the enormous symmetrical gash that runs through it. Climbing into the Upper Grove, the trail reaches the road again near four magnificent specimens. Paths split off in all directions—continue right on the posted Outer Loop Trail, following the road's upper loop. The Mariposa Grove Museum (open daily 9 AM–4 PM) is visible beyond the restrooms and has informative displays, books, and a welcome drinking fountain (2.2/6460´).

Continuing on the Outer Loop Trail, take time for a quick side trip inside the Telescope Tree. Without blemish on the outside, inside it's hollow and blue sky can be seen through the opening on top. The trail next loops to the famous Wawona Tunnel Tree (2.8/6600´), lying on its side below the trail. The final landmark tree on this hike is the Galen Clark Tree, named for the man who tirelessly promoted the grove and urged its protection in the late 1850s and 1860s.

Immediately past the Galen Clark Tree is the junction for Wawona Point Vista, which offers views across the South Fork Merced River to Wawona Dome. The return to the parking lot on Outer Loop Trail leaves the sequoias behind and passes instead through a quiet forest of sugar pines, incense cedars, white firs, and Jeffrey pines. Those wishing to return through the sequoias should backtrack to the museum and descend from there. Otherwise, continue straight at all junctions in the upper grove. Halfway down to the parking lot (4.5/6120´) the trail to Wawona splits off west, but you continue straight and bear right at the remaining junctions to reach the lot.

Nearest Visitors Center: Wawona Information Station, (209) 375-9501, is open daily 8:30 AM–4:30 PM (closed for lunch) in summer. From Hwy. 41 in Wawona take Chilnualna Falls Rd. to the first right-hand turn past the stables. For general recorded park information, call (209) 372-0200.

Backpacking Information: Camping is prohibited in the grove from April through October when the access road is open. Once snow closes the road, the grove becomes designated wilderness, and intrepid cold-weather backpackers can hike, ski, or snowshoe the access road and camp beneath the sequoias. A wilderness permit is required, available from the Wawona Information Station. Note that the highway from the Wawona area to the Valley is closed during the winter.

Nearest Campground: Wawona Campground is located near Wawona (93 sites, $20) and is open year-round. Reservations are required May through September and can be made up to five months in advance, in blocks of one month at a time, with the next block becoming available on the 15th of each month. To make reservations, call (877) 444-6777 between 7 AM and 9 PM or visit www.recreation.gov. It is recommended that you make reservations as early as possible. Also try Summerdale Campground (30 sites) in Sierra National Forest, located immediately south of the park on Hwy. 41. For the adventurous with a map of Sierra National Forest, secret Nelder Grove Campground (free) is not too far away.

Additional Information: www.nps.gov/yose

HIKE 90

Mammoth Crest

The Upper Crest

Highlights	Mammoth Lakes Basin and the Sierra Divide
Distance	4.5 miles round-trip
Total Elevation Gain/Loss	1700´/1700´
Hiking Time	4–6 hours
Optional Map	USGS 7.5-min. *Crystal Crag*
Best Times	June through October
Agency	Inyo National Forest
Difficulty	★★★

In the town of Mammoth Lakes you can buy fresh arugula at the grocery store. You can also hike to the top of Mammoth Crest, view the entire crystalline basin, and then stare west into the heart of the Sierra Nevada.

Mammoth Lakes occupies the western end of the Long Valley caldera, an enormous depression formed 760,000 years ago in a massive volcanic eruption that blew ash as far away as Missouri. After the eruption, the top of the volcano collapsed to create this 10-by-20-mile-wide elliptical basin. Volcanic activity continued here over the next 560,000 years, producing lava flows and the bulging dome of Mammoth Mountain. While the past 100,000 years have been quiet, a large body of magma is believed to still exist as close as 3 miles below the caldera surface. Between 1980 and 1986 swarms of earthquakes struck the area and were accompanied by ground uplift, an indicator of magma movement below and a warning of a potential eruption. Although the region quieted down after 1986, activity and uplift in portions of the caldera continue today, making this region California's greatest volcanic hazard.

The Hike climbs from Lake George to the top of the Sierra Divide, which separates the Mammoth Lakes Basin from the drainage of the San Joaquin River. Crystal Lake makes a nice stopover halfway up, and is the end destination for many hikers. Above it people are fewer, a pleasant contrast to the crowds that frequent Mammoth Lakes virtually year-round. September is your best bet for tranquility. Fishing is possible in Crystal Lake. Water and all the amenities are available at the trailhead.

To Reach the Trailhead: Take Hwy. 203 west to the town of Mammoth Lakes—the turnoff is on Hwy. 395 roughly midway between Lee Vining and Bishop. At the first stoplight, continue straight on Main St. At the second stoplight, bear left onto Lake Mary Rd. and proceed 3.7 miles to a junction near Lake Mary—continue straight toward Mamie Lake. By the Pokonobe Marina 0.4 mile farther turn left; drive 0.3 mile—immediately passing Lake Mary Campground—to a posted junction for Lake George. Turn right and go 0.3 mile to the large but often full lot by Lake George Marina and Campground.

Description: Begin by the entrance to the parking lot (0.0/9030´) in a forest of lodgepole pine, western white pine, and mountain hemlock. The jagged granite thumb of Crystal Crag (10,377´)—visible from the lot—juts above Lake George; watch your perspective on this landmark

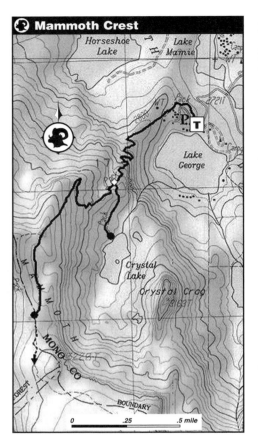

and McLeod Lake is farther west, just below Mammoth Pass (9360′). Traversing southeast near the ridgetop, you enter John Muir Wilderness (1.5/10,080′), where the rock changes from pale granite to red volcanics. You can see in the rocks behind the sign the turbulent flow currents and air bubbles preserved as they solidified. As you round the flank of a false crest, the true ridgetop becomes visible across a barren landscape dotted with krummholz trees. Once you've attained it, an off-trail stroll brings you to the western edge of the ridge where you can enjoy views into the San Joaquin drainage.

Raking the northern sky are the dark Minarets of the Ritter Range, remnants of volcanoes that erupted some 100 million years ago. Magma that fed those volcanoes is today's granite beneath your feet; it crystallized miles below the surface but later was exposed by erosion. The tallest mountains of the Ritter Range are Banner Peak (12,945′), seen farthest east, and adjacent Mt. Ritter (13,140′). The trail continues southeast along Mammoth Crest and offers ever-changing panoramic vistas, but this hike ends here after having conquered the Sierra Divide.

change dramatically over the course of the hike. Switchbacking west along the ridge above Lake George, the trail soon reaches the junction for Crystal Lake (0.9/9650′). A short spur leads down to this exquisite body of water, flanked by Crystal Crag on the east and Mammoth Crest on the west. A maze of use paths surround the lake.

After you've resumed climbing on the main trail, mountain hemlocks soon disappear in a predominantly lodgepole pine forest, and views of the basin below open up. Just beyond Lake George, a small flotilla of boats plies Lake Mary, the largest of the lakes. Mammoth Creek drains Lake Mary, passing through Lake Mamie and Twin Lakes on its way to Owens Valley. To the north, Horseshoe Lake lies between you and Mammoth Mountain (11,053′)

Nearest Visitors Center: Mammoth Lakes Visitors Center, (760) 924-5500, is located immediately east of town on Hwy. 203 and open daily 8 AM–5 PM.

Nearest Campground: There are six campgrounds in the Mammoth Lakes Basin, including one (16 sites, $18) by the trailhead at Lake George. They are all extremely popular and usually full, especially in July and August. A few of the sites can be reserved in advance by calling (877) 444-6777 or visiting www.recreation. gov. The remainder are first-come, first-served.

Additional Information: www. fs.fed.us/r5/inyo

HIKE 91

Balloon Dome

The Land of Balloon Dome

Highlights	Monolithic Balloon Dome and the mighty San Joaquin
Distance	9.9 miles round-trip
Total Elevation Gain/Loss	2300′/2300′
Hiking Time	8–10 hours
Optional Map	USGS 7.5-min. *Balloon Dome*
Best Times	May through October
Agency	Ansel Adams Wilderness
Difficulty	★★★★

A naked bubble of granite rising nearly 3000 feet from canyon bottom, Balloon Dome stands—a monolith, an inspiration, a companion on your descent to the sandy banks of the mighty San Joaquin River. Carving the Sierra Nevada between well-trod Yosemite and Kings Canyon national parks, the river pours through a delightful, less-visited landscape of abundant wildlife.

The Hike begins at the western border of Ansel Adams Wilderness and follows Cassidy Trail as it descends steadily to the San Joaquin River. A lower elevation hike, it makes an exciting option in spring and late fall when snow has closed the higher regions. Fishing and swimming are possible in the San Joaquin. Bring sun protection. Water is available at the trailhead from Granite Creek.

To Reach the Trailhead: Go 4.5 miles north on Hwy. 41 from the Hwy. 49 junction in Oakhurst and turn east on Bass Lake Rd. In 6 miles, turn left on Beasore

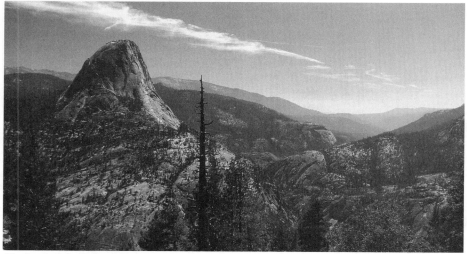

The land of the Balloon Dome

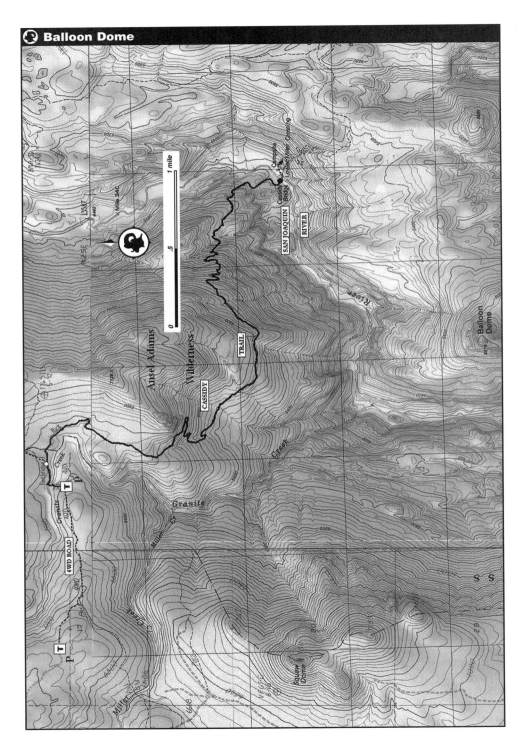

Rd. (Forest Service Rd. 7), which you'll follow for the next 30-plus miles. Cold Springs Summit is reached in 12.1 miles, where the road becomes a U.S. Forest Service Scenic Byway. Paved FSR 6S01 branches right 2.7 miles later—continue straight. The pavement ends 5 miles later just past a posted junction for Mugler Creek and Grizzly Rd. Continuing for another 11 miles on increasingly rough road (the last 2 miles are the worst), you reach a stop sign and the end of FSR 7. Go straight on FSR 5S30 for 1.1 miles, and turn right at the posted turnoff for Cassidy Trail. The first 1.7 miles is very rough but passable for all vehicles; then the access road drops steeply down a granite ramp. Park here if you can't go farther. The final 1.3 miles requires a high-clearance vehicle, and reaches the trailhead in an open parking area just before the road switchbacks down toward Granite Creek.

Description: From the parking area (0.0/6550´), descend north on Cassidy Trail to cross Granite Creek on a seasonal footbridge. The path curves right (downstream), slowly traverses upward, and passes a trail junction on the left. You next cross above a gully and head southwest, passing through a dense forest of large Jeffrey pines, sugar pines, white firs, and incense cedars. The bald hump of Squaw Dome (7818´) appears directly ahead before the trail begins to descend slowly and bend southeast. Suddenly you see Balloon Dome between the trees!

A granite dome occurs when a huge block of fracture-free granite is exposed at the surface after overlying layers have eroded away. Freed from the pressure of overlying rock, the dome begins slowly shedding giant curved layers of rock in a process known as exfoliation. Such an unusually solid mass of rock takes a long time to wear away and will stand sentinel over the landscape for eons. Half Dome (Hike 87) is the most famous example.

Changing views of Balloon Dome finally disappear as the trail begins a long arcing traverse to the east. Look for Sitting Hen Rock on the left, posted with the only sign you will encounter on this hike. At the upper elevation of their range, black oaks appear along this section. At the end of the traverse (2.7/5950´), the trail begins its 1500-foot descent to the river. Looking northeast, the Middle Fork San Joaquin can be seen curving west from Mammoth Crest (Hike 90) on the horizon. The South Fork flows just south of Balloon Dome and although you can't see it, the northern headwaters drain the peaks of the Silver Divide on the east skyline.

The descent to the river is rocky, often exposed to the sun, and comprises more than 40 switchbacks. Poison oak appears near the bottom. Finally a metal bridge comes into view and river sounds fill your ears (4.9/4410´). Helicoptered to this site in 1956, the bridge has sustained recent flood damage: Its bent central girders testify to the river's mind-boggling height that day. Exploration up- and downriver is easy and fishing holes are aplenty. While Cassidy Trail continues across the bridge toward Rattlesnake Lake, to keep this a dayhike you must return the way you came.

Nearest Visitors Center: Tiny Clover Meadow Ranger Station, (559) 877-2218 ext. 3136, is located 0.6 mile past the turnoff for Cassidy Trail on FSR 5S30 and open daily 8 AM–noon and 1–5 PM mid-June through mid-September. In the off-season try the Bass Lake Ranger District Office, (559) 877-2218, open year-round 8 AM–4:30 PM Monday through Friday.

Backpacking Information: Wilderness permits are required and are available at Clover Meadow. There is no quota for Cassidy Trail.

Nearest Campground: Clover Meadow (7 sites, free) almost always has space.

Additional Information: www. fs.fed.us/r5/sierra

HIKE 92

Kaiser Peak

The Riser to Kaiser

Highlights	A panoramic view of the central Sierra Nevada
Distance	10.0 miles round-trip
Total Elevation Gain/Loss	3200´/3200´
Hiking Time	6–8 hours
Optional Map	*Kaiser Wilderness* by the U.S. Forest Service
Best Times	Mid-June through September
Agency	Kaiser Wilderness
Difficulty	★★★★

Kaiser Peak stands alone—a western spur of the towering Sierra ridge that bounds the San Joaquin River. Ascend this peak and stand upon the lip of a great divide.

The Hike climbs steadily up the southern slope of Kaiser Peak (10,310´) and offers increasingly expansive views of the Huntington Lake basin, before reaching the summit crest and superlative vistas north. Despite its immediate proximity to popular Huntington Lake, Kaiser Wilderness attracts few hikers. A visit in late June or September will provide an unusual degree of solitude. Potable water is available at the pack station near the trailhead, and there are two sources along the trail—Deer Creek near the beginning and Bear Creek near the goal.

To Reach the Trailhead: Take Hwy. 168 east from Clovis to its end along the east shore of Huntington Lake; turn left at the T-junction. In 1.0 mile turn right at the posted turnoff for the D&F Pack Station (just before the entrance to Deer Creek Campground). Bear right on Upper Deer Creek Lane after 0.1 mile and right again onto Deer Lane after another 0.5 mile. While the dirt road horseshoes over a creek and into the pack station, you should park in the small lot before the creek. The trail-

head is at the north end of the pack station customer parking lot.

Description: At the trailhead (0.0/7200´) two trails split off—bear left toward Kaiser Peak. Ascending among large Jeffrey pines, you reach another junction 100 yards along—continue straight ahead. The trail narrows to single-track and slowly climbs to meet Deer Creek on the right (0.5/7600´). Briefly paralleling the creek, the trail then begins a long switchbacking ascent to College Rock among enormous, fantastically shaped granite boulders. Flowers abound in season, including lupine, paintbrush, and western hound's-tongue. The red cones of snow plants protrude from the litter of forest floor.

An ideal picnic spot, College Rock (2.5/9055´) can be surmounted with a bit of scrambling for some exciting views. Ringed by mountains, Huntington Lake is spread out below. If you look southwest into the Great Central Valley, the Coast Range outline often appears above the haze—a distance of more than 100 miles!

From here, several tight switchbacks lead up 200 feet before the trail slowly traverses to Bear Creek, joining it at a large flat meadow (3.0/9340´) among lodgepole and western white pines. Weaving to and

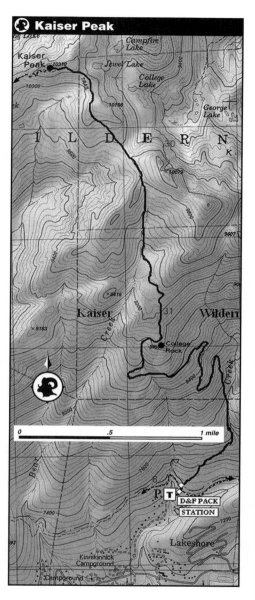

Kaiser Peak

Jewel Lake (closer) and Campfire Lake (farther) several hundred feet below. The summit (5.0/10,310´) is finally obtained via a very short, posted spur trail.

The view is exceptional. Before you drains the mighty San Joaquin. The prominent granite knob to the north poking out of the river valley is Balloon Dome (Hike 91). Farther north, the sawtoothed Minarets of the Ritter Range are easily identified, with the North Fork San Joaquin draining west below them. The Middle Fork wraps east around them, curving north below Mammoth Crest (Hike 90). The high peaks west of the Minarets form the southern border of Yosemite National Park. East-southeast, the South Fork San Joaquin drains the distant mountains of northern Kings Canyon National Park, visible along the skyline. Just below to the northwest is Bonnie Lake. The small twins of Bobby Lake lie nearly 1000 feet beneath you. Don't be so distracted by the view that you leave your food unattended—several marmots that make the summit rocks their home love to pilfer! Return the way you came.

Nearest Visitors Center: High Sierra Ranger District Office, (559) 855-5355, located in Prather on the way up Hwy. 168 and open daily 8 AM–4:30 PM.

Backpacking Information: A wilderness permit is required, obtainable in Prather during business hours. Due to a lack of good campsites on this hike, there is a quota of 8 people in effect for this trailhead from the last Friday in June through mid-September. This quota is seldom met, though you may want to reserve a permit for peak holiday weekends by contacting the district office.

Nearest Campground: Six campgrounds ($18–22) line the shores of Huntington Lake.

Additional Information: www.fs.fed.us/r5/sierra

from creekside, the trail passes below a massive fortress of granite as it ascends to a crest (4.0/9800´). Suddenly, the strange moonscape of upper Kaiser Ridge comes into view, devoid of all trees and only occasionally matted with plant life. Traversing around a false summit, you reach a small cleft below now-visible Kaiser Peak, with

HIKE 93

Dinkey Lakes

Mighty Dinkey

Highlights	Remote meadows, four lakes, and adventure road access
Distance	6.7 miles
Total Elevation Gain/Loss	850'/850'
Hiking Time	3–5 hours
Optional Map	*Dinkey Lakes Wilderness* by the U.S. Forest Service
Best Times	May through September
Agency	Dinkey Lakes Wilderness
Difficulty	★★

The bear charged. Dinkey attacked. Biting the hind leg of the massive brute, Dinkey was exterminated seconds later. Yet the bravery of this tiny dog saved its owner, giving him enough time to grab his gun and kill the bear. Although he was "no bigger than a rabbit" (according to a Kings River Ranger District brochure), local legend and appellation honor mighty Dinkey to this day.

The Hike gently climbs along sweetly flowing Dinkey Creek before weaving among four pleasant lakes. Wildflowers are abundant in the early summer—shooting stars can ring First Dinkey Lake with a pink halo, while mountain pride pensemons and crimson columbines lend color to quiet forest glades. Due to the boggy nature of the lake plateau, mosquitoes swarm in uncommon numbers throughout June and July, and are present to some degree all summer long. While there is no water available at the trailhead, Dinkey Creek is accessible over the first 1.2 miles.

To Reach the Trailhead: A high-clearance vehicle is all but essential. Although four-wheel-drive is not necessary, passenger cars with low clearance risk a bottom-scraping experience on the roughest access roads covered in this book. Take Hwy. 168 east from Clovis to the town of Shaver Lake and turn east onto Din-

key Creek Rd. In 9.5 miles, turn left onto posted Rock Creek Road (Forest Service Rd. 9S09)—mostly paved but dotted with treacherous potholes. In 6.4 miles, you reach a T-junction. Go right on marginally paved FSR 9S10 for 4.9 miles, until you reach a posted junction for FSR 9S62. Make the hard right, and jounce along for 2.4 miles (bearing left at all forks the final 1.4 miles) through a hellish section of roots and ruts to the substantial trailhead lot.

Description: From the information sign (0.0/8640'), the trail immediately drops down to Dinkey Creek and a small waterfall. The taffylike exposures of metamorphic rock here are part of the Dinkey Creek Roof Pendant, a remnant of the landscape that existed prior to the granite intrusion of the Sierra Nevada. A distinct interface between the layered metavolcanics and a marble outcrop's gray smoothness can

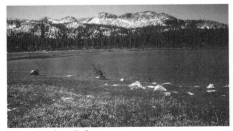

First Dinkey Lake

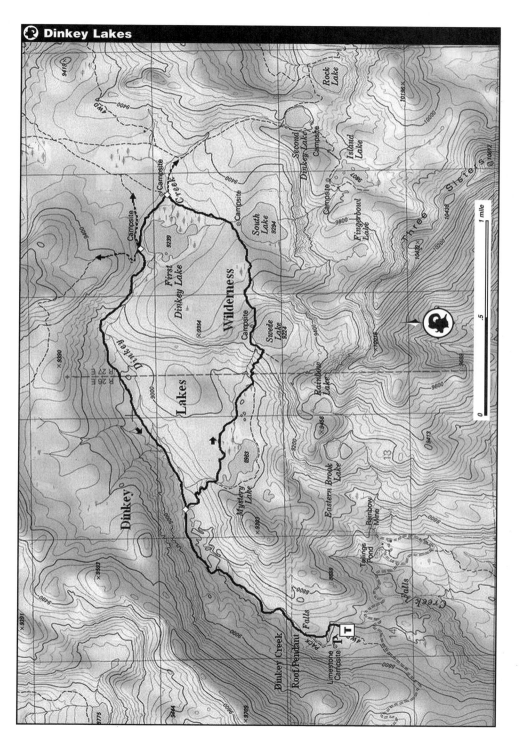

Dinkey Lakes

be seen on the opposite shore. This roof pendant is the likely metamorphosed remains of an ancient offshore volcanic island, similar to the one exposed near Boulder Creek in Kings Canyon National Park (Hike 96).

Recrossing the creek by another fountainlike waterfall, the level trail soon reaches the more typical granite of the Sierra. Here the trail climbs over a bouldery terminal moraine formed by the glacier that once filled this valley. Glacial polish can be identified intermittently from this point onward. Winding through lodgepole pines, the trail reaches the posted junction for Mystery Lake (1.2/8840′) and the start of the four-lake loop. While the hike can be completed in either direction, this description heads first to Mystery Lake, allowing you to reach the lakes in rough order of their increasing scenic beauty.

Bear right, cross Dinkey Creek, and make a gradual ascent to reach Mystery Lake near its outlet (1.5/8960′). Numerous use paths lead to the shores of this shallow, rather unexciting lake. The trail skirts the lake, passes through its boggy east end, and then crosses the outflow stream from Swede Lake. Climbing a dozen switchbacks, the trail regains the stream just prior to reaching Swede Lake itself (2.4/9220′). Backed by bare granite faces on its southeast shore, round Swede Lake presents better swimming and angling opportunities at its deeper north end. Past its north end, you quickly gain 150 feet before a mellow traverse and a slight drop bring you to South Lake (3.1/9300′). Bigger, deeper, and prettier, South Lake is fed by a waterfall rushing over an exposed granite ledge on its south side.

Beyond South Lake the trail becomes difficult to identify as use paths diverge in all directions. Most head down to the bogs around First Dinkey Lake's east shore, a very wet and soggy option. The actual trail crosses the lake's outflow creek and gradually traverses above the bogs to rejoin Dinkey Creek. Trees are blazed along the correct route but if you find yourself

off-track, continue traversing on the level until you reach Dinkey Creek and the very obvious trail alongside it. Upstream leads to further adventure and three more lakes (Second Dinkey, Rock, and Island lakes) less than a mile away. This hike heads downstream to the north shore of First Dinkey Lake (3.7/9240′). The lake is meadow-fringed and deep, with the studded granite ridge of the Three Sisters visible beyond its southern shore. Depending on the mosquito swarms, this is the nicest, most scenic picnic spot on the hike. From here, the trail arcs around the lake's north shore, reaching a junction just past the large boulders by the lake's outlet. Bear left and begin a gradual descent along or near Dinkey Creek. Look for the small but plentiful brook trout in the many limpid pools, as you return to the earlier junction for Mystery Lake and continue back to the trailhead.

Nearest Visitors Center: Dinkey Creek Ranger Station, located on Dinkey Creek Rd. 2.8 miles past the turnoff for Rock Creek Rd., is open 8 AM–4:30 PM daily mid-May through September, though the volunteered-managed facility may occasionally be closed due to limited staffing. A more reliable source of information is the High Sierra Ranger District Office, (559) 855-5355, in Prather on Hwy. 168 and open daily 8 AM–4:30 PM.

Backpacking Information: A wilderness permit is required, obtainable from either ranger station during business hours. The best campsites are found at Swede and South lakes. There is no quota in effect for this trailhead.

Nearest Campground: Dinkey Creek Campground (128 sites, $18) is located adjacent to Dinkey Creek Ranger Station.

Additional Information: www. fs.fed.us/r5/sierra

HIKE 94

Methusaleh Grove

Wizened

Highlights	Phantasmagoria and the oldest living things on Earth
Distance	4.2 miles
Total Elevation Gain/Loss	1000´/1000´
Hiking Time	2–3 hours
Optional Map	USGS 7.5-min. *Westgard Pass*
Best Times	Mid-June through September
Agency	Ancient Bristlecone Pine Forest, Inyo National Forest
Difficulty	★★★

Gnarled and twisted, sculpted and sublime, the bristlecone pines endure. Commune with trees more than 4000 years old.

The rocks of the White Mountains were deposited as sea-floor sediment approximately 600 million years ago, making them the oldest rocks described by this guidebook. Thrust into mountains about 350 million years ago, the rocks today contain numerous exposed pockets of dolomite, a form of metamorphic limestone that is highly alkaline and inhospitable to most plants. In this soil, at elevations from 9000 to 11,000 feet, the hardy bristlecone pine sets its roots.

Pinus longaeva (long-lived pine) is readily identified by its curved branchlets resembling long foxtails; its dark green, short needles growing in clusters of five; and its gooey sap-laden purple cones. The small bristle that appears at the end of mature cones gives the tree its name. Precipitation is minimal in the White Mountains. Between 12 and 15 inches fall annually, limiting the trees to only six to eight weeks of growth each year. The short growth cycle, coupled with the nutrient-poor dolomitic soil, allows the trees to produce only very small amounts of wood each year. Extremely dense and resinous, the wood is highly resistant to rot, pests,

and fire. Ironically, the oldest trees grow in the most inhospitable sites: steep slopes of poor soil that retain little water. These restricted conditions cause slower than normal growth, producing denser (up to 150 rings per inch) and more durable wood than trees growing in better spots. During times of adversity, a bristlecone can also

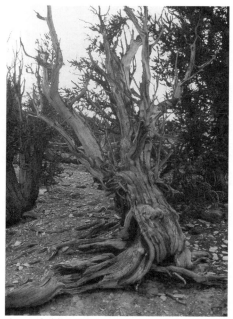

A gnarled bristlecone pine

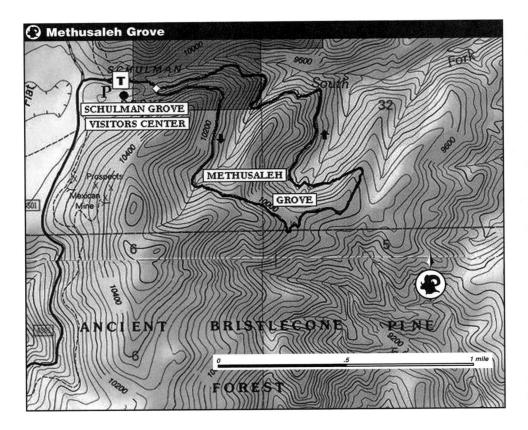

let entire limbs die, often maintaining adequate nutrient flow to only a single branch. Dead branches take thousands more years to decay, becoming sculpted into fantastical shapes by wind-blown sand and ice crystals. Tree roots are seldom deeper than 2 feet, and despite the slow rate of slope erosion (less than one foot per 1000 years), death by toppling over is a common end for the most ancient trees. Fallen trees can remain on the ground for up to 7000 years! A dendrochronologist's delight, bristlecone pines provide a nearly complete chronology of the past 10,000 years through living and dead wood samples.

The Hike winds down to Methuselah Grove, location of more than 20 trees older than 4000 years and home of Methuselah, at 4700 years the world's oldest living thing. In order to protect Methuselah, its exact location is kept secret. Throughout

this hike, it is critical that you stay on the trail—off-route hiking greatly increases the rate of erosion and can damage the root system of the trees. Additionally, the removal of any wood, living or dead, is strictly prohibited. Because trail elevation hovers around 10,000 feet, altitude sickness is a real concern, especially for those driving straight up from Owens Valley 6000 feet below. A morning start is best for solitude on the trail, as many day-trippers arrive in the early afternoon from Owens Valley. Weather can range unpredictably from cold to sudden thunderstorms to scorching sun. It can snow year-round.

To Reach the Trailhead: Take Hwy. 168 east from Hwy. 395 in Big Pine—the turnoff is 0.5 mile north of the Texaco station. After 13.5 miles, turn left onto White Mountain Road. With the exception of small bottles available for purchase at the visitors center, water and supplies are not available past this point—be prepared! The trailhead is at the Schulman Grove Visitors Center parking lot, a steep 10.7 miles past the entrance station, where a day-use fee is collected ($3 per person or $5 per vehicle).

Description: The trail begins left of the picnic tables, where a self-guiding trail brochure can be picked up for $1 (0.0/10,100'). After a short 0.2 mile, bear right at the fork. (You'll return from the left.) Curving along south slopes of a deep creek gully, the trail climbs to the first rest bench (0.5/10,220'), which provides views east far into Nevada. The trail brochure's Stop 7, past the second bench, overlooks Methuselah Grove, occupying a small, distinctly white ridgelet in the valley below. As you hike there, you cross a vegetation zone where sagebrush and mountain mahogany dominate, due to more hospitable sandstone soils.

Descending from the ridge, you soon begin passing through the ancient Methuselah Grove. With many of these trees predating the Pyramids of Egypt, there is an impalpable feeling of time. Are you walking softly? Departing the grove at the trail's lowest point (2.3/9730'), the trail bends west and gradually switchbacks up the creek canyon to return to the parking lot.

Nearest Visitors Center: Schulman Grove Visitors Center (no phone) is located at the trailhead and is open 10 AM–5 PM daily Memorial Day through mid-October, with reduced hours in spring and fall. For general information, contact the White Mountain Visitors Center in Bishop, (530) 873-2500.

Camping Information: There is no backpacking or backcountry camping allowed in the Methuselah Grove or anywhere within the designated Ancient Bristlecone Pine Forest, a 44-square-mile area straddling the White Mountains above 9000 feet. Backcountry camping is allowed with a valid campfire permit in the surrounding Inyo National Forest, however. The closest organized camping is at Grandview Campground (no water), a donation-based campground 5.1 miles beyond the entrance station on White Mountain Rd., which doesn't quite live up to its name.

Additional Information: www.fs.fed.us/r5/inyo

HIKE 95

Palisade Glacier

Granite Glory

Highlights	Emerald lakes and the Sierra Nevada's largest glacier
Distance	17.0 miles round-trip
Total Elevation Gain/Loss	5200´/5200´
Hiking Time	12–16 hours
Optional Maps	John Muir Wilderness by the U.S. Forest Service; USGS 7.5-min. Split Mountain, North Palisade, Mount Thompson, and Coyote Flat
Best Times	Mid-July through September
Agency	John Muir Wilderness
Difficulty	★★★★★

Stride the east side. Less than 5 miles from the trailhead, above an idyllic basin studded with emerald lakes and naked granite, the Sierra Divide splits the sky. Continuing upward to attain the edge of Palisade Glacier as a dayhike is the greatest challenge this book offers. It is a mile of vertical gain to an active glacier below a serrated ridge of 14,000-foot peaks. In this highest mountain zone, life is left behind for a land of rock and ice.

The Hike follows North Fork Big Pine Creek into a substantial basin and visits five spectacular lakes. From there, it climbs 1800 feet along an increasingly thin trail to reach the glacier. The final 700 feet of ascent are cross-country, and the hike tops out at over 12,000 feet. Due to the hike's high elevation, altitude sickness can be a problem and snow can linger deep into the summer, sometimes beyond mid-July. Wear your sturdiest and stiffest hiking boots for this hike, as loose rock and constant boulder-hopping can wreak havoc on your feet.

The limited trailheads of the Sierra's eastern slopes tend to funnel crowds into small geographic areas, and this hike is no exception. Obtaining a wilderness permit for overnight trips can be challenging

(see below), and the best time to visit is September when summer crowds begin to dwindle. Even then, don't expect solitude. Fishing is possible at all the lakes. No water is available at the trailhead, but the river is regularly accessible after the first mile.

To Reach the Trailhead: Take Crocker St. west from Hwy. 395 in Big Pine—the turnoff is between the Texaco and Mobil stations. Crocker St. becomes Glacier Lodge Rd., snaking upward 10 miles to the trailhead lot on the right, immediately past Upper Sage Flat and Sage Flat campgrounds. The road continues another 0.3 mile to Big Pine Creek Campground, but all hikers must leave their vehicles in the designated trailhead lot.

Description: Beginning by the outhouse (0.0/7750´), the single-track trail strikes west through open sage and passes above the Glacier Pack Station before gently climbing to First Falls Walk-In Campground (0.9/8250´). A short drop below the trail, the free campground has five sites with picnic tables and fire rings, though firewood is nonexistent. Unseen and inaccessible because of the brush, First Falls can only be heard.

On the next section from First Falls to the base of Second Falls, you have two options. The more scenic route traverses the creek's partly exposed northeast slopes, offering good views up-canyon. The alternative—along the valley floor from First Falls Campground—provides easy walking on a wide path, before it climbs steeply to rejoin the main trail. It is shadier and has regular access to water. The trails join at a junction for Baker Lake (1.7/8580′)—continue straight ahead toward impressive Second Falls. The trail switchbacks tightly near the top of the falls, where numerous overlooks let you view the tumbling river.

Now almost level, the trail meanders a dense riparian corridor of lodgepole pines, cottonwoods, and alders, with a few Jeffrey pines. Big Pine Wilderness Ranger Camp (2.6/9160′), an impressive granite building, soon encountered on the left, once belonged to actor Lon Chaney. The fluted massif of Temple Crag comes into full view south as the trail enters more open terrain. You soon reach the posted junction beginning your loop (4.2/10,000′)—continue straight toward First Lake.

The surreal color of First Lake (4.4/9960′) can be spotted through the trees and numerous use paths lead to the rocky shore. Like Second and Third lakes, First Lake is fed by meltwater from Palisade Glacier. Extremely fine sediment ground by the glacier (glacial flour) is suspended in the water, causing the startling green hue of the three lakes. From shore the rounded summits of Mt. Gayley (13,510′) and—farther—Mt. Sill (14,153′), just west behind landmark Temple Crag, can be identified. The serrated ridge visible on the southwest skyline includes (from south to north) North Palisade (14,242′), Mt. Winchell (13,775′), and Mt. Agassiz (13,893′).

The trail traverses some 100 feet above Second Lake (10,059′), the largest, before passing near Third Lake (10249). While both are readily accessed via a number of use paths, Second Lake provides the more impressive lakeshore. Paralleling much-diminished Big Pine Creek above Third Lake, the trail climbs quickly to a large meadow, where posted Glacier Trail splits off (6.0/10,640′).

To head to Palisade Glacier, cross the creek and follow Glacier Trail upward on numerous tight switchbacks. Paralleling an oft-hidden stream coursing beneath granite rubble, the trail eventually crests into Sam Mack Meadow (6.8/11,050′). Waving with shooting stars and paintbrush, the meadow contains a shallow creek whose blue-gray tint indicates its glacial origin. While an obvious trail continues through the meadow to a few high-elevation campsites, you should rock-hop across the creek near the foot of the meadow. Continue climbing on the opposite slope, where the trail is marked.

Increasingly rough and rocky, the trail passes krummholz whitebark pines, marking the upper limit of tree growth. As you attain the top of a small ridge and continue traversing upward on the far side, incredible views down-canyon of First, Second, and Third lakes open up. The distinctive linear heap of small stones and loose scree now visible above you is a lateral moraine left behind by receding Palisade Glacier. Wrapping around the base of the moraine (8.0/11,780′), the trail fades completely

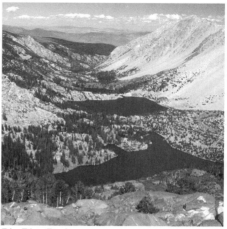

Big Pine Basin

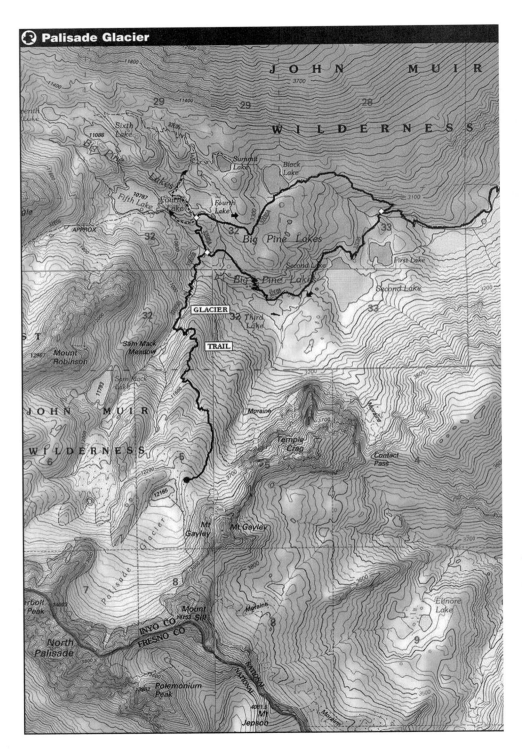

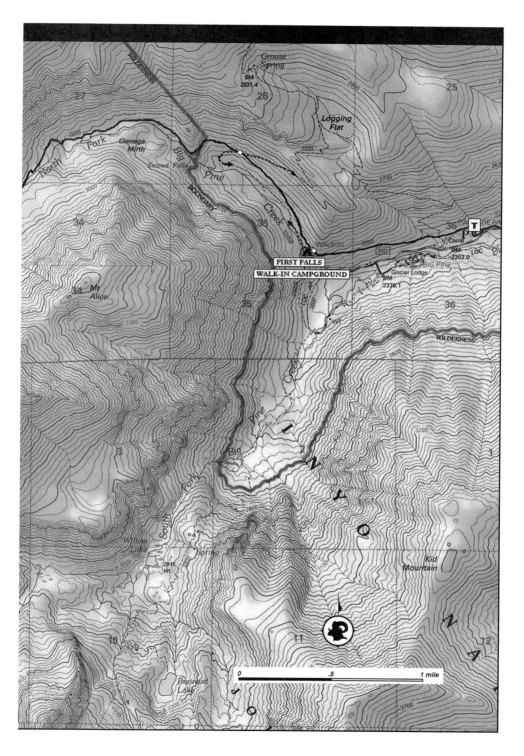

after crossing the loosest (and most maddening) rock of this trip. Indicated by numerous small cairns, the now completely cross-country route ascends the former glacier path, an undulating polished granite ramp. Sucking enough oxygen from the thin air is now the hardest part. When you finally crest the rubble of the terminal moraine (8.5/12,300′), you behold the great amphitheater of Palisade Glacier.

The glacier's snout terminates in an ice-choked pond 150 feet below you; the towering peaks scrape the sky 2000 feet above. Hidden from all angles but this one, Palisade Glacier gouges a barren alpine landscape. Time and energy permitting, scramble down the loose moraine slopes to walk on the glacier itself. Unlike its larger relatives, Palisade Glacier generally lacks crevasses or cracks that would pose serious risk—especially on its lower, boulder-strewn surface—but always exercise caution. The notable features from

south to north above the glacier are: Mt. Sill (14,153′), the prominent dome-shaped summit; V-notch and U-notch, two neighboring gaps in the ridge clearly resembling these letters; North Palisade (14,242′), though small and rounded immediately north of U-notch, the highest point; and Thunderbolt Peak (14,003′), the incisor-sharp spires above the glacier's far northwest corner. North beyond the glacier basin are the summits of Mt. Winchell (13,775′) and Mt. Agassiz (13,893′).

Savor the thickening air as you retrace your steps downward to the earlier junction in Big Pine Basin (11.0/10,640′). Bear left and ascend briefly to Fourth Lake (11.3/10,760′). Fed by snow rather than glacial ice, its water contrasts sharply with the Technicolor of the first three. The long descent home begins here. After dark Black Lake (11.8/10,680′), the trail then descends 500 feet via nine switchbacks to join the earlier trail. Return the way you came.

Nearest Visitors Center: White Mountain Visitors Center, (760) 873-2500, located on Hwy. 395 in downtown Bishop (across the road from Burger King), is open 8 AM–5 PM daily mid-June through mid-September. The rest of the year it's open 8 AM–noon and 1–4:30 PM Monday through Friday.

Backpacking Information: Wilderness permits are required and there is a quota of 24 people per day for this trailhead, effective from May 1 through November 1. Due to its deserved popularity, the quota is usually met. While 60 percent of the permits are reservable, with the remaining 40 percent available on a walk-in (first-come, first-served) basis on the day before or day of your trip. Reservations must be made at least 3 days in advance of your trip, after which it is walk-in only. The fee for reserved permits is $5 per person and reservations for the quota season can be made up to six months in advance of your trip date by calling (760) 873-2483. Permits, whether walk-in or reserved, may be picked up at the White Mountain Visitors Center.

You can also pick up permits at Mammoth Lakes Visitors Center, (760) 924-5500, located immediately east of town on Hwy. 203 and open daily 8 AM–5 PM. Another pickup location is the outstanding Mono Basin Scenic Area Visitors Center, (760) 647-3044, located on Hwy. 395 near Lee Vining, 1.3 miles north of the Hwy. 120 junction. It's open 9 AM–5:30 PM daily from May through October, with extended summer and weekend hours, and is closed in the off-season.

Nearest Campground: Big Pine Creek Campground (30 sites, $18) is located at the road's end. Also try Upper Sage Flat and Sage Flat campgrounds ($18) near the trailhead.

Additional Information: www.fs.fed.us/r5/inyo

HIKE 96

Boulder Creek

Leaves of Three

Highlights	Mountains of marble and secluded swimming spots
Distance	2.0 miles round-trip
Total Elevation Gain/Loss	300´/300´
Hiking Time	1–3 hours
Optional Map	USGS 7.5-min. *Wren Peak*
Best Times	May through September
Agency	Sequoia National Forest
Difficulty	★★★

Here, ancient coral reefs have been compressed and sutured, metamorphosed and thrust into the sky as mountains of marble. While a perilous sea of poison oak is an unfortunate obstacle, mellifluous Boulder Creek is a compelling attraction.

In a land of granite, the Windy Cliffs and surrounding peaks are a geologic island. Made of marble, this anomaly was once a coral reef ringing a volcanic island far off the coast of ancient North America. Heavily deformed fossils within the rock indicate that the reef formed between 190 and 220 million years ago. Through the action of plate tectonics, the volcanic island and its reef were mashed against and accreted to the North American continent approximately 160 million years ago. Subjected to intense pressures and temperature, the reef was transformed into marble, and the layered volcanic rocks folded like warm taffy into the metavolcanics of Boulder Creek. Sometime during the next 80 million years, rising magma solidified to granite, surrounding but not otherwise altering the marble. An isolated remnant of the pre-Sierra landscape such as this is referred to as a roof pendant. As land above was wasted away by erosion, the marble was exposed at the surface, forming the blank gray cliff faces of the Windy Cliffs region.

The Hike is short and moderate, following a gentle traverse above the Kings River and Boulder Creek to reach a great swimming hole. You can't avoid the poison oak, however, growing over, next to, and actually in the trail at times. Long pants and long sleeves are highly recommended, as well as some anti-poison-oak treatment for after the hike. The trail's poison oak, brushiness, and (a few) exposed slopes bump up the overall difficulty rating. While no potable water is available at the trailhead, snacks and bottled water can be purchased at the Boyden Cave souvenir shop and the Kings River rushes adjacent to the parking lot.

To Reach the Trailhead: Take Hwy. 180 east from Grant Grove Visitors Center in northern Kings Canyon National Park to the large parking lot for Boyden Cavern, located where the highway crosses the Kings River on its south bank. Although this hike is in Sequoia National Forest, access requires passage through Kings Canyon National Park where a $20 entrance fee per vehicle is collected at Big Stump Entrance Station.

Description: Begin by the souvenir shop, following the paved trail that leads to Boyden Cavern. After climbing 80 feet above the Kings River, the paved trail switchbacks by a metal gate—the unposted

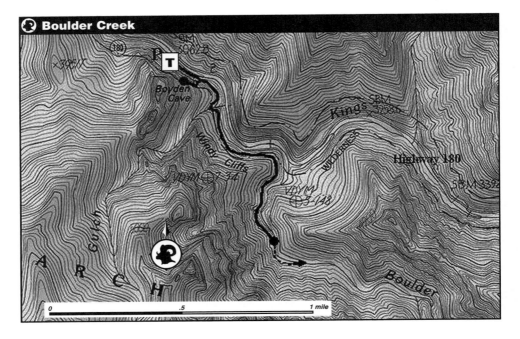

Boulder Creek

junction for this hike. Go through the gate and continue up the narrow trail over a mildly precarious rocky slope. A few railings provide intermittent security on the steep slopes above the Kings River. Poison oak soon appears in the shade of California bays and canyon live oaks, growing ever thicker as you continue.

The brushy, overgrown trail curves slowly south above the Boulder Creek drainage, providing exceptional views of the crenellated marble peaks soaring above you. Though the trail gets narrow and spotty, you finally reach the water at a prime swimming hole and picnic spot, accessed via a quick jog where the trail swings closest to the creek. Exploratory journeys await both up- and downstream, and native rainbow trout populate the many holes. Return the way you came and wash off that poison oak!

Nearest Visitors Center: Kings Canyon Visitors Center at Grant Grove, (559) 565-4307, located 2 miles past the park entrance station along Hwy. 180, is open 365 days a year. Although hours vary depending on the season, it's generally open 9 AM–5 PM May through June, 8 AM–6 PM July through Labor Day, and 9 AM–4:30 PM in winter. The nearest visitors center for Sequoia National Forest is the Hume Lake District Office, (559) 338-2251, 20 miles west of the Big Stump Entrance Station on Hwy. 180, which is open 8 AM–4:30 PM Monday through Friday.

Backpacking Information: While backpacking is permitted, the poison oak and lack of campsites make it an unappealing option. A campfire permit is required.

Nearest Campground: There are more than a dozen campgrounds in Kings Canyon National Park and adjacent Sequoia National Forest. Check at the visitors center for current availability.

Additional Information: www.fs.fed.us/r5/sequoia and www.nps.gov/seki

Yucca Point

King of Kings

Highlights	The deepest canyon in North America
Distance	3.4 miles round-trip
Total Elevation Gain/Loss	1150'/1150'
Hiking Time	2–3 hours
Optional Maps	USGS 7.5-min. *Hume* and *Wren Peak*
Best Times	Spring and fall
Agency	Sequoia National Forest
Difficulty	★★★

Though Hwy. 180 winds a stunning course above the Kings River, gaining perspective from your car on the immense depth of Kings Canyon is difficult. Luckily, your descent to the river below Yucca Point will remedy this.

The Hike descends quickly to the confluence of the Middle and South Forks of the Kings River, and provides spectacular views up both river canyons. Due to the lower elevation here, spring and fall provide the most agreeable temperatures and May offers the best wildflowers. Summer months can be sweltering. The trail is also a popular access point for anglers, although there are strict regulations governing this stretch of river. In order to protect its population of large wild trout, catch-and-release fishing applies and only artificial lures with barbless hooks may be used. Current regulations should be posted by the trailhead. The river is usually not fishable until July, when the raging waters of melting snowpack subside. No water is available at the trailhead.

To Reach the Trailhead: Take Hwy. 180 east from Grant Grove Visitors Center for 15 miles. On the left, a U.S. Forest Service sign for Yucca Point and a dirt lot with space for four vehicles mark your trailhead. This hike is in Sequoia National Forest but access requires passage through

Kings Canyon National Park, where a $20 entrance fee per vehicle (valid for seven days), is collected.

Description: From the trailhead (0.0/3380'), descend among manzanita, canyon live oaks, cottonwoods, California buckeyes, and California bays until you reach the first switchback (0.5/2900'). From here views of the South Fork canyon open up; the Windy Cliffs (Hike 96) are visible where the river bends out of sight. Look for wildflowers as you descend west to the second switchback. Along with the ubiquitous flowering yucca you can find western wallflower and farewell-to-spring—two wildflowers rarely seen at higher elevations.

Views along the upper section of trail are more expansive than from canyon bottom. Spanish Mtn. (10,051'), rising nearly 8000 feet from the opposite bank, offers a neck-craning exercise in topographic relief. The Middle Fork tumbles southwest through nearly 10 miles of inaccessible gorge and is overshadowed south by Monarch Divide, a steep ridge ushering the two forks together.

At the third switchback (0.9/2600') a cottonwood tree can be readily identified by its heart-shaped leaves. Below the fourth switchback (1.3/2430'), an unexpected and beautiful stream races over

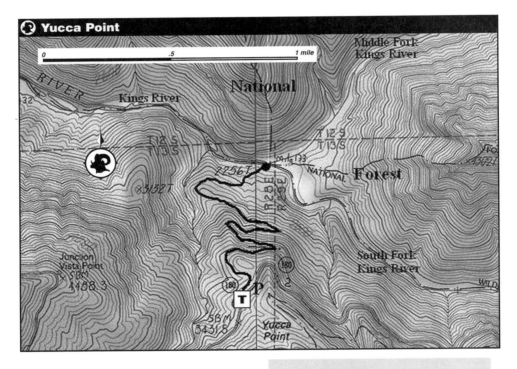

seven visible cascades—each one becoming progressively larger. Finally the water pours over a smooth granite face into a deep pool full of brook trout. This is Tenmile Creek, which drains the Hume Lake Reservoir 4 miles upstream. While pleasant in May and June, the water here gets funky as the flow decreases and Hume Lake receives its thousands of summer-camp visitors in July and August. Ten yards beyond where the falls first become visible, an unmarked spur trail leads down to a vantage point and a short scramble to the flat rocks at the base of the waterfall.

As you continue to Kings River, poison oak appears everywhere. The trail ends among the granite jumble of the riverbank (1.7/2250′). Many boulders include excellent examples of inclusions (overlying rocks absorbed and partially melted by rising molten bubbles of granite) some 100 million years old. Sparrows dart above the river in search of insects. Return the way you came.

Nearest Visitors Center: Kings Canyon Visitors Center at Grant Grove, (559) 565-4307, located 2 miles past the park entrance station along Hwy. 180, is open 365 days a year. Although hours vary depending on the season, it's generally open 9 AM–5 PM May through June, 8 AM–6 PM July through Labor Day, and 9 AM–4:30 PM in winter.

Backpacking Information: Backpacking is permitted, but the lack of campsites makes it an unappealing option. A campfire permit is required.

Nearest Campground: There are more than a dozen campgrounds in Kings Canyon National Park and adjacent Sequoia National Forest. Check at the visitors center for current availability.

Additional Information: www.nps.gov/seki and www.fs.fed.us/r5/sequoia

HIKE 98

Redwood Canyon

Sequoias

Highlights	Enchanted groves whose patriarchs dwarf your mind
Distance	10.0 miles
Total Elevation Gain/Loss	1900′/1900′
Hiking Time	5–7 hours
Optional Map	USGS 7.5-min. *General Grant Grove*
Best Times	June through September
Agency	Kings Canyon National Park
Difficulty	★★★

Redwood Canyon provides the opportunity to peacefully commune with giant sequoias in the largest grove on earth. One-on-one with these magnificent trees, while your mind gropes at scales of time and size, you feel the insignificance of humankind.

The Hike loops around the canyon slopes and ridges, dropping briefly to Redwood Creek and passing through numerous stands of giant sequoias. While it can readily be completed in either direction, this description covers the route clockwise. (A shorter, 7.5-mile loop can be created by using the trail that heads directly down-canyon.) Late June offers abundant flowering lupines and dogwood as well as fewer people; it is the ideal time

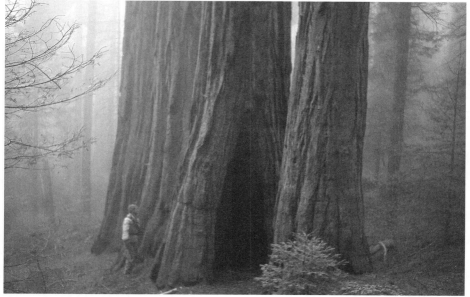

Giant sequoias dwarf your mind.

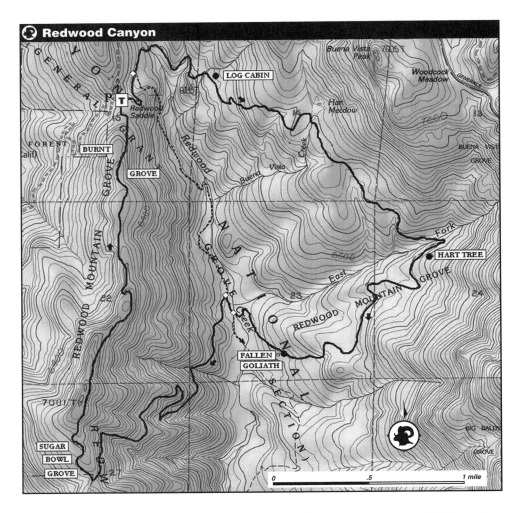

Redwood Canyon

to visit. While no water is available at the trailhead, an ample number of streams are encountered along the way.

To Reach the Trailhead: Take Hwy. 180 east from Fresno to Kings Canyon National Park. Continue 1 mile past the entrance station to a Y-junction—bear right onto Generals Hwy. heading south toward Sequoia National Park. In 3.8 miles you reach the posted turnoff for Hume Lake on the left. Instead, make a right here onto what appears to be a small dirt cul-de-sac. The bumpy dirt road to Redwood Canyon begins at this dirt lot and is easily navigable for all cars, although trailers and RVs

are definitely not recommended. Immediately beyond an ENTERING KINGS CANYON NATIONAL PARK sign, the road gradually descends 1.9 miles to the posted turnoff for the trailhead. There is a $20 entrance fee per vehicle for Kings Canyon and Sequoia national parks, valid for seven days.

Description: The trail begins at the information sign by the far end of the parking lot (0.0/6250′). Your return path winds in from the right but you head left down a 3-foot-wide loamy trail, immediately passing a fire hydrant and sign for REDWOOD CANYON-HART TREE TRAIL. You soon find yourself enveloped in the primeval giant sequoia forest, whose numerous large specimens dwarf the white firs, sugar pines, Jeffrey pines, and dogwoods also found here. The trail descends steadily via several lazy switchbacks and comes to a posted junction (0.4/6070´); bear left toward the Hart Tree. (Right takes you directly down-canyon to connect with the midpoint of the hike, shaving 2.5 miles off the hike.) From here the trail traverses the eastern slopes of the canyon, crossing three small tributaries of Redwood Creek before reaching a log cabin (1.1/6100´).

Nothing more than a single fallen sequoia log, the cabin was originally owned by woodcutter John Crose. Used in the 1890s for equipment storage, the log was modified in the early part of the century by Crose's son Jack and nephew Willis. Upon scraping out the log's insides, the pair enclosed it with shakes, a door, and a fireplace and chimney. The Barlow family purchased Crose's holdings in the late 1920s, and both families lived in the area well into the 1930s, inhabiting both Crose's log and a tiny cabin (now long gone) built atop a large sequoia stump. The federal government acquired the property in the late 1930s, bringing an end to this unique lifestyle.

From here you briefly leave the sequoias and ascend 400 feet among black oaks, incense cedars, and alders. The trail tops out at a large open space of bare granite, offering the only vista from the canyon's eastern slopes. Another undulating trail mile takes you past boggy Hart Meadow (and through another hollow sequoia log) to the East Fork Redwood Creek. Although it's too small to be fishable, keep an eye out for the small, native brook trout that populate its crystalline waters. A brief climb out of the creek gully brings you to a posted 100-yard spur trail to the Hart Tree (3.4/6200´).

Once thought to be the world's fourth largest tree, the Hart Tree is now recognized as only the sixteenth largest on Earth. As of 1990 it was 278´ tall, had a ground perimeter of 75.3´, a diameter of

21´, and was estimated to contain 34,407 cubic feet of wood. Back on the main trail, a gradual descent brings you to the Fallen Goliath (4.8/5700´), just beyond view from the trail. Moist, covered in moss, and nurse log to young sequoias sprouting from its crest, the Fallen Goliath probably sprouted more than 3000 years ago; it provides an excellent example of the incredible decay resistance of sequoia wood.

The trail now descends to Redwood Creek (5.3/5400´). Clear as glass, the creek flows through level surroundings studded with impressive sequoias. From mid-June through July, a sea of purple lupine washes the area, lapping at the cinnamon sequoia trunks. Just across the creek a signed junction indicates the route up-canyon to the right.

A short 0.1 mile upstream, the trail reaches another junction; head west up the canyon slope toward Sugar Bowl Grove.

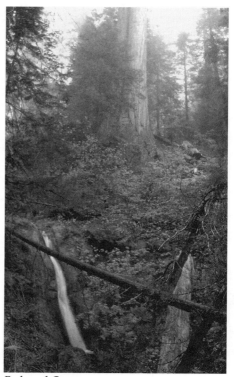

Redwood Canyon

(Those tired or short of time can take the shorter, more direct route up-canyon to reach the parking lot.) Climbing gradually to the ridgetop, the trail quickly breaks out of the dense forest after two quick switchbacks. The result of a recent fire, the clearing lets you see the proliferation of young sequoias whenever openings occur in the forest canopy. Extending spiny branches into the air, the young trees outgrow their neighbors to maximize sunlight. Extremely shade-intolerant, the trees shed any sickly yellow-green branches and will rapidly perish if overtopped by another tree. Beyond this clearing, thimbleberry, bear clover, paintbrush, and green-leaf manzanita are abundant, as the trail steadily climbs to the ridgetop.

Before attaining the ridgetop, you enter Sugar Bowl Grove (7.5/6600´), a thick stand of mature sequoias interspersed with several gnarled, ancient specimens of stupendous size. A cluster of more than 20 stand sentinel within a 75-yard radius at the heart of this enchanted grove. From here the trail follows the ridgetop, soon reaching its highest elevation of 1,500 feet above the canyon floor. Now slowly descending, you begin passing through Burnt Grove. Another thick stand of sequoias, Burnt Grove parallels the trail to the parking lot for the final mile.

Nearest Visitors Center: Kings Canyon Visitors Center at Grant Grove, (559) 565-4307, located 2 miles past the park entrance station along Hwy. 180, is open 365 days a year. Although hours vary depending on the season, it's generally open 9 AM–5 PM May through June, 8 AM–6 PM July through Labor Day, and 9 AM–4:30 PM in winter.

Backpacking Information: Redwood Canyon offers one of the few giant sequoia groves open to backpackers. A wilderness permit is required and can be obtained at Kings Canyon Visitors Center; there is a fee of $15 per permit. There is a quota of 15 people per day for this trailhead, though it seldom fills. You must camp at least a mile from the trailhead. Fires are prohibited in Redwood Canyon.

Nearest Campground: There are more than a dozen campgrounds in Kings Canyon National Park and adjacent Sequoia National Forest. Check at the visitors center for current availability.

Additional Information: www. nps.gov/seki

HIKE 99

Pear Lake

Sequoia High Sierra

Highlights	Shattered granite basins and the Watchtower
Distance	12.4 miles round-trip
Total Elevation Gain/Loss	2750'/2750'
Hiking Time	8–12 hours
Optional Map	USGS 7.5-min. *Lodgepole*
Best Times	July through September
Agency	Sequoia National Park
Difficulty	★★★★

Pear Lake's frigid green waters fill a granite bowl ringed by crenellated cliffs of fractured stone. En route are three choice Sierra lakes and the Watchtower, a titanic granite tower rising 2000 feet above Tokopah Valley.

The Hike climbs steeply to the Watchtower before making a gradual traverse above impressive Tokopah Valley to reach the lakes. For those seeking a shorter hike, the round-trip to the Watchtower is 7 miles, gains 1700 feet of elevation, and can be completed in 4–6 hours. Snow usually clears from the trail by late June and returns in November. July provides spectacular wildflowers. Water is available at the trailhead in the nearby restrooms.

To Reach the Trailhead: From Generals Hwy. in Sequoia National Park, take the road to Wolverton east to the parking lot at the road's end—your turnoff is 1.7 miles south of the one for Lodgepole Visitors Center and 0.7 mile north of the General Sherman Tree parking lot. The trail begins midway along its northern edge. Lockers provide the only safe storage of your foodstuffs while you're on the trail, because bears break into vehicles here all the time.

Description: Striking first through a forest dominated by white firs, the trail is quickly joined on the left by a small feeder trail from the Lodgepole complex (0.1/7400'), and then right by a short spur from the Wolverton area. The trail now slowly gains elevation traversing a forest whose lush understory includes numerous wildflowers: lupine, phlox, tiger lilies, shooting stars, and paintbrush. Beyond a junction for Alta Peak Trail (1.8/8060'), the path recrosses a small spring-fed creek before reaching the junction for the Hump (2.1/8160'). A right turn, taking you over the Hump, provides a slightly shorter, more direct, route to Heather Lake. But this shortcut is steeper, more strenuous, and lacks the exceptional views of the main trail. If you bear left instead, a gradually rising traverse leads you to the Watchtower (3.5/8973').

Take a memorable break on the Watchtower by scrambling to the top of this towering granite pillar, skirting its precipitous chasm. With Tokopah Valley visible in its entirety, even Lodgepole Visitors Center can be spotted down-canyon. Below where the Marble Fork Kaweah River tumbles down 1000 feet of granite chutes and faces are Tokopah Falls. Up-canyon, the high peaks on the southern rim overshadow your unseen destinations—Emerald and Pear lakes.

Views lost as the trail continues east become sweeping vistas as it heads southeast,

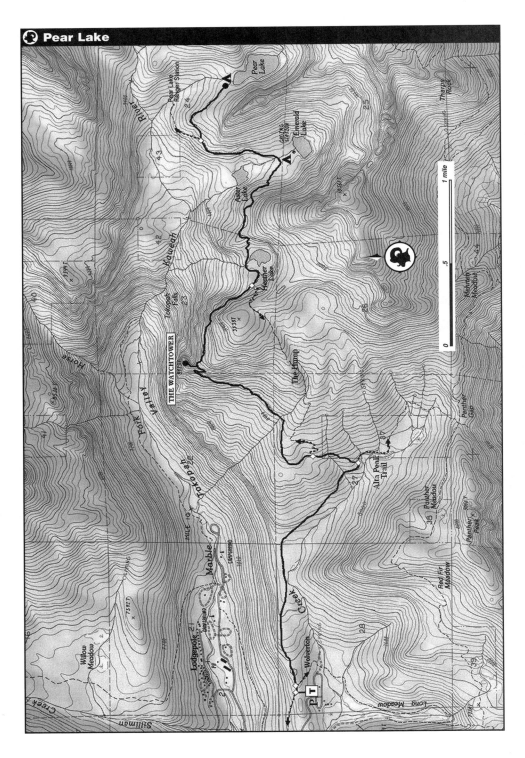

Pear Lake

now offering views of the Heather Lake basin. The lake remains hidden until you pass the junction where the Hump shortcut rejoins the main trail (4.1/9260′). Lodgepoles and western white pines are scattered about this day-use-only lake, whose facilities include California's most rudimentary outdoor toilet. Like the others on this hike, Heather Lake brims with brook trout up to 8 inches in length.

Continuing to even prettier lakes, the trail briefly climbs before descending into the granite amphitheater of the Emerald Lake basin. Aster Lake can be seen north of the trail, but there is no established access trail. Approaching Emerald Lake, you reach the organized campsites near its north shore (5.1/9030′). Both food lockers and a downright luxurious restroom are provided. Glacial polish and striations on the rock are evidence of the glacier that once carved this cirque. The summit visible southeast across the lake is Alta Peak (11,204′).

Striking north, the trail winds among granite slabs and vibrant patches of seasonal wildflowers such as mountain pride, paintbrush, and meadow penstemon. Look here for Coville's columbine, a large cream-colored flower with five petals, extending into backward-projecting spurs up to 1 inch long. Found only at rocky, high elevations in the southern Sierra Nevada, it is closely related to, and can hybridize with, the crimson columbine, according to Richard Spellenberg in *National Audubon Society Field Guide*. Magnificent examples of the rosy palette created by this cross-pollination can be found here soon after snowmelt—usually in late June and the first half of July. Do not pick the wildflowers.

Wrapping east, the trail passes a spur to seasonally staffed Pear Lake Ranger Station before turning southeast to reach the appropriately shaped Pear

Lake (6.2/9550′). A few lodgepole pines are sprinkled about the sloping granite shoreline; soaring ramparts of the basin heighten your sense of grandeur. The trail ends among the designated campsites near the lake's north shore (the "stem"), where food lockers and another plush outhouse can be found. Return the way you came.

Nearest Visitors Center: Lodgepole Visitors Center, (559) 565-4436, located on the road to Wolverton 1.6 miles east of Generals Hwy., is open daily 8 AM–6 PM mid-June to mid-September, with reduced hours in early June and late September.

Backpacking Information: The hike to Pear Lake makes for an ideal (and popular) two-day trip. Wilderness permits are required and can be obtained from an office next to the visitors center entrance, (559) 565-4408. There is a fee of $15 per permit, and the office is open 7 AM–4 PM daily June through September. There is a trail quota of 25 people per day, but space is usually available except for the busiest weekends and holidays. Wilderness permits can be reserved (by mail only) starting March 1; call (559) 565-4307 for more information. Due to heavy use, no fires are allowed, and camping is permitted in designated sites only.

Nearest Campground: Lodgepole Campground (214 sites, $20) is located adjacent to the visitors center. Reservations are recommended in summer, and can be made by calling (877) 444-6777 or visiting www.recreation.gov.

Additional Information: www.nps.gov/seki

HIKE 100

Moro Rock

The Granite Fin

Highlights	Surmounting a precipitous granite fin and enjoying views of the Great Western Divide
Distance	0.6 mile round-trip
Total Elevation Gain/Loss	250´/250´
Hiking Time	1 hour
Optional Map	USGS 7.5-min. *Giant Forest*
Best Times	June through September
Agency	Sequoia National Park
Difficulty	★★

A sharp granite nubbin extending from the lip of the Giant Forest plateau, Moro Rock protrudes thousands of feet above the Kaweah River gorge. A narrow runway atop its prow offers superlative views of the jagged Great Western Divide.

The Hike climbs to the top of Moro Rock along precipitous ledges and up steps dynamited out of the rock. Among all the trails of Giant Forest with their ubiquitous crowds, this short climb to a unique viewpoint should not be missed. Giant sequoias grow elsewhere in greater seclusion (Hike 98), but there is only one Moro Rock. Crowds are always heavy. Water is available at the trailhead.

To Reach the Trailhead: Take Generals Hwy. to Giant Forest Village and turn east on Crescent Meadow Rd.; the turnoff is located at the southern end of the complex. In 1.3 miles turn right onto the posted one-way loop for Moro Rock; park in the often crowded parking lot 0.4 mile farther along. There is a $20 entrance fee per vehicle for Sequoia National Park, valid for seven days.

Description: Because Jeffrey pines, incense cedars, white firs, and sugar pines are thick at the outset, bare granite views through the trees provide little hint of the grandeur that awaits you. At step 21, a

sign cries out WARNING—AREA OF EXTREME DANGER! Respect the warning about lightning strikes and postpone your ascent if thunderstorms threaten. Past this sign, the magic begins.

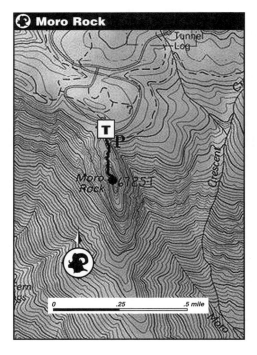

Overhanging sections, narrow cracks, and concrete stairs allow almost everybody—be they sprinters and climbers, walkers and talkers, or huffers and puffers—to surmount the rock. Two of the many informative placards en route identify the peaks of the Great Western Divide (including Sawtooth Peak, Hike 101) and detail the history of Generals Hwy., seen twisting tortuously below where it climbs 4000 feet in 19 miles. The pink flowers of mountain pride penstemon can be spotted in season sprouting from cracks in the rock. Climbers might also be seen clambering up the rock's steeper faces. At the summit, a 4-foot-wide level walkway with the trail's only bench distinguishes the edge of this precipitous granite blade.

Nearest Visitors Center: The Giant Forest Museum in Giant Forest Village is open year-round, though hours vary by season. It's generally open 9 AM–5 PM daily May through June, 8 AM–6 PM July through Labor Day, and 9 AM–4:30 PM in winter.

Other park visitor centers include the following: Kings Canyon Visitors Center at Grant Grove, (559) 565-4307, located 2 miles past the park entrance station along Hwy. 180, is open 365 days a year. Although hours vary depending on the season, it's generally open 9 AM–5 PM May through June, 8 AM–6 PM July through Labor Day, and 9 AM–4:30 PM in winter. Lodgepole Visitors Center, (559) 565-4436, located on the road to Wolverton 1.6 miles east of Generals Hwy., is open 8 AM–6 PM daily mid-June to mid-September, with reduced hours in early June and late September.

Nearest Campground: There are more than a dozen campgrounds in Kings Canyon National Park and adjacent Sequoia National Forest. Check at the Kings Canyon Visitors Center in Grant Grove for current availability.

Additional Information: www.nps.gov/seki

HIKE 101

Sawtooth Peak

Knife's Edge

Highlights	A towering summit of the Great Western Divide
Distance	13.0 miles round-trip
Total Elevation Gain/Loss	4500'/4500'
Hiking Time	12–16 hours
Optional Map	USGS 7.5-min. *Mineral King*
Best Times	July through September
Agency	Sequoia National Park
Difficulty	★★★★★

The Great Western Divide towers more than 4000 feet above the small hamlet of Mineral King in southern Sequoia National Park. The trail climbs up, straight up the divide's flanks, providing sweeping views of the soaring mountains and precipitous valleys. Beautiful Monarch Lake awaits at the base of 12,343-foot Sawtooth Peak, a jagged, trail-less summit that offers magnificent and far-reaching views of the Sierra Crest, the Kern River Canyon, and the Great Western Divide.

The Hike ascends Sawtooth Peak from Mineral King. Epic but brutal, it gains 4500 feet in less than 6 miles. Exceptional fitness and an early start are required for a one-day ascent. Lower Monarch Lake nestles at the mountain's base and provides a rest stop, or overnight campsite, 4.4 miles and 2500 feet up from the trailhead. Some degree of acclimatization is important for the rarefied air above 10,000 feet; gaiters are useful for keeping grit out of your boots on the mountain's loose slopes. The last 1500 feet of elevation gain is off-trail and involves considerable boulder-hopping and scrambling—wear the stiffest boots you own. No water is available at the trailhead; there is a faucet in front of the ranger station (see below). The first convenient trailside source is 1.3 miles distant and nearly 1000 feet up.

To Reach the Trailhead: From Hwy. 198 at Hammond, take the road to Mineral King—the turnoff is 4 miles northeast of the town of Three Rivers and 2 miles southwest of the Ash Mountain Entrance Station to Sequoia National Park. While only 23 miles long, the narrow, winding Mineral King Rd. can take upward of 90 minutes to drive. You reach the park entrance station 12 miles past the turnoff, where a $20 entrance fee per vehicle is collected. After another 6 miles, the road's surface alternates between dirt and pavement. The road soon passes through the tiny settlement of Silver City; a small general store here provides last-minute supplies. You pass Mineral King Ranger Station, where two large parking lots, an outhouse, and a pay phone are located, a short 0.9 mile before the desired trailhead.

Beware of lactating marmots! Throughout June and most of July, these critters develop a peculiar craving for antifreeze and brake fluid. Marmots will chew through coolant hoses, brake lines, and even spark plug wires seeking salts from this odd cocktail. Some people fence off the underside of their vehicles with chicken wire to avoid disaster. Some park in a less-risky lot, while others just risk it. A safe parking alternative is the Tar Gap lot located

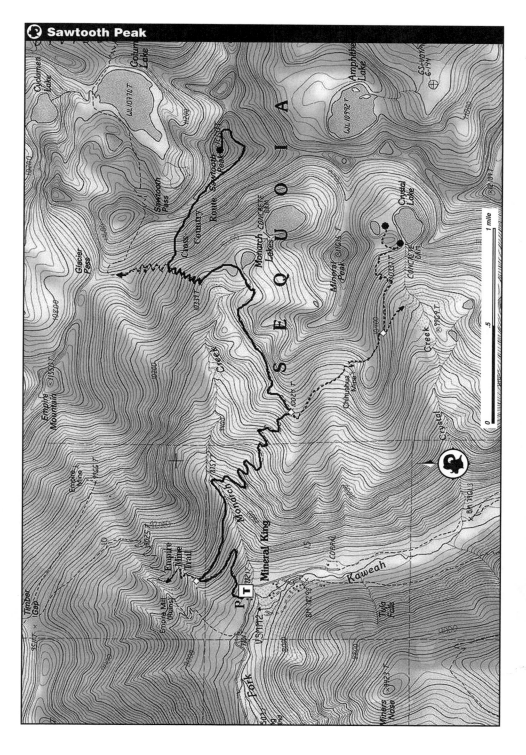

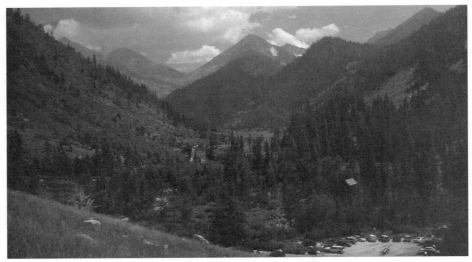

Looking south from Mineral King

0.1 mile east of the ranger station, but it means a 0.7-mile road walk to the trailhead. Most active in June, marmots become more lethargic as July progresses. Ask at the ranger station for the most current marmot report.

Description: The trail begins at the end of the north parking lot (0.0/7820´), where current trail conditions are posted. The East Fork Kaweah River turns sharply west here, and views south toward its headwaters are highlighted by the striking parabola made by Farewell Gap (10,586´), bordered west by the red metamorphic pyramid of Vandever Mtn. (11,947´).

Immediately climbing, the trail's first mile is the steepest, passing through open sage grassland with a few Sierra juniper. The distant pinnacle of Sawtooth Peak dominates the skyline east above Monarch Creek. Bouldery staircases help you ascend to a waterfall overlook. Now the trail traverses west and then—at the junction for Empire Mine Trail (0.6/8320´)—east back toward the creek. Ponderosa pines appear here and corn lilies, yarrow, Indian paintbrush, and lupine can be spotted underfoot. Climbing along the stream again, you pass a mossy spring gushing from the opposite hillside before the trail

reaches creek level (1.3/8760´). Imposing cliffs north, which tower 1500 feet, actually represent only the lower southwest face of Empire Mountain, whose hidden slopes rise another 1300 feet to the summit. Refill your water bottles here as this is your last opportunity before Monarch Lake.

Cross the stream and commence switchbacking up the slopes. At the fourth switchback Western white pines appear, and by the thirteenth you've already ascended 700 feet above the creek. Traversing south, you cross a small ridgetop and then climb east below the ridgeline to reach the posted junction for Crystal Lake (2.6/9860´). (The idyllic basin offers some exceptionally nice campsites near the south end of Crystal Lake, a 1.8-mile one-way journey from here.)

Continuing toward Sawtooth Peak, proceed straight on the main trail to begin a dramatic traverse beneath the lower flanks of Mineral Peak. Lower Monarch Lake remains hidden until you're almost upon it, when the red jutting molar of Mineral Peak (11615) also becomes visible for the first time south of the lake.

Lower Monarch Lake (4.4/10,380´) straddles a geologic divide. The distinctive rock interface across the lake marks where overlying volcanic rocks have been intruded by Sierra Nevada granite. Rarely is this geologic divide so pronounced. North, the granite mass of Sawtooth Peak rises dramatically above the lake, its summit just visible as the highest point on the ridge more than 2000 feet above you. Several good campsites are scattered around the western shore with food storage lockers for bear and marmot protection. The lake, which can be circumnavigated with some scrambling, boils with small brook trout. Upper Monarch Lake is easily accessed by a use trail at the lake's far shore, north of the small inlet creek.

Briefly winding northwest away from the lake at the base of Sawtooth's slope, the posted trail to Sawtooth Pass begins climbing in an obvious spot. It completes five switchbacks before reaching a long swath of grit and dust extending upslope. The trail ascends this via numerous steep switchbacks, gaining 500 feet above the lake before—near the top of the loose sandy slope—spinning off various paths. While the actual trail over Sawtooth Pass heads upward and to the left from here, you should begin slowly bearing right as you ascend toward the summit. The last stand of foxtail pine, above you to the right, provides a good landmark for climbing and for the return descent.

Continue upward until you are nearly level with these trees, and then climb above and slightly to the right of them until you reach the ridge—a gain of around 1000 feet from the top of the sandy slope. Incredible views east open up here, but they're better from the top. The peak is now clearly visible southeast, jutting from the ridge. To climb it, traverse below and then approach it from the south; the final scramble to the top is considerably easier from this direction. The last 100 feet require the most scrambling.

The view is epic. East lies the Kern River Canyon and its serrated eastern rampart, the Sierra Divide. Mt. Whitney (14,494´) can be spotted east-northeast.

Looking north, barren and oft-frozen Columbine Lake (10,970´) lies below you. The Great Western Divide strikes northeast beyond. On the divide's western slopes, Black Rock Pass Trail zigzags insanely up to its namesake. The large plateau that is home to Sequoia's Giant Forest is visible farther north-northwest, with the seemingly small knob of Moro Rock (Hike 100) on its western edge. On a good day the Minarets and Ritter Range are visible on the northern horizon, a distance of more than 75 miles.

You should find the summit register in an ammo can among the giant slabs of granite. On your return, don't be tempted by sandy routes that drop directly down Sawtooth toward Upper Monarch Lake, because the unseen slope steepens precipitously below. Look for that foxtail pine stand (pointed out earlier) to guide your descent as you retrace your steps to the trailhead.

Nearest Visitors Center: Mineral King Ranger Station, (559) 565-3768, is open 7 AM–3:30 PM daily from Memorial Day until early October.

Backpacking Information: Wilderness permits are required and may be obtained only from the ranger station during open hours. A quota of 20 persons per day is enforced for this trailhead, although capacity is typically only exceeded in late August and on the busiest summer holidays. There is a fee of $15 per permit, regardless of trip length or group size.

Nearest Campground: Cold Springs Campground (40 sites, $12) is 0.1 mile west of the ranger station. If it's full, try Atwell Mills Campground (21 sites, $12) 4.1 miles farther west. Neither is open before Memorial Day.

Additional Information: www.nps.gov/seki

Selected Sources and Recommended Reading

Atlases

Benchmark California Road & Recreation Atlas. 5th ed., Benchmark Maps, 2005.

Northern California Atlas & Gazetteer. 6th ed., Yarmouth, ME: DeLorme, 2003.

Southern California Atlas & Gazetteer. 4th ed., Yarmouth, ME: DeLorme, 1998.

Plant and Animal Identification

Johnson, Sharon G., Pamela C. Muick, Bruce M. Pavlik, and Marjorie Popper. *Oaks of California.* Los Olivos, CA: Cachuma Press, 1991.

Johnston, Verna R. *California Forests and Woodlands.* Berkeley, CA: University of California Press, 1994.

Keator, Glenn, Ruth M. Heady, and Valerie R. Winemiller. *Pacific Coast Fern Finder.* Rochester, NY: Nature Study Guild, 1981.

Lanner, Ronald M. *Conifers of California.* Los Olivos, CA: Cachuma Press, 1999.

Little, Elbert L. *National Audubon Society Field Guide to North American Trees, Western Region.* New York, NY: Alfred A. Knopf, 1998.

Lyons, Kathleen, and Mary Beth Cooney-Lazaneo. *Plants of the Coast Redwood Region.* Boulder Creek, CA: Looking Press, 1988.

Peterson, Roger Tory. *Western Birds.* New York, NY: Houghton Mifflin, 1998.

Spellenberg, Richard. *National Audubon Society Field Guide to North American Wildflowers, Western Region.* New York, NY: Alfred A. Knopf, 2001.

Watts, Tom. *Pacific Coast Tree Finder.* 2nd ed. Rochester, NY: Nature Study Guild, 2004.

Geology

General California Geology

Alt, David D., and Donald W. Hyndman. *Roadside Geology of Northern and Central California.* 2nd ed. Missoula, MT: Mountain Press Publishing Company, 2000.

Harden, Deborah R. *California Geology.* Upper Saddle River, NJ: Prentice-Hall, 1998.

McPhee, John. *Assembling California.* New York, NY: Farrar, Straus, and Giroux, 1993.

USGS. *Geologic Map of California.* 1:750,000. 1977.

Regional Geology

Durrell, Cordell. *Geologic History of the Feather River Country, California.* Berkeley, CA: University of California Press, 1987.

Galloway, Alan J. *Geology of the Point Reyes Peninsula.* Bulletin 202. California Division of Mines and Geology, 1977.

Konigsmark, Ted. *Geologic Trips: San Francisco and the Bay Area.* GeoPress, 1998.

Moore, James G., Warren J. Nokleburg, and Thomas W. Sisson. *Geologic Road Guide to Kings Canyon and Sequoia National Parks,* 1994.

Wahrhaftig, Clyde. *A Streetcar to Subduction and Other Plate Tectonic Trips by Public Transport in San Francisco.* Rev. ed. Washington, D.C.: American Geophysical Union, 1984.

Regional Information

The Central Coast, Bay Area, and Coast Ranges

California Coastal Resource Guide. *California Coastal Commission.* Berkeley, CA: University of California Press, 1987.

Cassady, Stephen. *Spanning the Gate.* Santa Rosa, CA: Squarebooks, 1986.

Elliot, Analise. *Hiking and Backpacking Big Sur: A Complete Guide to the Trails of Big Sur, Ventana Wilderness, and Silver Peak Wilderness.* Berkeley, CA: Wilderness Press, 2005.

Golden Gate National Recreation Area Guide to the Parks. San Francisco, CA: Golden Gate Conservancy, 2000.

Lage, Jessica. *Point Reyes: The Complete Guide to the National Seashore and Surrounding Area.* Berkeley, CA: Wilderness Press, 2004.

Paddison, Joshua. *A World Transformed: Firsthand Accounts of California Before the Gold Rush.* Berkeley, CA: Heyday Books, 1999.

Vanderwerf, Barbara. *The Coastside Trail Guidebook.* El Granada, CA: Gum Tree Lane Books, 1995.

Weintraub, David. *East Bay Trails: Hiking Trails in Alameda and Contra Costa Counties.* Berkeley, CA: Wilderness Press, 2005.

White, Peter. *The Farallon Islands: Sentinels of the Golden Gate.* San Francisco, CA: Scottwall Associates, 1995.

The North Coast and Klamath Mountains

Linkhart, Luther, and Mike White. *The Trinity Alps: A Hiking and Backpacking Guide.* Berkeley, CA: Wilderness Press, 2004.

Shasta and the Modoc Plateau

Boze, M. Jeanne. *The Nature of Bidwell Park.* 2nd ed. B. C. Publications, 1998.

Selters, Andy, and Michael Zanger. *The Mt. Shasta Book: A Guide to Hiking, Climbing, Skiing, and Exploring the Mountain and Surrounding Area.* Berkeley, CA: Wilderness Press, 2006.

White, Mike. *Lassen Volcanic National Park and Vicinity: A Complete Hiker's Guide.* Berkeley, CA: Wilderness Press, 2008.

The Sierra Nevada

Dinkey Creek: A Bridge from Past to Present. [pamphlet] Kings River Ranger District, 1997.

Browning, Peter. *Place Names of the Sierra Nevada.* Berkeley, CA: Wilderness Press, 1991.

Jenkins, J. C., and Ruby Johnson Jenkins. *Exploring the Southern Sierra: West Side.* Berkeley, CA: Wilderness Press, 1995.

Lamela, Susan, and Hank Meals. *Yuba Trails.* 1993.

Lekisch, Barbara. *Tahoe Place Names.* Lafayette, CA: Great West Books, 1988.

Moore, James G., Warren J. Nokleburg, and Thomas W. Sisson. *Geologic Road Guide to Kings Canyon and Sequoia National Parks,* 1994.

Morey, Kathy. *Hot Showers, Soft Beds, and Dayhikes in the Sierra.* Berkeley, CA: Wilderness Press, 2008.

———, Mike White, et al. *Sierra North: Backcountry Trips in California's Sierra Nevada.* 9th ed. Berkeley, CA: Wilderness Press, 2005.

———, Mike White, et al. *Sierra South: Backcountry Trips in California's Sierra Nevada.* 8th ed. Berkeley, CA: Wilderness Press, 2006.

Schaffer, Jeffrey P. *Desolation Wilderness and the South Lake Tahoe Basin: A Guide to Lake Tahoe's Finest Hiking Area.* Berkeley, CA: Wilderness Press, 2003.

———. *The Tahoe Sierra: A Natural History Guide to 112 Hikes in the Northern Sierra.* Berkeley, CA: Wilderness Press, 1998.

———. *Yosemite National Park: A Complete Hiker's Guide.* Berkeley, CA: Wilderness Press, 2006.

Schifrin, Ben. *Emigrant Wilderness and Northwestern Yosemite.* Berkeley, CA: Wilderness Press, 2004.

Secor, R. J. *The High Sierra, Peaks, Passes, and Trails.* Seattle, WA: The Mountaineers, 1999.

Whitney, Stephen. *The Sierra Nevada.* San Francisco, CA: Sierra Club Books, 1979.

Index

About the Author

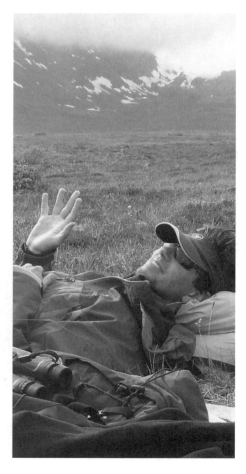

Matt Heid is the author of *Camping & Backpacking the San Francisco Bay Area, Best Backpacking Trips in New England,* and is a contributor to *Backpacking California*. He holds a degree in earth and planetary science from Harvard University and stays busy pursuing a passion for outdoor writing and remote wilderness adventure in Northern California, Alaska, and New England. He currently lives in Anchorage, Alaska.